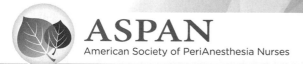
American Society of PeriAnesthesia Nurses

Certification Review for
PERIANESTHESIA NURSING

Fourth Edition

Theresa Clifford, MSN, RN, CPAN, CAPA
Manager of Perioperative Services
Mercy Hospital
Portland, Maine
Nurse Liaison for Special Projects
American Society of PeriAnesthesia Nurses
Cherry Hill, New Jersey

Denise O'Brien, DNP, RN, ACNS-BC, CPAN, CAPA, FAAN
Perianesthesia Clinical Nurse Specialist
Department of Operating Rooms/PACU
Michigan Medicine
University of Michigan
Adjunct Clinical Instructor
University of Michigan School of Nursing
Ann Arbor, Michigan

ELSEVIER

ELSEVIER

3251 Riverport Lane
St. Louis, Missouri 63043

CERTIFICATION REVIEW FOR PERIANESTHESIA NURSING, Fourth Edition   ISBN: 978-0-323-39940-1

Copyright © 2018, Elsevier Inc. All Rights Reserved.
Previous editions copyrighted 2013, 2008, 1996.

No part of this publication may be reproduced or transmitted in any form or by any means, electronic or mechanical, including photocopying, recording, or any information storage and retrieval system, without permission in writing from the publisher. Details on how to seek permission, further information about the Publisher's permissions policies and our arrangements with organizations such as the Copyright Clearance Center and the Copyright Licensing Agency, can be found at our website: www.elsevier.com/permissions.

This book and the individual contributions contained in it are protected under copyright by the Publisher (other than as may be noted herein).

Notice

Knowledge and best practice in this field are constantly changing. As new research and experience broaden our understanding, changes in research methods, professional practices, or medical treatment may become necessary.

Practitioners and researchers must always rely on their own experience and knowledge in evaluating and using any information, methods, compounds, or experiments described herein. In using such information or methods, they should be mindful of their own safety and the safety of others, including parties for whom they have a professional responsibility.

With respect to any drug or pharmaceutical products identified, readers are advised to check the most current information provided (i) on procedures featured or (ii) by the manufacturer of each product to be administered to verify the recommended dose or formula, the method and duration of administration, and contraindications. It is the responsibility of practitioners, relying on their own experience and knowledge of their patients, to make diagnoses, to determine dosages and the best treatment for each individual patient, and to take all appropriate safety precautions.

To the fullest extent of the law, neither the Publisher nor the authors, contributors, or editors assume any liability for any injury and/or damage to persons or property as a matter of products liability, negligence or otherwise, or from any use or operation of any methods, products, instructions, or ideas contained in the material herein.

Library of Congress Cataloging-in-Publication Data

Names: Clifford, Theresa, editor. I O'Brien, Denise, RN, editor. I Preceded
    by (work): Putrycus, Barbara. Certification review for perianesthesia
    nursing. I American Society of PeriAnesthesia Nurses.
Title: Certification review for perianesthesia nursing / [edited by] Theresa
    Clifford, Denise O'Brien.
Description: Fourth edition. I St. Louis, Missouri : Elsevier, [2018] I
    Preceded by Certification review for perianesthesia nursing / Barbara
    Putrycus, Jacqueline Ross. 3rd ed. c2013. I At head of title: American
    Society of Perianesthesia Nurses. I Includes bibliographical references
    and index.
Identifiers: LCCN 2016056069 I ISBN 9780323399401
Subjects: I MESH: Anesthesia--nursing I Nursing Process I Examination
    Questions
Classification: LCC RD82.3 I NLM WY 18.2 I DDC 617.9/60231--dc23 LC record available at
https://lccn.loc.gov/2016056069

Executive Content Strategist: Tamara Myers
Senior Content Development Manager: Laurie Gower
Associate Content Development Specialist: Elizabeth Fifer
Publishing Services Manager: Deepthi Unni
Book Project Manager: Maria Luisa P. Ordonio/Divya Krishna Kumar
Designer: Margaret Reid

Working together
to grow libraries in
developing countries

www.elsevier.com • www.bookaid.org

Printed in the United States of America

Last digit is the print number: 9   8   7   6   5   4

*In honor and memory of my mother, Lorraine,
who taught me by her loving example both the
joys and heartaches that come with being a nurse.
To my family, friends, colleagues, and mentors
who have supported my amazing
personal and professional adventures, my deepest thanks.*

Terry

*This book would not be possible without my family: my husband Mike, who offers
support, encouragement, and love in whatever I choose to do; my children Matt
and Bridget, who keep me grounded and real; my grandson Evan, who helps me
find joy and happiness every day; and especially my mother Donna, who is my
hero as a nurse and a woman. Thank you always.*

Denise

Contributors

Sylvia Baker, MSN, RN, CPAN
Clinical Education
Clinical Education Specialist
Mercy Health
Rockford, Illinois

**Kathy Daley, MSN, RN, ACNS-BC,
CCRN-CMC-CSC, CPAN**
Critical and Procedural Care Clinical Nurse
    Specialist
Charles George VA Medical Center
Asheville, North Carolina

Marie A. Evans, BSN, RN, CPAN
Perianesthesia Orientation Team Leader
Pre- & Post-Operative Services Department
MedStar Georgetown University Hospital
Washington, D.C.

**Tanya LeCompte Hofmann, MSN, APRN,
ACNS-BC, CPAN**
Clinical Case Manager
Integrated Case Management
Sarasota Memorial Health Care System
Sarasota, Florida

Vallire D. Hooper, PhD, RN, CPAN, FAAN
Manager: Nursing Research
Nursing Practice, Education, and Research
Mission Health
Asheville, North Carolina

Carolyn Kiolbasa, BSN, RN, CAPA
Staff Nurse, Outpatient Surgery
Lurie Children's Outpatient Center in Westchester
Ann and Robert H. Lurie Children's Hospital of
    Chicago
Chicago, Illinois

Janice Lopez, BSN, RN, CPAN, CAPA
PACU
St. Luke's Hospital
Kansas City, Missouri

Bonnie Niebuhr, MS, RN, CAE
Chief Executive Officer
ABPANC
New York, New York

Susan Norris, BSN, RN, CAPA
Staff Nurse
PreAdmission Testing Center
Baylor St Luke's Medical Center
Houston, Texas

Valerie Pfander, MSN, RN, ACCNS-AG, CPAN
Clinical Nurse Specialist
Perianesthesia
Munson Medical Center
Traverse City, Michigan

Renee Smith, MS, BSN, RN, CPAN, CAPA
Clinical Nurse Educator
PACU and Same Day Surgery
Geisinger Medical Center
Danville, Pennsylvania

Nancy Strzyzewski, MSN, RN, CPAN, CAPA
Supervisor, Department of PACU Education
Department of Operating Rooms/PACU
Michigan Medicine
University of Michigan
Adjunct Clinical Instructor
University of Michigan School of Nursing
Ann Arbor, Michigan

Diane Swintek, MSN, RN, CPAN
Staff Nurse
Phase 1 PACU
Medstar Franklin Square Medical Center
Baltimore, Maryland

Charlotte West, BSN, RN, CPAN
Clinical Supervisor
OPS, PACU, SEC
St. Vincent Carmel Hospital
Sheridan, Indiana

Reviewers

Linda Beagley, MS, RN, CPAN
Clinical Nurse Educator/Quality Coordinator
Swedish Covenant Hospital
Chicago, Illinois

Melanie Chichester, BSN, RN-OB, CPLC
Staff Nurse, Clinical Level III, Labor and Delivery
Christiana Care Health Services
Newark, Delaware

Susanne DeBell, RN, BSN, MCIS, CAPA, ONC
Registered Nurse
Department of Presurgical Services
Inova Fair Oaks Hospital and Inova Fairfax
    Hospital
Fairfax, Virginia

Jean M. Johnson, BSN, RN, CAPA
Inova Fairfax Hospital
Falls Church, Virginia

Kathleen J. Menard, PhD, RN-BC, CPAN, CAPA
Perianesthesia Nurse Education Specialist
UMass Memorial Medical Center
Assistant Professor of Nursing
University of Massachusetts, Worcester
Graduate School of Nursing
Worcester, Massachusetts

Debby Niehaus, BSN, RN, CPAN
Clinical Nurse
Cincinnati, Ohio

Teresa Passig, BSN, RN, CPAN, CAPA, CCRN
Learning Specialist
Arnold Palmer Medical Center PACU
Orlando Health
Orlando, Florida

Allyson Petosa, BSN, RN
Registered Nurse
University of Delaware
Newark, Delaware

Carol Salter, RN, CPAN
Registered Nurse
Banner Gateway Hospital
Department of Perianesthesia
Gilbert, Arizona

Kathleen Sarkin, MSN, RN, CPAN
Learning Consultant Perianesthesia Care Units
Department of Learning and Development
Orlando Health
Orlando, Florida

Allan Schwartz, DDS, CRNA
Assistant Clinical Professor
The Center for Advanced Dental Education
Department of Periodontics
Saint Louis University
St. Louis, Missouri

Twilla Shrout, BSN, MBA, RN, CAPA
Past President of ASPAN, 2013-2014
Staff Nurse, Same Day Surgery
Harry S Truman Memorial Veterans' Hospital
Columbia, Missouri

Brendan M. Walsh, BSN, CPAN, CAPA
Staff RN
Lahey Clinic, PACU
Burlington, Massachusetts

Preface

Since its inception in 1980, the American Society of PeriAnesthesia Nurses (ASPAN) supported specialty nursing certification. From the first Certification Committee to the incorporation of the American Board of PeriAnesthesia Nursing Certification, Inc. (ABPANC) and in subsequent years, ASPAN has promoted certification through education, scholarships, and product development. This book, now in its fourth edition, represents one aspect of ASPAN's commitment to advancing certification across the perianesthesia nursing specialty.

In the first examination for certification of postanesthesia nurses in November 1986, 172 nurses were certified. Today over 12,000 nurses are certified. The specialty remains unique and diverse. Nurses preparing for certification practice in settings ranging from a few beds to hundreds of beds, from specialty-focused freestanding facilities to multispecialty teaching medical centers. But the knowledge and experience of all of these nurses center around a solid foundation of specialized knowledge and proficiencies, shared across all settings and sizes of organizations. These are the domains of practice that are validated through the certification process.

Previous editions of this book include a purpose statement, which remains pertinent in this edition. The purpose of the *Certification Review for PeriAnesthesia Nursing* is "to articulate the knowledge base that underlies perianesthesia nursing." To the editors of this edition, this means that we are, as in past editions, clarifying and distinguishing the knowledge needed to prepare for the certification examination, in a manner that helps the nurse test critical thinking and clinical experience.

Meeting the criteria (www.cpancapa.org) to apply to test for certification is one of the initial steps on the certification journey. Once the decision is made by the nurse and the criteria met, preparation begins. Preparation is essential, and using tools designed to stimulate and challenge the critical thinking of the test taker encourage the test taker to confirm current knowledge and explore content areas where greater knowledge is needed to be successful on the examination.

This "question and answer book" remains, in this fourth edition, a useful resource, which is expected to be used along with other recommended references, as perianesthesia nurses prepare for the certification examination. This resource has been redesigned and questions revised, rewritten, or created new and formatted to follow the certification blueprint and study plan (www.cpancapa.org).

It is our sincere desire that all who use this resource in their preparation for perianesthesia certification are successful in achieving the goal of CPAN® and CAPA® certification!

Acknowledgments

This text, much like the certification exam, provides an opportunity for perianesthesia nurses to validate the foundation of knowledge, clinical experience, and capacity to provide high-quality best practice in perianesthesia care. The chapters follow the actual test blueprints, identifying key physiological, behavioral (or cognitive), and safety needs of perianesthesia patients. The questions and their rationales will provide perianesthesia nurses an opportunity to demonstrate test-taking strategies and will help the nurse identify areas of strength and opportunities for additional learning.

We wish to acknowledge those who saw talent in our collaboration to bring you a completely revised, up-to-date version of this book.

We would like to acknowledge the following individuals:

- First, we would like to thank ASPAN for giving us the opportunity to co-edit this coveted resource.
- To the perianesthesia nurse who strives for recognition for their clinical expertise and knowledge in daily perianesthesia practice—their dedication to perianesthesia practice inspires us.
- To Kathy Carlson, who as the first editor for the *Certification Review for Perianesthesia Nursing,* had the vision to improve the education for perianesthesia nurses through the first edition of this text. Thank you for following your passion!
- To Barbara Putrycus and Jacqueline Ross, who served as the co-editors of the second and third editions of this text. Thank you for your work to support the goals and aspirations of perianesthesia nurses seeking certification.

- For each contributing author who provided countless hours of time writing questions and providing grounded rationales. Perianesthesia nurses can be assured that this text represents the formatting of the certification exam in terms of all phases of care and the wide scope of perianesthesia practice.
- For each respected perianesthesia reviewer of this text—each of them took time from their busy schedules to read over the content, seek clarification, and promote a well-developed text.
- To our perianesthesia colleagues who offered suggestions and support for revisions and updates to this edition.
- To Elizabeth Fifer, Laurie Gower, Maria Luisa Ordonio, Divya Krishna Kumar, and Tamara Myers for their support and understanding during the process of publishing this book. Their ongoing assistance, patience, encouragement, and expertise provided us the motivation to follow our vision to create a comprehensive text that will guide nurses through the certification process.
- To the numerous other members of the Elsevier team who helped us throughout the many stages of this edition, we extend our sincere gratitude.

With sincere appreciation,

Terry and Denise

Contents

1

Certification of Perianesthesia Nurses

Bonnie Niebuhr

CPAN® AND CAPA® CERTIFICATION PROGRAMS

The American Board of Perianesthesia Nursing Certification, Inc. (ABPANC) is a not-for-profit corporation established in 1985 for the purpose of sponsoring specialty nursing certification programs for registered nurses (RNs) caring for perianesthesia patients. Its mission is "to assure a certification process for perianesthesia nurses that validates the achievement of knowledge gained through professional education and experience, ultimately promoting quality patient care."[1] The mission and related activities of ABPANC are aimed at achieving its compelling vision: "Recognizing and respecting the unequaled excellence in the mark of the CPAN and CAPA credentials, perianesthesia nurses will seek it, managers will require it, employers will support it and the public will demand it!"[1]

ABPANC is the organization that is responsible for the Certified Post Anesthesia Nurse (CPAN) and Certified Ambulatory Perianesthesia Nurse (CAPA) Certification Programs. **All questions about the CPAN and CAPA programs should be referred to ABPANC.**

ABPANC Resources

For the most up-to-date information about the CPAN and CAPA certification programs, visit the website at www.cpancapa.org; e-mail abpanc@proexam.org; or call the American Board of Perianesthesia Nursing Certification, Inc. (ABPANC) directly at 800-6ABPANC and press Option 2 or 3.

Definition of Certification

ABPANC has adopted the following definition of certification as defined by the American Board of Nursing Specialties (ABNS): "Certification is the formal recognition of the specialized knowledge, skills, and experience demonstrated by the achievement of standards identified by a nursing specialty to promote optimal health outcomes."[2] *State licensure* provides the legal authority for an individual to practice professional nursing.[3] Private, voluntary certification, as sponsored by ABPANC, reflects achievement of a standard *beyond* licensure for specialty nursing practice.

CPAN and CAPA Credentials

CPAN and CAPA credentials, granted to qualified RNs by ABPANC, are federally registered certification marks and are protected by law. RNs who have not achieved CPAN or CAPA certification status or whose certification status has lapsed are not authorized to use these credentials.

CPAN AND CAPA CERTIFICATION PROGRAMS

ABSNC Accreditation

Both CPAN and CAPA certification programs are accredited by the Accreditation Board for Specialty Nursing Certification, Inc. (ABSNC). Accreditation status must be renewed every 5 years.

ABSNC is a nationally recognized standard-setting body for specialty nursing certification programs and offers a stringent and comprehensive accreditation process. ABPANC must provide extensive documentation demonstrating that it has met the 18 ABSNC standards of quality. ABSNC accreditation signifies that a nationally recognized accrediting body has determined that CPAN and CAPA credentials are based on a valid and reliable examination process. Additionally, the structures in place to administer the examinations meet and exceed the standards of the certification industry from a legal, regulatory, and association management perspective.

For further information about ABSNC and the accreditation process and standards, visit their website at www.nursingcertification.org.

Basis for CPAN and CAPA Examinations—A Role Delineation Study

The CPAN and CAPA examinations are each based on the results of a role delineation study (RDS), also called a *job analysis* or *study of practice*. This type of study must be conducted (per accreditation standards) every 5 years to ensure that examination content remains relevant and current to the practice specialty. A variety of methods may be employed to gather data, the findings of which are reflected in the Test Blueprint. The Blueprint can be found in ABPANC's *Certification Candidate Handbook* on the ABPANC website (www.cpancapa.org) under the Certification tab.

The most recent RDS was conducted from August 2015 to February 2016 and resulted in *minor* updates to the listing of patient needs and nursing knowledge and a revision to the percentage of examination questions asked in each of the three domains of patient needs. These changes will be incorporated into the test blueprints beginning with the fall 2017 CPAN and CAPA examinations. The revised test blueprints will be published in the *Certification Candidate Handbook* released in early 2017.

Test Blueprints

The CPAN and CAPA examinations are organized around the following three domains of perianesthesia patient needs:

1. Physiological Needs
2. Behavioral and Cognitive Needs[1]
3. Safety Needs

Specific patient needs are listed under each domain in the Test Blueprint. The specific knowledge required of perianesthesia nurses in order to meet these patient needs is also identified for each of the three domains.

The CPAN and CAPA test Blueprints are based on data from the RDS. Although it was determined that patient needs and the knowledge base of the nurse to meet those needs are the same, the percentage of questions asked in each domain or category of patient need varies, depending on whether the candidate is taking the CPAN or CAPA examination. A complete listing of the most current patient needs and related nursing knowledge that make up the test Blueprints can be found on the ABPANC website (www.cpancapa.org) in the Resources tab under study tools.

Examination Questions

Examination questions are written by practicing CPAN and CAPA certified nurses. The Item Writer/ Reviewer Committee (IWRC) and Examination Review Committee (ERC) for CPAN and CAPA

programs are made up of individuals who currently practice in a variety of settings in various roles throughout the United States; this ensures that the examination reflects the diversity of practice around the country. Each question is reviewed a minimum of three times before use on an examination. Each question is judged against the criteria of relevance, currency, and criticality to the care of perianesthesia patients. Each question must also have a current, related reference no older than 5 years. In addition, test developers and psychometricians at PSI Services LLC, the testing company used by ABPANC, review each question for proper format as a multiple-choice question and ensure that item bias is not present. This complex process ensures that CPAN and CAPA examinations are current and relevant to perianesthesia nursing and are reflective of the content identified in the most recent RDS.

In addition, examination questions are written at various cognitive levels based on a condensed version of Bloom's taxonomy.[4] The three cognitive levels used by ABPANC are as follows:

- **Level I**—Knowledge and Comprehension: Questions examine one's ability to recall a fact or understand a principle.
- **Level II**—Application and Analysis: Questions examine one's ability to relate two or more facts to a situation or analyze a group of facts.
- **Level III**—Synthesis and Evaluation: Questions examine one's ability to evaluate a situation using facts or make recommendations based on analysis and evaluation of facts.

Most CPAN and CAPA questions are focused at levels II and III.

Each CPAN and CAPA examination is a 3-hour test consisting of 175 questions. In addition to the 140 questions that are scored, 35 questions are being pretested (piloted) and do not count toward the candidate's final score. These 35 piloted questions are randomly distributed through the examination and are not specifically identified. Each scored question is carefully written, referenced, and validated to ensure accuracy and correctness.

Determining Which Examination to Take

Determining which examination is most relevant to an examination candidate's practice is based on patient needs and the amount of time patients spend in the specific phases described by the Perianesthesia Continuum of Care (as defined in ASPAN's Scope of Practice, Perianesthesia Nursing).[5] Regardless of the setting in which the examination candidate practices,

---

[1] Based on the results of the 2015 RDS, this domain will be called Behavioral Health and Cognitive Needs.

if most of the examination candidate's time is spent caring for patients in Phase I, the CPAN examination is most relevant. If most of the examination candidate's time is spent caring for patients in the Preanesthesia Phase, Day of Surgery/Procedure, Postanesthesia Phase II, and/or Extended Care, the CAPA examination is more relevant.

Eligibility Requirements

To sit for either the CPAN or the CAPA certification examination, the applicant must:

- Possess a current, unrestricted RN license in the United States or any of its territories that use the National Council Licensure Examination (NCLEX) as the basis for determining RN licensure
- Have at least 1800 hours of direct clinical experience caring for patients in Phase I (if taking the CPAN examination) or Preanesthesia Phase, Day of Surgery/Procedure, Postanesthesia Phase II, and/or Extended Care (if taking the CAPA examination) in the two years prior to applying for initial certification

To be eligible to sit for *both* the CPAN and CAPA exams, a candidate must meet the licensure and direct care requirements and have:

- At least 1800 hours of direct clinical experience caring for patients in Postanesthesia Phase I
- At least 1800 hours of direct clinical experience caring for patients in Preanesthesia Phase, Day of Surgery/Procedure, Postanesthesia Phase II, and/or Extended Care

and

- Submit a complete application and fee

A complete description of eligibility requirements is found on the ABPANC website (www.cpancapa.org) and in the *Certification Candidate Handbook*. The policy of ABPANC is that no individual shall be excluded from the opportunity to participate in the CPAN or CAPA certification programs on the basis of age, sex, race, religion, national origin, ethnicity, disability, marital status, sexual orientation, and gender identity.

Online Examination Application and Computer-Based Testing

Candidates register for CPAN and CAPA examinations online. The online application is accessed through the ABPANC website. The examinations are given by computer at hundreds of test sites offered by the testing vendor, Prometric. There are many advantages of computer-based testing, including the ability to receive a preliminary, unofficial score on the site. Visit the ABPANC website for further information about this testing modality.

Certification Period

To ensure that certified perianesthesia nurses possess the most up-to-date knowledge and current experience, CPAN and CAPA certification status is granted for a period of 3 years and must be renewed. To renew credentials, CPAN and CAPA certified nurses must meet certain RN licensure and clinical experience eligibility requirements and either successfully complete the examination or earn contact hours related to continual learning. Acceptable activities for obtaining contact hours are described in the Recertification Handbook, found on the ABPANC website.

STUDYING FOR CPAN AND CAPA CERTIFICATION EXAMINATIONS

The ABPANC website provides a variety of study resources for the CPAN and CAPA examinations at http://cpancapa.org/resources/study-tools/.

The *Certification Candidate Handbook* provides important information regarding preparation and testing (e.g., registration process, dates and deadlines, Prometric test centers).

Certification Review Courses are available online or by live seminar. When choosing a review course, ensure the course content covers what is listed on the CPAN/CAPA Test Blueprint. Ask about the qualifications of the instructor teaching the review course. Is he or she CPAN and/or CAPA certified? ABPANC does not endorse any particular courses.

ABPANC Study Resources

• *Certification Candidate Handbook*
   • Test Blueprints
   • Study References—in Appendix D
   • Sample Questions
 • CPAN and CAPA Study Question of the Week
 • Four Practice Exams (for purchase)
 • Webinars
   • Test-Taking Strategies
   • Fear of Failure
 • Study Tips Brochure
 • Mind Mapping Study Guide

After the Test

A preliminary, unofficial pass/fail score is given to the candidate at the Prometric test center. ABPANC will mail an official, final score report within 2 to 3 weeks, along with a wallet identification card and wall certificate.

CELEBRATE!

Is the test over? The successful candidate can now plan a celebration. Congratulations are in order for taking the next step in one's professional career. The study process, in and of itself, is a wonderful opportunity. The journey helps recognize the best perianesthesia nurses!

REFERENCES

1. ABPANC. About Us. http://cpancapa.org/about-abpanc/. Accessed February 22, 2016.
2. ABNS. Definition of Certification. www.nursing certification.org. Accessed February 22, 2016.
3. Niebuhr B, Muenzen P. A study of perianesthesia nursing practice: the foundation for newly revised CPAN and CAPA certification examinations. *J Peri-Anesth Nurs.* 2001;16(3):163-173.
4. Armstrong P. *Bloom's Taxonomy*; 2016. Available at https://cft.vanderbilt.edu/guides-sub-pages/blooms-taxonomy/. Accessed August 11, 2016.
5. ASPAN. *2015-2017 Perianesthesia Nursing Standards Practice Recommendations and Interpretive Statements.* Cherry Hill, NJ: ASPAN; 2014.

2

Respiratory, Cardiovascular, Peripheral Vascular, and Hematological Systems

Valerie Pfander, Kathy Daley, Marie A. Evans, and Renee Smith

2-1. A patient is admitted to the Phase I PACU after a dilation and curettage for retained placenta. Postoperatively, the surgeon is concerned that the patient has disseminated intravascular coagulation (DIC). The nurse receives an order for heparin to be given. What is the rationale for giving heparin to a patient with DIC?

    a. Heparin blocks the fibrinolytic system so that stable clots are not degraded

    b. Heparin reestablishes normal hemostatic potential

    c. Heparin decreases the amount of fibrin split products that act as anticoagulants

    d. Heparin prevents further microclots and prevents platelet aggregation

2-2. A patient arrives in the Phase I PACU after placement of an inferior vena cava (IVC) filter using a right femoral approach. The insertion site was infiltrated with local anesthetic at the end of the case. On initial assessment the patient's vital signs are stable and the dressing to the puncture site is dry and intact. After 1 hour the nurse reassesses the patient and notices that the right leg is slightly cooler than the left leg. In addition there is now firmness on the skin around the puncture site. What might the nurse conclude?

    a. This is a normal postoperative finding

    b. A hematoma may be forming and the physician should be informed

    c. The firmness and coolness can be attributed to the infiltration of local anesthetic at the puncture site

    d. The puncture site should be observed an additional 60 minutes for any further expansion of the area of firmness

Consider this scenario for questions 2-3, 2-4, and 2-5.

    A 72-year-old patient undergoes a four-vessel coronary artery bypass graft with a left internal mammary artery graft (LIMA). He is admitted to the Phase I PACU, intubated, mechanically ventilated and has a pulmonary artery catheter, radial arterial line, three mediastinal chest tubes, and atrial and ventricular pacing wires. He also has an indwelling urinary catheter. The quantity of drainage from his chest tubes on initial assessment was 200 mL of sanguineous fluid. Fifteen minutes later, there is another 100 mL.

2-3. The Phase I PACU nurse knows that this type of drainage is:

    a. Normal chest tube drainage postcardiac surgery

    b. When chest tubes should be stripped to prevent clotting

    c. Excessive chest tube drainage

    d. When suction on chest tubes should be decreased to −10 cm

2-4. The bleeding is now controlled after administration of protamine sulfate. The patient is intubated, and the nurse received instructions to extubate the patient within 4 hours of arrival to recovery. Which of the following is an acceptable extubation parameter?

    a. FiO_2 65%

    b. Negative inspiratory force (NIF) of −30 cm water

    c. Respiratory rate 40 breaths per minute

    d. PaO_2 60 mm Hg

2-5. The cardiac monitor shows a sinus rhythm of 84, BP is 86/45, pulmonary artery pressure (PA) is 15/4, and cardiac output is now at 3.8. The initial action to correct the patient's hemodynamic status would be to:

a. Start an epinephrine drip at 0.5 mcg/kg

b. Initiate temporary pacing at a rate of 95

c. Decrease sedation

d. Administer a volume bolus

Consider this scenario for questions 2-6 and 2-7.

A patient is in the Phase I PACU after repair of an abdominal aortic aneurysm. On admission the abdominal dressing is dry and intact with a small amount of sanguineous drainage in the bulb drain. An arterial line has been placed in the left radial artery to monitor blood pressure and for obtaining labs and has been appropriately zeroed on admission. The bilateral 18-gauge intravenous catheters in place in both hands have crystalloids infusing.

2-6. The waveform on the arterial line now appears dampened. Which of the following is a possible cause of this change in the waveform?

a. Stopcock turned off to the patient

b. Pressure bag inflated to 300 mm Hg

c. Transducer positioned above the phlebostatic axis

d. Air bubbles in the tubing

2-7. The blood pressure readings of the arterial line indicate hypotension confirmed by cuff pressure. The anesthesiologist has ordered hetastarch. An advantage of using hetastarch instead of dextran is:

a. This infusion does not require a central line for infusion

b. The risk of communicable disease is less

c. Hetastarch has minimal effects on coagulation

d. They have similar hypersensitivity reactions

2-8. After a left rotator cuff repair a 64-year-old male patient arrives in the Phase II PACU once transfer criteria have been met. Fifteen minutes after arrival the patient complains of an ache in his jaw. The nurse observes that the patient is pale, diaphoretic, and has become increasingly anxious. The nurse places the patient on monitor and calls for help. The nurse anticipates that the anesthesia provider will most likely order the following laboratory tests:

a. Troponin level

b. Electrolytes

c. Magnesium

d. C-reactive protein

2-9. The Phase I PACU nurse receives a patient status post exploratory laparotomy from an abdominal wound. The patient was transfused 6 units of blood before surgery and during surgery for blood loss. The nurse closely observes the electrocardiogram for changes associated with banked blood infusions including:

a. Prolongation of the QT

b. Tall-peaked T waves

c. Atrioventricular block

d. Torsades de point

2-10. All of the following actions are involved in achieving hemostasis EXCEPT:

a. Local vasoconstriction to reduce blood flow

b. Inauguration of the clot after tissue repair is complete

c. Formation of a fibrin mesh to strengthen the plug

d. Platelet aggregation at the injury site and formation of a platelet plug

2-11. The nurse receives an order to monitor a patient's atrial pressure after coronary artery bypass grafting (CABG) surgery to evaluate the patient's preload status. The nurse understands that afterload refers to the:

a. Percentage of blood in the ventricle

b. End-diastolic pressure

c. Amount of blood ejected by the ventricle

d. Resistance to ejection of blood from the ventricle

2-12. Patients who have gastric resection should be observed carefully for nutritional-deficiency anemia related to malabsorption. Evidence of nutritional-deficiency anemia includes which of the following?

a. Bone pain

b. Dark yellow or bronze skin

c. Numbness and tingling of extremities

d. Steatorrhea

2-13. Signs and symptoms associated with obstructive sleep apnea include all of the following EXCEPT:

a. Impotence

b. Nocturia

c. Hypotension

d. Loud snoring

2-14. In the preoperative holding area, a patient is being prepared for coronary artery bypass graft (CABG) surgery. The nurse notes a "do not resuscitate" (DNR) status. The nurse should:

a. Support clarification of the patient and family wishes about resuscitation

b. "Flag" the DNR status on the chart or electronic health record

c. Contact a member of the risk management team for code status interpretation

d. Inform the patient and family that DNR is not recognized in surgery and in the immediate postoperative period

2-15. A patient is going to the operating room (OR) to have his diabetic stasis ulcers debrided. He admits he has read on the Internet about an "ankle block" that can be done for a patient who undergoes this type of surgery. His history includes congestive heart failure (CHF), type II diabetes (DMII) controlled with oral medications, peripheral vascular disease (PVD), and a surgical history of a femoral-popliteal bypass for claudication. What medical condition in his history would make the providers decline to do an ankle block?

a. CHF

b. DMII

c. PVD

d. Femoral-popliteal bypass

2-16. A postoperative patient with a significant cardiac history becomes tachycardic and has increased central venous pressures (CVPs), muffled heart tones, and pulsus paradoxus. The Phase I PACU nurse notifies the physician that she suspects:

a. Bleeding from the surgical site

b. Cardiac tamponade

c. A complete heart block

d. Tension pneumothorax

2-17. A 26-year-old male dialysis patient arrives in the Phase II PACU after having a thrombectomy of his right atrioventricular (AV) fistula. On initial assessment the nurse notices that the patient has 2+ bilateral radial pulses and capillary refill time of less than 3 seconds. As the surgical site is assessed, it is noted that the dressing is dry and intact and the graft has a thrill, but a bruit cannot be heard. What would be the next course of action that the nurse should take?

a. Continue with Phase II care and gather discharge instructions for the patient

b. Offer fluids and crackers to the patient in anticipation of discharge home

c. Keep patient NPO and call the physician

d. Apply a soft pressure dressing to decrease the development of a hematoma

2-18. Signs and symptoms of bronchospasm include:

a. Cough, expiratory wheezing, and dyspnea

b. Bradycardia, inspiratory wheezing, and tachypnea

c. Crowing respirations, fever, and use of accessory muscles

d. Cough, sneezing, and bradycardia

2-19. A patient has been on heparin therapy and has been diagnosed with heparin-induced thrombocytopenia (HIT). What would be the drug of choice for reversing HIT?

a. Vitamin K

b. Clopidogrel

c. Argatroban

d. Protamine

2-20. Early signs and symptoms associated with acute noncardiogenic pulmonary edema include:

a. Crowing, stridor, and wheezing

b. Decreased chest excursion

c. Decreased capillary permeability

d. Dyspnea, cough, and tachypnea

2-21. The nurse is caring for a patient in the Phase I PACU after open abdominal aortic aneurysm repair. Over the last hour the urine output has dramatically decreased, the patient has hypotension not responsive to fluids or vasopressors, abdominal girth has increased, and there are increased ventilator requirements. The nurse suspects that the patient may be experiencing:

a. Leaking of the aortic graft

b. Abdominal compartment syndrome

c. Thrombosis of the graft

d. Sepsis

2-22. A patient arrives in the Phase I PACU after a right total hip replacement. Preoperative medications include atenolol, atorvastatin calcium, hydrochlorothiazide, and fluvoxamine. In spite of an estimated blood loss of 400 mL, his heart rate is 80 bpm. The Phase I PACU nurse knows that which of these medications prevent him from responding with tachycardia?

a. Atorvastatin calcium

b. Hydrochlorothiazide

c. Atenolol

d. Fluvoxamine

2-23. Some patients who have been intubated for surgery may complain of a sore throat postoperatively. The perianesthesia nurse should:

a. Administer oxygen to soothe the throat

b. Observe the oropharynx and auscultate the chest

c. Inform the patient that it is normal for a sore throat to last at least 7 days

d. Apply heat to the patient's neck to relieve the symptoms

2-24. Raynaud's disease is usually seen in all of the following EXCEPT:

a. Exposure to extreme cold

b. Exposure to extreme heat

c. Women over 30 years of age

d. Times of emotional stress

2-25. A patient's recovery from vascular surgery is uneventful and the patient has been started on heparin intraoperatively for the prevention of thromboembolism. On routine assessment of the patient the nurse notes the patient has developed bleeding gums. The nurse reviews the labs and notes that the platelet count is 98,000. What should the nurse do?

a. Nothing as this is an expected side effect of heparin therapy

b. Call the physician and ask if he or she would like to decrease the heparin dose

c. Call the physician and ask if he or she would like to increase the heparin dose

d. Call the physician and ask if he or she would like to discontinue the heparin

2-26. A patient has a platelet count of 50,000 and is diagnosed with immune thrombocytopenic purpura. The nurse would expect initial treatment to include:

a. Splenectomy

b. Corticosteroids

c. Administration of platelets

d. Immunosuppressive therapy

2-27. Laboratory values for a patient with hypotension and abdominal bleeding include a hematocrit of 30%, platelets 50,000/mm^3, and international normalized ratio (INR) 1.3. In addition to administering a fluid bolus of 250 mL of normal saline, the nurse anticipates administration of which of the following?

a. 1 unit of packed red blood cells (RBCs)

b. 6 units/300 mL of platelets

c. Fresh-frozen plasma 4 units/250 mL

d. 50 mL of salt-poor albumin/25% albumin

2-28. A 73-year-old patient arrives in the procedural Phase II PACU after his fistulogram. He has been assessed by the nurse, and his vital signs are stable. He has a good thrill and bruit on his left atrioventricular (AV) fistula. Preoperatively he was not assessed to be a fall risk. The patient tells the nurse that he needs to urinate and cannot urinate in a supine position. What should the nurse do?

a. Because the patient needs to remain supine for 1 hour, provide a urinal

b. Offer to raise the head of the bed so that the patient can try to urinate in a sitting position

c. Assist the patient to ambulate to the bathroom to urinate

d. Allow the patient to stand at the bedside with the curtain pulled for privacy

2-29. Three initial responses to vascular injury include:

a. Inflammation, hemodilution, and vasoconstriction

b. Necrosis, platelet adhesion, and thrombin generation

c. Vasoconstriction, platelet adhesion, and thrombin generation

d. Thrombin generation, inflammation, and vasoconstriction

2-30. What is the most common site of pulmonary aspiration?

a. Right lung

b. Left lung

c. Left bronchus

d. Pharynx

2-31. A patient in the Phase I PACU after repair of an abdominal aortic aneurysm is receiving a low-dose intravenous ketamine infusion as part of the pain management plan. The nurse recognizes that addition of ketamine to the regimen is associated with all the following EXCEPT:

a. Improved pain control

b. Lower opioid requirements

c. Less nausea

d. Increased psychotomimetic effects

2-32. On physical assessment of the patient with severe anemia the nurse would expect to find:

a. Nervousness and agitation

b. Fever and tenting of the skin

c. Systolic murmur and tachycardia

d. Bluish mucous membranes and reddened tissues

2-33. After a minor vascular procedure the nurse is reviewing discharge instructions with the patient. The physician has ordered acetaminophen with oxycodone tablets for pain management. Which of the following medications would concern the nurse the most if it appeared on the patient's home medication list?

a. Celecoxib

b. Ibuprofen

c. Acetaminophen with hydrocodone

d. Diclofenac sodium

Consider this scenario for questions 2-34 and 2-35.
The anesthesia provider administered a nondepolarizing neuromuscular blocking agent (NMBA) during induction. A reversal agent was given immediately before admission to the Phase I PACU. The patient is awake and talking. After 20 minutes the patient becomes unarousable, with shallow respirations at 6/minute, BP 90/60, and HR 70.

2-34. The initial nursing intervention for this patient is:

a. Apply O_2 by nasal cannula at 4 liters/minute

b. Administer a repeat dose of the NMBA reversal agent

c. Apply a bag-valve-mask device for ventilation support

d. Initiate cardiopulmonary resuscitation (CPR)

2-35. The anesthesia provider returns to the patient's bedside and prepares to administer:

a. Neostigmine and epinephrine

b. Phenylephrine or glycopyrrolate

c. Phenylephrine or atropine

d. Neostigmine and glycopyrrolate

2-36. A patient with thrombocytopenia with active bleeding has 2 units of platelets prescribed. To administer the platelets, the nurse:

a. Checks for ABO compatibility

b. Agitates the bag periodically during the transfusion

c. Takes vital signs every 15 minutes during the procedure

d. Refrigerates the second unit until the first unit has transfused

2-37. A 24-year-old patient with no previous medical history develops a moist cough, dyspnea, and pink frothy sputum after extubation. Lung auscultation reveals bilateral coarse crackles at the bases. An appropriate treatment plan would include:

a. Esmolol 1 gm intravenously piggyback immediately

b. Furosemide 1 mg intravenously push now; follow with a furosemide drip

c. 1 liter bolus of 0.9% normal saline

d. Bumetanide 1 mg intravenously push now; follow with a bumetanide drip

2-38. Anesthesia affects the mechanical properties of the lungs and chest wall. Patients emerging from anesthesia have:

a. Decreased lung volumes and increased lung capacity

b. Decreased lung volumes and decreased lung capacity

c. Increased lung volumes and decreased lung capacity

d. Increased lung volumes and increased lung capacity

2-39. A 57-year-old male patient has had a left iliac thrombectomy. He has been in the Phase I PACU for 45 minutes. The nurse caring for him has to give a handoff report. Included in the handoff of care should be the condition of the surgical site dressing and:

a. Pulses and temperature of the lower extremities

b. Color and pulses of the left lower extremity

c. Color, warmth, and pulses of the affected extremities

d. Color, warmth, sensation, and pulses of both lower extremities

2-40. Assessment findings associated with laryngospasm may include all of the following EXCEPT:

a. Absence of breath sounds

b. Continuous musical rhonchi

c. Paradoxic rocking motion of chest wall

d. Diminished breath sounds

2-41. An elderly patient with a history of congestive heart failure (CHF) in the Phase I PACU develops an abnormal breathing pattern of rhythmic waxing and waning of the depth of respirations along with regularly recurring periods of apnea. This abnormal breathing pattern is known as:

a. Tachypnea

b. Kussmaul breathing

c. Cheyne-Stokes breathing

d. Biot's breathing

2-42. When using any form of assisted ventilation, the most harm can be caused by delivering:

a. Excessive volume

b. Insufficient volume

c. Excessive liters per minute

d. Insufficient rate

2-43. Signs and symptoms associated with pneumothorax include:

a. Crowing, stridor, and wheezing

b. Chest pain, tracheal deviation, and dyspnea

c. Hyperthermia, tachycardia, and flushing

d. Decreased work of breathing and increased fremitus

2-44. When there is a left shift in the oxyhemoglobin dissociation curve, this is indicative of:

a. Acidosis

b. Hypercapnia

c. Hypothermia

d. Increased levels of 2,3-diphosphoglycerate (2,3-DPG)

2-45. A 34-year-old dialysis patient has undergone a thrombectomy of his right arteriovenous fistula under general anesthesia. He is now in the Phase II PACU with his wife. Before the patient is given his discharge instructions, the nurse rechecks the fistula. The assessment reveals that the fistula may have developed another thrombus, which warrants that the patient return to the operating room (OR). The surgeon is notified and comes to speak to the patient about reexploration of the fistula. Who will consent for the patient for this new procedure?

a. Because the patient is ready for discharge, he can sign his own consent

b. The consent is covered under his original consent

c. The situation is an emergency and implied consent will be used

d. The wife as next of kin will sign for the patient

2-46. After general anesthesia, while the patient is in the Phase I PACU, cardiac rate and rhythm are monitored:

a. Continuously

b. For 30 minutes

c. For 1 hour

d. For 4 hours

2-47. A patient complains of itching all over his body 30 minutes after a unit of packed red blood cells (RBCs) is started transfusing. The vital signs obtained are normal. The most appropriate initial intervention is to:

a. Assess for glottal edema

b. Administer IV diphenhydramine as ordered

c. Stop the transfusion

d. Continue to observe the patient

2-48. After a splenectomy for treatment of immune thrombocytopenic purpura (ITP), the nurse would expect the patient's laboratory results to reveal:

a. Decreased red blood cells (RBCs)

b. Decreased white blood cells (WBCs)

c. Increased platelets

d. Decreased platelets

2-49. The Phase I PACU nurse is caring for a patient who has had a cervical sympathectomy as palliative treatment of peripheral vascular disease. Horner's syndrome is common after this procedure. The nurse would expect to see the following signs EXCEPT:

a. Ptosis of the upper eyelid

b. Dilation of the affected pupil

c. Increased salivation

d. Drooping of the mouth on the affected side

2-50. Risks and complications specific to pulmonary artery (PA) catheter monitoring include:

a. Perforation of the left ventricle

b. Rupture of the aorta

c. Perforation of the aorta

d. Perforation of the right ventricle

2-51. A postoperative patient develops symptomatic bradycardia that does not resolve, and a temporary pacemaker is applied. When troubleshooting a temporary pacemaker that is experiencing failure to capture, the Phase I PACU nurse should anticipate:

a. Turning up the sensitivity

b. Turning down the sensitivity

c. Turning up the rate

d. Turning up the milliamperage (mA)

2-52. An involuntary partial or complete closure of the vocal cords, caused by irritation during emergence, is a postoperative complication known as:

a. Laryngospasm

b. Bronchospasm

c. Subglottic edema

d. Aspiration

2-53. Myocardial changes in the older adult include:

a. Left ventricular hypertrophy

b. Decreased myocardial irritability

c. Endocardial thinning

d. Improved valve competence

2-54. Soon after a postextubation laryngospasm, the patient becomes hypoxic and tachypneic and produces frothy sputum. This assessment can be a sign of:

a. Pulmonary embolism

b. Postobstructive pulmonary edema (POPE)

c. Cardiogenic pulmonary edema

d. Subglottic edema

2-55. During a plasma transfusion, the nurse keeps in mind:

a. It must be ABO compatible and used within 24 hours after thawing

b. Unconcentrated plasma contains all coagulation factors

c. 1 unit is equivalent to 300 to 500 mL

d. It is incompatible to the patient with antithrombin III deficiency

2-56. Known cardiovascular effects from the volatile inhalation agent isoflurane include:

a. Transient bradycardia

b. Increased coronary blood flow

c. Peripheral vasoconstriction

d. Impaired myocardial function

2-57. Preoperative patient and family education for an implantable cardioverter-defibrillator (ICD) include all of the following EXCEPT:

a. Information regarding how the ICD is programmed to function

b. Actions to take if a shock occurs

c. Antidysrhythmic and heart failure medications will be discontinued in 24 to 48 hours

d. Activity limitations related to driving and avoiding strong magnetic fields

Consider this scenario for questions 2-58, 2-59, and 2-60.

Mr. L, a 62-year-old businessman, arrives in the Phase I PACU. The report from the anesthesia care provider is that Mr. L sustained a myocardial infarction while on the operating table and now appears to be in cardiogenic shock.

2-58. Cardiogenic shock is caused by:

a. Loss of intravascular fluid volume

b. Impairment of cardiac contractility

c. Solid organ injury

d. Increased cardiac output

2-59. While assessing Mr. L, the perianesthesia nurse focuses interventions of care to include:

a. Increasing cardiac afterload with fluid boluses

b. Decreasing cardiac output by administration of diuretics

c. Supporting oxygenation and tissue perfusion

d. Decreasing myocardial oxygen supply requirements

2-60. All of the following pharmacologic agents are most likely initial treatment options for Mr. L EXCEPT:

a. Adrenergic blocking agents

b. Beta blockers

c. Vasodilators

d. Vasopressors

2-61. Respiratory acidosis is characterized by:

a. A $PaCO_2$ above the normal range of 36 to 44 torr

b. A $PaCO_2$ below the normal range of 36 to 44 torr

c. A PaO_2 below 90%

d. A PaO_2 between 90% and 100%

2-62. When the patient has recovered from the effects of anesthesia and is ready for transfer to the nursing unit or discharge area, the perianesthesia nurse should ensure all of the following has been completed EXCEPT:

a. A licensed practitioner has seen the patient or the name of the responsible physician has been documented in the patient record

b. The patient received an initial dose of opioid within the last 10 minutes to ensure comfort level during transport

c. The patient has regained a satisfactory level of consciousness to the point of being oriented and being able to call for assistance, if necessary

d. The patient is dressed in a clean, dry, appropriate hospital gown

2-63. The nurse is performing a neurologic check on a patient in the Phase I PACU after endovascular carotid stent placement. The patient exhibits poor swallowing, inadequate gag reflex, and vocal difficulties. The nurse suspects damage to which nerve:

a. Glossopharyngeal

b. Hypoglossal

c. Recurrent laryngeal

d. Facial

2-64. The nurse is beginning her reassessment of a 24-year-old male patient who has had a venogram with a femoral approach. He has been on bed rest for an hour and is now complaining to the nurse that he thinks he has been incontinent and has "wet himself." What might the nurse want to do first?

a. Prepare to scan the bladder and offer a urinal

b. Reassure the patient that due to his procedure it is an expected temporary outcome

c. Check the surgical site dressing for potential bleeding

d. Verify medications given during the procedure because incontinence can be a common side effect in vascular procedures

2-65. What selective laboratory tests are used for assessment of the coagulation cascade before surgery?

a. Prothrombin time and partial thromboplastin time

b. Platelet count and bleeding time

c. Fibrinogen and platelet count

d. Clotting time and fibrinogen

2-66. Which of the following patient care instructions would be most appropriate to give to a patient being discharged after placement of an implantable cardioverter-defibrillator (ICD)?

a. Driving is typically restricted for 6 months

b. Upper extremity motion will be limited for 3 months

c. Bed rest required for the first 48 hours in a monitored setting

d. A magnetic resonance imaging (MRI) will be scheduled 4 to 6 weeks postoperatively

2-67. When a laryngeal mask airway (LMA) is in place, lifting of the jaw could:

a. Improve the patient's work of breathing

b. Cause a laryngospasm

c. Assist with the removal of the LMA

d. Ensure the LMA is correctly placed

2-68. Common causes of excessive carbon dioxide elimination and respiratory alkalosis include all of the following EXCEPT:

a. Decreased body temperature

b. Anxiety

c. Aspirin

d. Central nervous system lesions

2-69. The ambulatory perianesthesia nurse is giving a patient discharge instructions after recovering from skin biopsy. The patient is also newly diagnosed with leukemia with low platelet count. Patients with low platelet counts need to be instructed to avoid:

a. Aspirin

b. Fresh fruits

c. Green, leafy vegetables

d. Prednisone

2-70. Cardiac dysrhythmias can occur in patients undergoing anesthesia. The cardiovascular effect of inhalation agents includes:

a. Slowing the rate of sinus atrial (SA) node discharge

b. Increasing the bundle of His-Purkinje fibers

c. Increasing ventricular conduction times

d. Increasing the rate of SA node discharge

2-71. Early clinical signs of acute hypoxemia in the postoperative patient include:

a. 8 to 10 regular respirations per minute

b. Pulse oximetry measurement of 91% to 93%

c. Restlessness and anxiety

d. Bright red flushing of the skin

2-72. An accumulation of air or gas in the pleural space causing sharp ipsilateral chest pain and dyspnea is indicative of:

a. Bronchospasm

b. Pulmonary edema

c. Pneumothorax

d. Aspiration

2-73. When placing defibrillator/automated external defibrillator (AED) pads on a patient with an implanted defibrillator/pacemaker:

a. Place the defibrillator/AED pad directly on top of the implanted device to override it during shock administration

b. Place the defibrillator/AED pad to either side of the implanted device

c. Place the defibrillator/AED pad in the same location as you would for any patient regardless of an implanted device

d. Never place a defibrillator/AED pad on a patient who has an implanted defibrillator/ pacemaker

2-74. What is the primary stimulus to ventilation?

a. Oxygen

b. Alveolar dead space

c. Carbon dioxide

d. Carbon monoxide

2-75. A 62-year-old male patient recovering from a cholecystectomy reports new chest pain. What actions have the highest priority?

a. Administer an IV fluid bolus and obtain arterial blood gas

b. Start dopamine at 2 mcg/kg/min and obtain a chest x-ray

c. Obtain a 12-lead electrocardiogram (ECG) and administer aspirin if not contraindicated

d. Send blood to the laboratory for chemistry and cardiac enzymes

2-76. A 16-year-old male patient is recovering in the Phase I PACU after a right knee arthroscopy and develops sudden onset of narrow-complex tachycardia at a rate of 220/minute. His BP is 128/58 and pulse oximetry reading is 98%. He has vascular access and has not been given any vasoactive drugs. A 12-lead electrocardiogram (ECG) confirms a supraventricular tachycardia (SVT) with no evidence of ischemia or infarction. The heart rate has not responded to vagal maneuvers. Due to the age of the patient, what is the next recommended intervention?

a. Amiodarone 300 mg IV push

b. Adenosine 6 mg IV push

c. Synchronized cardioversion at 50 joules

d. Synchronized cardioversion at 200 joules

Consider this scenario for questions 2-77, 2-78, and 2-79.

A patient in the Phase I PACU becomes hypertensive. A right radial arterial line is in place. The most recent blood pressure is 210/160. The physician orders a nitroprusside drip.

2-77. The medication nitroprusside is classified as a:

a. Peripheral vasoconstrictor

b. Dopamine-receptor antagonist

c. Potent antiarrhythmic

d. Peripheral vasodilator

2-78. When given intravenously, the onset of this medication is:

a. 3 to 5 minutes

b. 15 to 20 minutes

c. 30 to 40 minutes

d. 30 to 60 seconds

2-79. The patient continues to receive nitroprusside as ordered in the Phase I PACU and is beginning to complain of headache and dizziness. Current BP is 140/83 and heart rate is 125. The PACU nurse is aware that prolonged use or high dosages of nitroprusside may result in:

a. Antihistamine release

b. Ethanol toxicity

c. Carbon monoxide poisoning

d. Cyanide toxicity

2-80. A patient arrives in the surgery center for an outpatient procedure. The patient relayed a history of sickle cell disease. The nurse is aware that a number of factors trigger a sickle cell crisis and knows that the most common type of sickle cell crisis is:

a. Vasoocclusive

b. Aplastic

c. Sequestration

d. Hemolytic

Answers and Rationales for Chapter 2, Respiratory, Cardiovascular, Peripheral Vascular, and Hematological Systems

2-1. *Correct answer:* **d**
Slowing consumption of coagulation factors by inhibiting the processes involved in clot formation is another strategy used in treating disseminated intravascular coagulation (DIC). Heparin has been beneficial in obstetric emergencies such as retained placenta or incomplete abortion, severe arterial occlusions, or multiple organ dysfunction syndrome (MODS) caused by microemboli. Thrombosis of small vessels has the greatest effect on morbidity and mortality in DIC, not hemorrhage. (Urden L, Stacy K, Lough M. *Critical Care Nursing, Diagnosis and Management.* 7th ed. St. Louis, MO: Elsevier; 2014:997-1016.)

2-2. *Correct answer:* **b**
According to the Association for Radiologic and Imaging Nurses (ARIN) resource in the ASPAN *Standards*, the firmness at the puncture site could be an indication of the formation of a hematoma. The slightly cooler temperature of the limb in comparison to the other limb, as well as the firmness, are potential indications of a hematoma that may be compromising circulation. (American Society of PeriAnesthesia Nurses. *2015-2017 PeriAnesthesia Nursing Standards, Practice Recommendations and Interpretive Statements.* Cherry Hill, NJ: ASPAN; 2014:145.)

2-3. *Correct answer:* **c**
Postoperative bleeding from the mediastinal chest tubes can be caused by inadequate hemostasis, disruption of suture lines, or coagulopathy associated with cardiopulmonary bypass or hypothermia. Bleeding is more likely to occur with internal mammary artery (IMA) grafts as a result of the extensive chest wall dissection required to free the IMA. If bleeding in excess of 150 mL/hr occurs early in the postoperative period, clotting factors (fresh-frozen plasma, fibrinogen,

and platelets), protamine, or desmopressin may be administered. (Urden L, Stacy K, Lough M. *Critical Care Nursing, Diagnosis and Management.* 7th ed. St. Louis, MO: Elsevier; 2014:412-466.)

2-4. *Correct answer:* **b**
Extubation weaning criteria generally include a temperature of 36.8°C, ability to lift head on request, spontaneous respirations, and hemodynamic stability. Acceptable extubation parameters include alertness and ability to follow commands, respiratory rate less than 30 breaths per minute, tidal volume greater than 50%, positive end-expiratory pressure (PEEP) less than 5 cm H_2O, negative inspiratory force (NIF) less than −20 cm of water, SaO_2 greater than 91%, FiO_2 less than 40%, pH 7.33 to 7.46, $PaCO_2$ greater than 33 to 49 mm Hg, and PaO_2 greater than 65 mm Hg. (Schick L, Windle PE. *Perianesthesia Nursing Core Curriculum: Preprocedure, Phase I and Phase II PACU Nursing.* 3rd ed. St. Louis, MO: Saunders; 2015:562-641. Odom-Forren J. *Drain's Perianesthesia Nursing: A Critical Care Approach.* 6th ed. St. Louis, MO: Saunders; 2013:489-525. Urden L, eds. *Critical Care Nursing, Diagnosis and Management.* 7th ed. St. Louis, MO: Elsevier; 2014:549-586.)

2-5. *Correct answer:* **d**
In most patients, reduced preload is the cause of low postoperative cardiac output. The most common causes of decreased preload are due to hypovolemia from bleeding and fluid shifts caused by the systemic inflammatory response. To enhance preload, volume may be administered in the form of crystalloid, colloid, or packed red cells. (Urden L, Stacy K, Lough M. *Critical Care Nursing, Diagnosis and Management.* 7th ed. St. Louis, MO: Elsevier; 2014:412-466.)

2-6. *Correct answer:* **d**
Air bubbles in the system can cause it to be overdampened. Carefully backflush any bubbles away from the patient. Make sure that all connections are tight, and use needleless blood access systems to reduce the risk of air entry into the system. (Lough ME. *Hemodynamic Monitoring: Evolving Technologies and Clinical Practice.* St. Louis, MO: Elsevier-Mosby; 2015:70-72. Urden L, Stacy K, Lough M. *Critical Care Nursing, Diagnosis and Management.* 7th ed. St. Louis, MO: Elsevier; 2014:246.)

2-7. *Correct answer:* **c**
Neither solution requires a central line for infusion or carries risk of communicable diseases. The hetastarch actually has less likelihood to produce hypersensitivity reactions. The main reason to use the hetastarch is that it has minimal coagulation effects, and the dextran interferes with platelet function and may cause prolonged bleeding time. (Schick L, Windle PE. *PeriAnesthesia Nursing Core Curriculum: Preprocedure, Phase I and Phase II PACU Nursing.* St. Louis, MO: Saunders; 2016:1241.)

2-8. *Correct answer:* **a**
Common laboratory tests for the patient experiencing chest pain include serial troponins and cardiac enzymes (including creatine kinase and creatine kinase-MB isoenzyme, which are cardiac specific laboratory tests.) (Schick L, Windle PE. *PeriAnesthesia Nursing Core Curriculum: Preprocedure, Phase I and Phase II PACU Nursing.* 3rd ed. St. Louis, MO: Saunders; 2016:578).

2-9. *Correct answer:* **b**
Banked blood is high in potassium because of hemolysis. Look for tall-peaked T waves and widening of the QRS complex. Other considerations with transfusion of banked blood are hypocalcemia, hypothermia, and decreased tissue oxygen delivery caused by decreased levels of 2,3-diphosphoglycerate. (Urden L, Stacy K, Lough M. *Critical Care Nursing, Diagnosis and Management.* 7th ed. St. Louis, MO: Elsevier; 2014:997-1016.)

2-10. *Correct answer:* **b**
Hemostasis, the ability of the body to control bleeding and clotting, is an intricate balancing act between the coagulation mechanism and fibrinolysis. Four major actions are involved in achieving hemostasis: 1) local vasoconstriction to reduce blood flow; 2) platelet aggregation at the injury site and formation of a platelet plug; 3) formation of a fibrin mesh to strengthen the plug; and 4) dissolution of the clot after tissue repair is complete. Disruption of the normal hemostatic balance can result in devastating hemorrhagic or thrombotic conditions. (Urden L, Stacy K, Lough M. *Critical Care Nursing, Diagnosis and Management.* 7th ed. St. Louis, MO: Elsevier; 2014:997-1016.)

2-11. *Correct answer:* **d**
Afterload is the resistance to the ejection of blood from the ventricle. It is increased by peripheral arterial vasoconstriction, obstruction of flow from valvular stenosis or pulmonary embolus, increased ventricular diameter (e.g., congestive heart failure [CHF]), and blood viscosity (e.g., increased hematocrit). It is decreased by peripheral arterial vasodilation, incompetent valves, or hemodilution. (Urden L, Stacy K, Lough M. *Critical Care Nursing, Diagnosis and Management.* 7th ed. St. Louis, MO: Elsevier; 2014:562-641.)

2-12. *Correct answer:* **c**
The patient who has had a gastric resection is at risk for anemia because intrinsic factors may decrease, leading to vitamin B_{12}-deficiency anemia with associated neurologic deficits such as numbness and tingling of extremities. The other symptoms are not related to nutritional-deficiency anemia. (Schick L, Windle PE. *PeriAnesthesia Nursing Core Curriculum: Preprocedure, Phase I and Phase II PACU Nursing.* 3rd ed. St. Louis, MO: Saunders; 2016:820-838.)

2-13. *Correct answer:* **c**

Signs and symptoms associated with obstructive sleep apnea include impotence, nocturia, esophageal reflux, depression, high blood pressure, loud snoring, and excessive sleepiness. (Odom-Forren J. *Drain's Perianesthesia Nursing: A Critical Care Approach.* 6th ed. St. Louis, MO: Saunders; 2013:179, Box 12-5.)

2-14. *Correct answer:* **a**

The American Society of PeriAnesthesia Nurses (ASPAN) recommends that at the time of surgery and before receiving any anesthetic medications a patient with an active "do not resuscitate" (DNR) advance directive be asked to clarify wishes about resuscitation during the perianesthesia period. To limit potential for ethical dilemmas, the patient's informed consent includes discussion of the advance directive, living will, or physician order that specifies DNR or "do not intubate" (DNI) and well-documented conversation with physician. Each facility establishes and communicates a policy that identifies resources and procedures that detail the management of a patient's DNR/DNI status during the perianesthesia period. (Schick L, Windle PE. *PeriAnesthesia Nursing Core Curriculum: Preprocedure, Phase I and Phase II PACU Nursing.* 3rd ed. St. Louis, MO: Saunders; 2016:562-641. American Society of PeriAnesthesia Nurses. *2015-2017 PeriAnesthesia Nursing Standards, Practice Recommendations and Interpretive Statements.* Cherry Hill, NJ: ASPAN; 2014:90-93.)

2-15. *Correct answer:* **c**

The patient has severe peripheral vascular disease (PVD), which has already resulted in the need for a femoral-popliteal bypass. Although severe diabetes is a contraindication for peripheral nerve blocks, the patient's diabetes is controlled with oral medications. (Odom-Forren J. *Drain's Perianesthesia Nursing: A Critical Care Approach.* 6th ed. St. Louis, MO: Saunders; 2013:339.)

2-16. *Correct answer:* **b**

Fluid accumulation within the pericardial space has the classic findings of Beck's triad, which includes increased central venous pressure (CVP), muffled heart tones, and pulsus paradoxus. Pulsus paradoxus, also called *paradoxical pulse,* is a fall of systolic blood pressure of greater than 10 mm Hg during the inspiratory phase. (Schick L, Windle PE. *PeriAnesthesia Nursing Core Curriculum: Preprocedure, Phase I and Phase II PACU Nursing.* 3rd ed. St. Louis, MO: Saunders; 2016:638-639.)

2-17. *Correct answer:* **c**

Keep the patient NPO and call the physician in anticipation that the patient may need to return to surgery. The lack of a bruit denotes that another occlusion may be occurring and repeat intervention is necessary. (American Society of PeriAnesthesia Nurses. *2015-2017 PeriAnesthesia Nursing Standards, Practice Recommendations and Interpretive Statements.* Cherry Hill, NJ: ASPAN; 2014:145.)

2-18. *Correct answer:* **a**

Signs and symptoms of bronchospasm include cough, expiratory wheezing, dyspnea, use of accessory muscles, and tachypnea. (Odom-Forren J. *Drain's Perianesthesia Nursing: A Critical Care Approach.* 6th ed. St. Louis, MO: Saunders; 2013:396.)

2-19. *Correct answer:* **d**

Protamine is the direct treatment for heparin. Protamine reverses the anticoagulant effects of heparin by binding to it. The expected reaction time is 5 minutes within administration of Protamine. (Odom-Forren J. *Drain's Perianesthesia Nursing: A Critical Care Approach.* 6th ed. St. Louis, MO: Saunders; 2013:528.)

2-20. *Correct answer:* **d**
Dyspnea, cough, and tachypnea are early signs of noncardiogenic pulmonary edema. Later signs include fatigue, pedal edema, and paroxysmal nocturnal dyspnea. With severe alveolar edema, diminished breath sounds and pink, frothy sputum may be seen. (Schick L, Windle PE. *PeriAnesthesia Nursing Core Curriculum: Preprocedure, Phase I and Phase II PACU Nursing.* 3rd ed. St. Louis, MO: Saunders; 2016:517.)

2-21. *Correct answer:* **b**
Abdominal compartment syndrome can be a result of prolonged surgery with fluid resuscitation that results in edema of the abdominal organs and compression of the inferior vena cava. Treatment is emergency decompression laparotomy with packing of the abdominal wound and delayed closure. (Stannard D, Krenzischek DA, eds. *PeriAnesthesia Nursing Care: A Bedside Guide for Safe Recovery.* Sudbury, MA: Jones and Bartlett Learning; 2011:311. Urden L, Stacy K, Lough M. *Critical Care Nursing, Diagnosis and Management.* 7th ed. St. Louis, MO: Elsevier; 2014:877.)

2-22. *Correct answer:* **c**
Several conditions render certain patients unable to respond with tachycardia. These include patients taking beta-blocker medications as well as patients with transplanted hearts (which are denervated and therefore lack capacity for autonomic responses). (Schick L, Windle PE. *PeriAnesthesia Nursing Core Curriculum: Preprocedure, Phase I and Phase II PACU Nursing.* 3rd ed. St. Louis, MO: Saunders; 2016:562-641.)

2-23. *Correct answer:* **b**
Throat discomfort may persist for 1 to 3 days, especially if a traumatic intubation occurred. An ice bag can be applied for comfort and to decrease inflammation. Medication such as dexamethasone can be given to reduce inflammation. An assessment should be performed and abnormal findings reported to the anesthesiologist. (Odom-Forren J.

Drain's Perianesthesia Nursing: A Critical Care Approach. 6th ed. St. Louis, MO: Saunders; 2013:423.)

2-24. *Correct answer:* **b**
Raynaud's is seen more prevalent in women than in men, between the ages of 30 and 50. Exposure to cold and stress can cause an exacerbation of symptoms to include cold fingers or toes, color changes to skin, as well as numb and prickly sensations in the digits. (Schick L, Windle PE. *PeriAnesthesia Nursing Core Curriculum: Preprocedure, Phase I and Phase II PACU Nursing.* 3rd ed. St. Louis, MO: Saunders; 2016:1086.)

2-25. *Correct answer:* **d**
The patient may be experiencing heparin-induced thrombocytopenia (HIT), and another anticoagulant should be used in place of heparin. HIT is characterized by a platelet count less than 100,000 or a decrease of 40% to 50% from a baseline platelet count. Another consequence of HIT is the potential increased risk for bleeding. (Odom-Forren J. *Drain's Perianesthesia Nursing: A Critical Care Approach.* 6th ed. St. Louis, MO: Saunders; 2013:528.)

2-26. *Correct answer:* **b**
Corticosteroids suppress phagocytic response of splenic macrophages, decreasing platelet function; they also depress autoimmune antibody formation and reduce capillary fragility and bleeding time. (Urden L, Stacy K., Lough M. *Critical Care Nursing, Diagnosis and Management.* 7th ed. St. Louis, MO: Elsevier; 2014:997-1016.)

2-27. *Correct answer:* **b**
The nurse would anticipate administration of platelets to decrease bleeding in this patient. The normal platelet count is 200,000 to 450,000/mm^3. (Odom-Forren J. *Drain's Perianesthesia Nursing: A Critical Care Approach.* 6th ed. St. Louis, MO: Saunders; 2013:194-206.)

2-28. *Correct answer:* **c**

Per the Association for Radiologic and Imaging Nurses (ARIN), the patient may get up ad lib after this procedure as long as the patient is hemodynamically stable. (American Society of PeriAnesthesia Nurses. *2015-2017 PeriAnesthesia Nursing Standards, Practice Recommendations and Interpretive Statements.* Cherry Hill, NJ: ASPAN; 2014:145.)

2-29. *Correct answer:* **c**

Platelets are activated by the arrival of thrombin at the site of injury. Local platelets change shape, become sticky, and begin to aggregate along the vessel wall. Activated platelets undergo degranulation, releasing several factors to assist in clot formation. Serotonin and histamine, two potent vasoconstrictors, help limit blood loss while the clot is forming. The prostaglandin thromboxane A2 (TXA2) contributes to vasoconstriction and promotes further platelet degranulation. Adenosine diphosphate (ADP) recruits platelets by increasing adherence and degranulation, and the process continues. (Urden L, Stacy K, Lough M. *Critical Care Nursing, Diagnosis and Management.* 7th ed. St. Louis, MO: Elsevier; 2014:997-1016.)

2-30. *Correct answer:* **a**

The most common site of pulmonary aspiration is the right lung, because the right primary bronchus is wider and has a straighter angle than the left bronchus. (Schick L, Windle PE. *PeriAnesthesia Nursing Core Curriculum: Preprocedure, Phase I and Phase II PACU Nursing.* St. Louis, MO: Saunders; 2016:492.)

2-31. *Correct answer:* **d**

When a low-dose ketamine infusion was added to the multimodal pain management plan, patients had improved control of pain, used less opioid, and experienced less nausea and fewer psychotomimetic effects. (Pasero C, McCaffery M, eds. *Pain Assessment and Pharmacologic Management.* St. Louis, MO: Elsevier-Mosby; 2011:714.)

2-32. *Correct answer:* **c**

Tachycardia occurs in severe anemia as the body compensates for hypoxemia and the low viscosity of the blood contributes to the development of systolic murmurs and bruits. Depression of the central nervous system is common with fatigue, lethargy, and malaise; poor skin turgor may be present, but fever is not associated with anemia. Skin and membranes are pale with blue-tinged sclera. (Urden L, Stacy K, Lough M. *Critical Care Nursing, Diagnosis and Management.* 7th ed. St. Louis, MO: Elsevier; 2014:997-1016.)

2-33. *Correct answer:* **c**

Because both compounds contain acetaminophen, if the patient continues to take both pain medications, the 4000 mg maximum daily dose of acetaminophen may be exceeded and place the patient at risk of liver damage. (Pasero C, McCaffery M, eds. *Pain Assessment and Pharmacologic Management.* St. Louis, MO: Elsevier-Mosby; 2011:256.)

2-34. *Correct answer:* **c**

The duration of the nondepolarizing neuromuscular blocking agent (NMBA) could be longer than the duration of the neostigmine and glycopyrrolate (commonly used NMBA reversal agents), necessitating additional airway support once the reversal agent has worn off. Once ventilation is supported, the patient is assessed and additional reversal agent may be given. (Schick L, Windle PE. *PeriAnesthesia Nursing Core Curriculum: Preprocedure, Phase I and Phase II PACU Nursing.* 3rd ed. St. Louis, MO: Saunders; 2016:397-400.)

2-35. *Correct answer:* **d**

Neostigmine and glycopyrrolate is the preferred combination of medications for reversing the effects of nondepolarizing neuromuscular blocking agent (NMBA). (Schick L, Windle PE. *PeriAnesthesia Nursing Core Curriculum: Preprocedure, Phase I and Phase II PACU Nursing.* 3rd ed. St. Louis, MO: Saunders; 2016:397-400.)

2-36. *Correct answer:* **b**

Platelets adhere to plastic bags and should be gently agitated throughout the transfusion. Platelets do not have A, B, or Rh antibodies, and ABO compatibility is not a consideration. Baseline vital signs should be taken before the transfusion is started, and the nurse should stay with the patient during the first 15 minutes. Platelets are stored at room temperature and should not be refrigerated. (Urden L, Stacy K, Lough M. *Critical Care Nursing, Diagnosis and Management.* 7th ed. St. Louis, MO: Elsevier; 2014:1016.)

2-37. *Correct answer:* **d**

The symptoms describe pulmonary edema of a noncardiogenic nature. Treatment includes albumin, diuretics, and continuous positive airway pressure. The dose for the furosemide is incorrect. (Odom-Forren J. *Drain's Perianesthesia Nursing: A Critical Care Approach.* 6th ed. St. Louis, MO: Saunders; 2013:165.)

2-38. *Correct answer:* **b**

The major factor that contributes to this reduction in lung volumes in patients after surgery is a shallow, monotonous, sighless breathing pattern caused by general inhalation anesthesia, pain, and opioids. (Odom-Forren J. *Drain's Perianesthesia Nursing: A Critical Care Approach.* 6th ed. St. Louis, MO: Elsevier; 2013:180-181.)

2-39. *Correct answer:* **d**

Assessment of the affected limbs should include the color, warmth, sensation, movement, and pulses. The most recent and comprehensive assessment of these should be included in handoff of care. (Odom-Forren J. *Drain's Perianesthesia Nursing: A Critical Care Approach.* 6th ed. St. Louis, MO: Elsevier; 2013:526-539.)

2-40. *Correct answer:* **b**

Patients with a partial or complete airway obstruction such as laryngospasm usually have a paradoxic rocking motion of the chest wall. Stridor and high-pitched crowing respirations indicate partial obstruction, and absent breath sounds indicate total obstruction. The perianesthesia nurse should auscultate breath sounds and check for chest wall motion. (Odom-Forren J. *Drain's Perianesthesia Nursing: A Critical Care Approach.* 6th ed. St. Louis, MO: Saunders; 2013:154. Schick L, Windle PE. *PeriAnesthesia Nursing Core Curriculum: Preprocedure, Phase I and Phase II PACU Nursing.* St. Louis, MO: Saunders; 2016:470-471.)

2-41. *Correct answer:* **c**

Cheyne-Stokes is a rhythmic waxing and waning of the depth of breathing with regularly recurring periods of apnea secondary to central nervous system (CNS) disease and CHF. Biot's breathing is irregular breathing interspersed with variable periods of apnea secondary to stroke, trauma, and increased intracranial pressure, and Kussmaul breathing is rapid, deep breathing that may be secondary to metabolic acidosis. (Schick L, Windle PE. *PeriAnesthesia Nursing Core Curriculum: Preprocedure, Phase I and Phase II PACU Nursing.* St. Louis, MO: Saunders; 2016:505.)

2-42. *Correct answer:* **a**

Excessive ventilation can be harmful because it increases intrathoracic pressure, decreases venous return to the heart, and diminishes cardiac output. (American Heart Association. *Advanced Cardiovascular Life Support. Provider Manual.* Dallas, TX: AHA; 2016:41.)

2-43. *Correct answer:* **b**

Signs and symptoms of pneumothorax include dyspnea, tachypnea, chest pain, increased work of breathing, decreased fremitus, tracheal deviation to the contralateral side, and decreased or absent breath sounds. (Schick L, Windle PE. *PeriAnesthesia Nursing Core Curriculum: Preprocedure, Phase I and Phase II PACU Nursing.* St. Louis, MO: Saunders; 2016:517.)

2-44. *Correct answer:* **c**

The oxyhemoglobin dissociation curve describes the relationship between available oxygen and amount of oxygen carried by hemoglobin. When there is a shift to the left, less oxygen is available to the tissues; an example of this would be a patient with hypothermia. (Schick L, Windle PE. *PeriAnesthesia Nursing Core Curriculum: Preprocedure, Phase I and Phase II PACU Nursing.* St. Louis, MO: Saunders; 2016:500. Odom-Forren J. *Drain's Perianesthesia Nursing: A Critical Care Approach.* 6th ed. St. Louis, MO: Saunders; 2013:356-357.)

2-45. *Correct answer:* **d**

The patient has undergone anesthesia and is not able to sign consent for himself due to his impaired capacity. The next of kin would be the person to consent. (Odom-Forren J. *Drain's Perianesthesia Nursing: A Critical Care Approach.* 6th ed. St. Louis, MO: Saunders; 2013:89.)

2-46. *Correct answer:* **a**

In the immediate postoperative period, cardiac dysrhythmias are likely because of light anesthesia during emergence or due to the administration of drugs that alter sympathetic activity. (Odom-Forren J. *Drain's Perianesthesia Nursing: A Critical Care Approach.* 6th ed. St. Louis, MO: Saunders; 2013:134. American Society of PeriAnesthesia Nurses. *2015-2017 PeriAnesthesia Nursing Standards, Practice Recommendations and Interpretive Statements.* Cherry Hill, NJ: ASPAN; 2014.)

2-47. *Correct answer:* **c**

Hypersensitivity response accounts for 1% to 3% of transfusion reactions. It occurs as a result of antibodies to donor-blood foreign proteins, often in a patient with significant allergy history. Reaction may progress unpredictably, so the transfusion must be stopped. One should assess for glottal swelling. An intravenous antihistamine is administered. (Schick L, Windle PE. *PeriAnesthesia Nursing Core Curriculum: Preprocedure, Phase I and Phase II PACU Nursing.* 3rd ed. St. Louis, MO: Saunders; 2016:820-838.)

2-48. *Correct answer:* **c**

Splenectomy may be indicated for treatment of immune thrombocytopenic purpura (ITP), and when the spleen is removed platelet counts increase significantly in most patients in any of the disorders in which the spleen removes excessive blood cells; splenectomy will most often increase peripheral RBCs, WBCs, and platelet counts. (Urden L, Stacy K, Lough M. *Critical Care Nursing, Diagnosis and Management.* 7th ed. St. Louis, MO: Elsevier; 2014:997-1016.)

2-49. *Correct answer:* **b**

Horner's syndrome exhibits ptosis of the upper eyelid, elevation of the lower eyelid, contraction of the pupil on the affected side, increased salivation, and drooping of the mouth on the affected side. (Schick L, Windle PE. *PeriAnesthesia Nursing Core Curriculum: Preprocedure, Phase I and Phase II PACU Nursing.* St. Louis, MO: Saunders; 2016:1101.)

2-50. *Correct answer:* **d**

Pulmonary artery (PA) catheters carry the same risks and complications of an arterial line and central venous line, plus some that are unique to PA catheters, such as PA rupture, perforation of the right ventricle, and dysrhythmias. (Schick L, Windle PE. *PeriAnesthesia Nursing Core Curriculum: Preprocedure, Phase I and Phase II PACU Nursing.* 3rd ed. St. Louis, MO: Saunders; 2015:623.)

2-51. *Correct answer:* **d**

Turning up the sensitivity is appropriate when there is failure to sense; turning up the rate and turning down the sensitivity are appropriate strategies for failure to pace. Turning up the milliamperage supports appropriate capture. (Schick L, Windle PE. *PeriAnesthesia Nursing Core Curriculum: Preprocedure, Phase I and Phase II PACU Nursing.* 3rd ed. St. Louis, MO: Saunders; 2016:632.)

2-52. *Correct answer:* **a**
A laryngospasm is an involuntary partial or complete closure of the vocal cords, caused by secretions or stimulation or irritation of the laryngeal reflexes during emergence. (Odom-Forren J. *Drain's Perianesthesia Nursing: A Critical Care Approach.* 6th ed. St. Louis, MO: Saunders; 2013:395-396.)

2-53. *Correct answer:* **a**
Myocardial changes in the geriatric patient include left ventricular hypertrophy, increased myocardial irritability, endocardial thickening and rigidity, and calcification of the valves. (Schick L, Windle PE. *PeriAnesthesia Nursing Core Curriculum: Preprocedure, Phase I and Phase II PACU Nursing.* 3rd ed. St. Louis, MO: Saunders; 2016:289.)

2-54. *Correct answer:* **b**
Post obstructive pulmonary edema (POPE), a form of noncardiogenic pulmonary edema, may follow a postextubation laryngospasm, epiglottitis, croup, choking, or endotracheal tube obstruction. Patients with POPE can exhibit hypoxemia, cough, failure to maintain oxygen saturation levels, tachypnea, and frothy sputum. (Odom-Forren J. *Drain's Perianesthesia Nursing: A Critical Care Approach.* 6th ed. St. Louis, MO: Saunders; 2013:397-398.)

2-55. *Correct answer:* **a**
Fresh-frozen plasma transfusion treats disseminated intravascular coagulation (DIC), antithrombin III deficiency, coagulation deficiencies secondary to liver disease, and dilutional coagulopathy after massive blood replacement. One unit is equivalent to 125 to 260 mL. It must be ABO compatible and used within 24 hours after thawing. Unconcentrated plasma contains all coagulation factors except platelets (Schick L, Windle PE. *PeriAnesthesia Nursing Core Curriculum: Preprocedure, Phase I and Phase II PACU Nursing.* 3rd ed. St. Louis, MO: Saunders; 2016:820-838.)

2-56. *Correct answer:* **b**
Isoflurane only slightly affects myocardial function. It can cause possible tachycardia and peripheral vasodilation. Isoflurane increases coronary blood flow and may promote "coronary steal" phenomenon. Coronary steal phenomenon refers to the phenomenon in which small vessel dilation and an increase in flow to an area already well-perfused leads to a decrease in flow to another area of myocardium with borderline perfusion and limited coronary reserve. (Schick L, Windle PE. *PeriAnesthesia Nursing Core Curriculum: Preprocedure, Phase I and Phase II PACU Nursing.* 3rd ed. St. Louis, MO: Saunders; 2016:379-380.)

2-57. *Correct answer:* **a**
Preoperative teaching for the "implantable cardioverter-defibrillator (ICD)" patient includes information about how the device works and what to expect during the implantation procedure. After implantation, education is focused on aspects of living with an ICD. Patients need information pertaining to scheduled device follow-up and instructions about what to do if they experience a shock. Many institutions have successfully used family support groups for this patient population. Finally, because the ICD is an adjunctive treatment rather than a cure for heart failure, patients need to understand the importance of continued risk-factor modification and prescribed medications. Pathophysiology of the underlying disease process includes sudden cardiac death, ventricular dysrhythmias, and heart disease. (Urden L, Stacy K, Lough M. *Critical Care Nursing, Diagnosis and Management.* 7th ed. St. Louis, MO: Elsevier; 2014:412-466.)

2-58. *Correct answer:* **b**

Cardiogenic shock is circulatory failure caused by impairment of cardiac contractility, not by a loss of intravascular fluid volume. A lack of oxygen-rich blood reaching the brain, kidneys, skin, and other parts of the body causes the signs and symptoms of cardiogenic shock. Some of the typical signs and symptoms of shock include at least two or more of the following: confusion, loss of consciousness, a sudden and ongoing rapid or weak pulse, diaphoretic and pale skin, weak pulse, tachypnea, low urine output, and cool hands and feet. (Odom-Forren J. *Drain's Perianesthesia Nursing: A Critical Care Approach.* 6th ed. St. Louis, MO: Saunders; 2013:762-763.)

2-59. *Correct answer:* **c**

Prompt improvement of myocardial oxygen supply and tissue perfusion with a decrease in myocardial oxygen demand is vital to minimize heart damage during cardiogenic shock. (Odom-Forren J. *Drain's Perianesthesia Nursing: A Critical Care Approach.* 6th ed. St. Louis, MO: Saunders; 2013:762-763.)

2-60. *Correct answer:* **b**

The goals of treatment for cardiogenic shock include pharmacologic support to improve or correct cardiac rhythm and to decrease afterload, which may be accomplished by lowering peripheral vascular resistance. Beta blockers suppress myocardial contractility and can lead to cardiogenic shock, and are not used for management. (Odom-Forren J. *Drain's Perianesthesia Nursing: A Critical Care Approach.* 6th ed. St. Louis, MO: Saunders; 2013:762-763.)

2-61. *Correct answer:* **a**

Respiratory acidosis is characterized by an increased $PaCO_2$. Some common causes of carbon dioxide retention and respiratory acidosis include sedation, anesthesia, pulmonary edema, bronchospasm, laryngospasm, chronic obstructive pulmonary disease (COPD), and cardiac arrest. (Odom-Forren J. *Drain's Perianesthesia Nursing: A Critical Care Approach.* 6th ed. St. Louis, MO: Saunders; 2013:170.)

2-62. *Correct answer:* **b**

When preparing to transfer a patient from the Phase I PACU, the patient should be recovered from the effects of anesthesia, regained a satisfactory level of consciousness, and assessed for an appropriate amount of time after an initial dose of opioids to monitor for adverse side effects. (Odom-Forren J. *Drain's Perianesthesia Nursing: A Critical Care Approach.* 6th ed. St. Louis, MO: Saunders; 2013:392.)

2-63. *Correct answer:* **c**

Damage to the recurrent laryngeal nerve can cause vocal cord paralysis, inadequate gag reflex, stridor, and airway obstruction. (Schick L, Windle PE. *PeriAnesthesia Nursing Core Curriculum: Preprocedure, Phase I and Phase II PACU Nursing.* St. Louis, MO: Elsevier; 2016:1090.)

2-64. *Correct answer:* **c**

A potential complication of this procedure would be bleeding at the puncture site. The prudent nurse would check the dressing to ensure there was not bleeding, and if bleeding was found, he or she would apply pressure and notify the physician. (American Society for PeriAnesthesia Nurses. *2015-2017 PeriAnesthesia Nursing Standards, Practice Recommendations and Interpretive Statements.* Cherry Hill, NJ: ASPAN; 2014:145.)

2-65. *Correct answer:* **a**

Selective screening tests are commonly performed before surgery and particularly for any patient with a history of bleeding problems. These tests include platelet count and bleeding time for assessment of platelet function and prothrombin time and partial thromboplastin time for assessment of the coagulation cascade. (Odom-Forren J. *Drain's Perianesthesia Nursing: A Critical Care Approach.* 6th ed. St. Louis, MO: Saunders; 2013:194-206 94-206.)

2-66. *Correct answer:* **a**

Appropriate instructions would include driving which is typically restricted for 6 months, limited arm movement on the affected side until site is healed, bed rest for 6 to 18 hours in a monitored setting, and a magnetic resonance imaging (MRI) is prohibited. (Schick L, Windle PE. *PeriAnesthesia Nursing Core Curriculum: Preprocedure, Phase I and Phase II PACU Nursing.* 3rd ed. St. Louis, MO: Saunders; 2016:634.)

2-67. *Correct answer:* **b**

Manual airway support is usually not necessary when a laryngeal mask airway (LMA) is in place. In fact, lifting the jaw may displace the LMA cuff and cause laryngospasm, malposition, or obstruction of the airway. (Odom-Forren J. *Drain's Perianesthesia Nursing: A Critical Care Approach.* 6th ed. St. Louis, MO: Saunders; 2013:424-426.)

2-68. *Correct answer:* **a**

Respiratory alkalosis is characterized by a reduced $PaCO_2$. Hyperventilation is a frequent cause, as well as anxiety, fever, central nervous system lesions, and aspirin. (Odom-Forren J. *Drain's Perianesthesia Nursing A Critical Care Approach.* 6th ed. St. Louis, MO: Saunders; 2013:170.)

2-69. *Correct answer:* **a**

This patient should avoid taking aspirin because both aspirin and a low platelet count predispose the patient to potential bleeding. Green, leafy vegetables need to be avoided when a patient is on warfarin, not aspirin. Individuals on reverse isolation for leukemia may have fruit restriction, but this patient's immediate concern is the low platelet count. Prednisone is not prohibited with a low platelet count. (Alspach JG, ed. *Core Curriculum for Critical Care Nursing.* 6th ed. St. Louis, MO: Saunders; 2006:641-689. Odom-Forren J. *Drain's Perianesthesia Nursing: A Critical Care Approach.* 6th ed. St. Louis, MO: Saunders; 2013:194-206.)

2-70. *Correct answer:* **a**

Anesthetic agents slow the rate of sinus atrial (SA) node discharge and prolong the bundle of His-Purkinje and ventricular conduction times. Cardiac dysrhythmias are likely because of light anesthesia during emergence, which causes alterations in the balance of the autonomic nervous system between the parasympathetic and sympathetic systems. (Odom-Forren J. *Drain's Perianesthesia Nursing: A Critical Care Approach.* 6th ed. St. Louis, MO: Saunders; 2013:133.)

2-71. *Correct answer:* **c**

Clinical signs of acute hypoxemia include shallow respirations, tachypnea, dyspnea, oxyhemoglobin saturation less than 90%, anxiety, restlessness, confusion, diaphoresis, and cyanosis. (Schick L, Windle PE. *Perianesthesia Nursing Core Curriculum: Preprocedure, Phase I and Phase II PACU Nursing.* 3rd ed. St. Louis, MO: Saunders; 2016:537.)

2-72. *Correct answer:* **c**

A pneumothorax is an accumulation of air or gas in the pleural space. Signs and symptoms include sharp ipsilateral chest pain, dyspnea, decreased breath sounds, and hyperresonance on the affected side. (Odom-Forren J. *Drain's Perianesthesia Nursing: A Critical Care Approach.* 6th ed. St. Louis, MO: Saunders; 2013:397.)

2-73. *Correct answer:* **b**

The presence of an implanted defibrillator/pacemaker is not a contraindication to attaching and using an automated external defibrillator (AED). Avoid placing the electrode pads directly over the device because the devices may interfere with each other. (Sinz E, Navarro K, Soderberg ES. *Advanced Cardiovascular Life Support Provider Manual.* American Heart Association; Dallas, TX: AHA; 2011:58.)

2-74. *Correct answer:* **c**
Respiratory control determines breathing rate and quality to facilitate adequate oxygenation and rapid homeostatic balance of pH. The drive to breathe comes from the need to remove CO_2, not to inhale oxygen. (Odom-Forren J. *Drain's Perianesthesia Nursing: A Critical Care Approach.* 6th ed. St. Louis, MO: Saunders; 2013:174-175.)

2-75. *Correct answer:* **c**
The 12-lead electrocardiogram (ECG) is at the center of the decision pathway in the management of ischemic chest discomfort. It is the only means of identifying ST-elevation myocardial infarction (STEMI) and should be done within the first 10 minutes of a patient having chest pain. If there is no history of true aspirin allergy and no evidence of recent gastrointestinal (GI) bleeding, give the patient aspirin (160–325 mg) to chew. Use rectal aspirin suppositories (300 mg) for patients with nausea, vomiting, active peptic ulcer disease, or other disorders of the upper GI tract. (American Heart Association. *Advanced Cardiovascular Life Support Provider Manual,* Dallas, TX: AHA; 2016:63.)

2-76. *Correct answer:* **b**
Supraventricular tachycardia refers to the sudden interruption of the sinus rhythm by an atrial ectopic focus that fires repetitively at a rate of 150 to 250 bpm and eventually stops as suddenly as it began. Supraventricular tachycardia is often a normal compensatory response to surgical stress, pain, anxiety, bladder distention, hypovolemia, fever, or reaction to medications. The patient is asked to bear down as if going to the bathroom. If this measure is unsuccessful, the next step usually is use of IV drugs if the patient is hemodynamically stable. Adenosine is usually sufficient to restore normal sinus rhythm. Adenosine is contraindicated in patients with severe asthma. Another IV medication that may be used to slow the rate is amiodarone. If the patient becomes unstable, the next step is an elective cardioversion. (American Heart Association. *Advanced Cardiovascular Life Support Provider Manual.* Dallas,

TX: AHA; 2016:126. Schick L, Windle PE. *PeriAnesthesia Nursing Core Curriculum: Preprocedure, Phase I and Phase II PACU Nursing.* 3rd ed. St. Louis, MO: Saunders; 2016:562-641.)

2-77. *Correct answer:* **d**
Sodium nitroprusside is a peripheral vasodilator used for management of hypertension by reducing afterload. The principal pharmacologic action of sodium nitroprusside is relaxation of vascular smooth muscle and consequent dilatation of peripheral arteries and veins. (Odom-Forren J. *Drain's Perianesthesia Nursing: A Critical Care Approach.* 6th ed. St. Louis, MO: Saunders; 2013:146, 147, 246.)

2-78. *Correct answer:* **d**
The onset of nitroprusside is 30 to 60 seconds. The peak action is 1 to 2 minutes and the duration 2 to 5 minutes. (Odom-Forren J. *Drain's Perianesthesia Nursing: A Critical Care Approach.* 6th ed. St. Louis, MO: Saunders; 2013:147, 246.)

2-79. *Correct answer:* **d**
Because of the unique chemical structure of nitroprusside, cyanide is released into the bloodstream when the drug is used. The cyanide then gets converted to thiocyanate by the liver. Signs and symptoms of thiocyanate toxicity include fatigue, nausea, anorexia, muscle spasms, and disorientation. (Odom-Forren J. *Drain's Perianesthesia Nursing: A Critical Care Approach.* 6th ed. St. Louis, MO: Saunders; 2013:147.)

2-80. *Correct answer:* **a**
Vasoocclusive crisis is the most common type and is characterized by tissue ischemia, infarction, and necrosis. The bones, tendons, synovia, spleen, liver, and intestine are the common sites of occlusion. Infections, dehydration, high altitudes, extreme physical exertion, and emotional upsets can trigger this type of crisis. (Odom-Forren J. *Drain's Perianesthesia Nursing: A Critical Care Approach.* 6th ed. St. Louis, MO: Saunders; 2013:194-206.)

3

Neurologic and Gastrointestinal Systems

Diane Swintek, Carolyn Kiolbasa, and Kathy Daley

Consider this scenario for questions 3-1 to 3-5.

A 54-year-old male patient is brought to the Phase I PACU following right L4–S1 microdiscectomy and partial hemilaminectomy for a herniated disk. The injury, L4 disk herniation, occurred 3 months earlier, when a motor vehicle in which the patient was the driver was struck from behind. Initial treatment was physical therapy for back pain with radiculopathy and an uneven gait. Although the physical therapy helped alleviate the intensity of the pain, the patient experienced progressive loss of motor coordination of the right foot and exhibited progressive signs of foot drop.

3-1. A Phase I PACU admission assessment of this patient would include vital signs and:

   a. Respiratory effort, pain intensity, Glasgow coma scale, skin temperature

   b. Level of consciousness (LOC), reflexes, dermatome level, motor function of lower extremities

   c. Lumbar numbness, urinary continence, breath sounds, cardiac rhythm

   d. Sensation in lower extremities, motor function of lower extremities, pedal pulses, skin color and temperature

3-2. The patient reports numbness and tingling in the right leg. A focused neurologic assessment is best completed every:

   a. 20 minutes

   b. 15 minutes

   c. 5 minutes

   d. 10 minutes

3-3. When testing for sensation corresponding to the L4 surgical site, the perianesthesia nurse focuses attention to the _____ dermatome level.

   a. Anterior, medial thigh

   b. Anterior, medial calf

   c. Posterior, lateral thigh

   d. Posterior, lateral calf

3-4. This patient experienced foot drop preoperatively. After microdiscectomy with partial hemilaminectomy, the Phase I PACU nurse wants to test ability and strength to:

   a. Dorsiflex

   b. Invert

   c. Evert

   d. Plantarflex

3-5. The strength of motor function is assessed as 4 points. This means:

   a. Able to lift extremity against gravity, but wavers and cannot sustain

   b. Full strength, no deficit or weakness

   c. Able to lift extremity against gravity and maintain position without wavering

   d. Able to slide along support surfaces such as a bed or chair

3-6. Pain and fear that activate the sympathetic nervous system have which effect on the stomach?

   a. Rapid emptying

   b. Increase in gastric secretions and increased motility

   c. Decreased gastric secretions and emptying

   d. Increase in gastric secretions and decreased emptying

3-7. The perianesthesia nurse understands that postoperative nausea and vomiting (PONV) can precipitate surgical site disruption, esophageal tears, electrolyte imbalance, airway compromise with aspiration, and fatigue. These types of complications are:

    a. Typical

    b. Exceptional

    c. Physiologic consequences

    d. Bothersome

Consider the following scenario for questions 3-8, 3-9, and 3-10.

The Phase I PACU nurse has just received a 4-week-old male infant, status postlaparoscopic pyloromyotomy. The infant's clinical history is significant for a birth weight of 3.8 kg and a normal spontaneous vaginal delivery (NSVD). The infant had a history of frequent projectile emesis despite multiple feeding changes, ranitidine, and thickened feedings. The infant presented to the emergency department two days ago, with lethargy, decreased urine output, sunken fontanelle, and a weight of 3.4 kg. His admission laboratory values demonstrated hypochloremic, hypokalemic metabolic alkalosis, which has normalized during his rehydration in the hospital.

3-8. The infant's admission vital signs are HR of 168, RR of 36, BP of 82/palpated, and temperature of 35.8° C temporal; his central color is pink, and extremities are mottled. He has a saphenous IV in place and received two 20-mL/kg boluses of Lactated Ringer's during the case. His surgical site is clean and dry. The nurse is most concerned at this point about:

    a. His temperature of 35.8° C and mottled extremities

    b. His HR of 168

    c. His RR of 36

    d. His BP of 82/P

3-9. The nurse understands that it is important to correct the infant's alkalosis prior to receiving general anesthesia, as alkalosis increases the risk for:

    a. Feeding intolerance

    b. Occurrence of apnea

    c. Poor wound healing

    d. Hyperkalemia

3-10. The nurse notes in her postoperative orders that the infant's IV fluid is to be switched from Lactated Ringer's to a maintenance IV of D5.2NS with 20 KCL at 24 mL/hour. She is concerned with this order because:

    a. The rate is too low for this infant

    b. The rate is too high for this infant

    c. The dextrose content is too high for this infant

    d. The dextrose content is too low for this infant

3-11. The preoperative nurse is admitting a 16-year-old male patient with eosinophilic esophagitis (EOE) for an esophagogastroduodenoscopy (EGD). The patient does not respond to admission questions and continues to play with his cell phone when the nurse attempts to engage with the patient. Mom states that her son refuses to follow the diet prescribed by his physician and has had multiple episodes of choking on food. The patient responds, "I'm not bringing special food to school when I eat with my friends."

The nurse understands that her patient's responses are reflective of a difficulty adjusting to his diagnosis and of which of Erickson's developmental stages?

    a. Industry vs. inferiority

    b. Initiative vs. guilt

    c. Identity vs. role confusion

    d. Intimacy vs. isolation

3-12. When discussing lifestyle changes with the patient who will undergo gastric bypass surgery, the perianesthesia nurse must be aware that this patient will need to:

    a. Eat frequent, small (less than 90 mL) calorie-rich meals

    b. Eat meals that are low in protein

    c. Choose liquids that are high in calories

    d. Eat frequent, small (less than 30 mL) low-calorie meals

Consider this scenario for questions 3-13, 3-14, and 3-15.

After a 4hour esophagogastrectomy secondary to carcinoma, a 56-year-old male patient is admitted to the Phase I PACU. His initial temperature is 35° C (95° F). He has a nasogastric tube that has initial brightred drainage in small volumes, two chest tubes, and a urinary catheter. He is placed in a semi-Fowler's position on arrival. An epidural catheter was placed at the end of the case for pain management.

3-13. Perioperative hypothermia is defined as:

a. Patient's subjective complaint

b. Oral temperature 2% less than admission temperature

c. Core body temperature less than 36° C

d. Skin feels cool to touch

3-14. Postanesthesia Phase I priorities for this patient include pain management and ensuring that the nasogastric tube is:

a. Irrigated with normal saline until clear

b. Placed to high-pressure continuous suction

c. Patent and the position is maintained

d. Repositioned for better drainage

3-15. When performing the preoperative phone call to the parent of an 18-month-old patient with an umbilical hernia repair, the nurse encourages the parent to have two adults present for the discharge home. The most important reason to have two adults present is:

a. One adult can hold the patient while the other receives discharge instructions

b. It is better for two adults to receive discharge instructions, in case there are questions

c. Because this patient requires a car seat, it is recommended that two adults be in the vehicle

d. The patient may require care during the ride home and another adult can help

3-16. Cranial nerve (CN) XI, the spinal accessory, is a mixed type nerve, although primarily it provides motor function signals. In the cranial portion it sends impulses to and from the voluntary muscles of the:

a. Pharynx

b. Tongue

c. Abdominal viscera

d. Trapezius

3-17. The nurse is admitting a 2-year-old for an umbilical hernia repair. The child is alert and active, but cries and states "no" when approached by staff. After obtaining vital signs and weight, the nurse and anesthesiologist discuss the use of a premedication with the family. What is a safe dose of oral midazolam for this patient?

a. 0.1 to 0.2 mg/kg

b. 0.25 to 0.50 mg/kg

c. 0.5 to 1.0 mg/kg

d. 1.0 to 1.5 mg/kg

3-18. After lumbar spine surgery, it is important to protect the patient from deep vein thrombosis (DVT) by:

a. Use of sequential compression devices

b. Frequent passive range of motion

c. Positioning with stabilization pillows

d. Use of a foot board

3-19. The preadmission nurse is interviewing a patient scheduled for arthroscopic knee surgery. The patient's history is significant for female gender, nonsmoker, who has had one previous surgery, of which she states: "The surgery went well, but I had a lot of vomiting after my anesthesia." With further questioning the nurse also determines that the patient suffers from motion sickness.

Given this screening of the patient, her percentage of risk of postoperative nausea and vomiting (PONV) would be:

a. 0% to 10%

b. 10% to 30%

c. 30% to 50%

d. 60% to 80%

3-20. Chronic subdural hematomas are seen most often in older adults. Treatment consists of:

a. Craniectomy to relieve pressure

b. Low-dose anticoagulant therapy

c. Continued monitoring for cognitive deficit

d. Evacuation through burr holes

3-21. A baseline preoperative neurologic assessment must include vital signs, level of consciousness (LOC), and:

a. Pupillary response, skin color, and temperature

b. Motor function of extremities and eye movement

c. Orientation and speech

d. Proprioception and sensory function of extremities

3-22. When preparing a patient at severe risk for postoperative nausea and vomiting (PONV), the perianesthesia nurse may include which of these interventions for PONV prophylaxis?

a. Inform the patient to avoid all food and clear liquids for at least 8 hours prior to surgery

b. Encourage the patient not to be afraid of PONV; thinking about it will only make it worse

c. Encourage the patient to look for an over-the-counter acupressure device

d. Inform the patient to avoid heavy, greasy foods the day before surgery

3-23. Pupil size and reaction are controlled by cranial nerve (CN) III and the brainstem. Which anesthetic agent may cause the patient to exhibit photosensitivity in the Phase I PACU?

a. Ketamine

b. Neostigmine

c. Midazolam

d. Glycopyrrolate

3-24. For patients undergoing anterior cervical discectomy it is important to monitor the patient for:

a. Headache

b. Rhonchi

c. Tracheal edema

d. Coughing

3-25. The mechanism of injury to the spinal cord and spine is often a result of all EXCEPT:

a. Hyperflexion

b. Rotational forces

c. Decompression

d. Hyperextension

3-26. The Phase I PACU nurse receives a patient status posthiatal hernia repair who has a dual lumen stomach tube in place with an order for low-pressure intermittent suction. The tube is taped to the nose and forehead. The nurse is aware this will:

a. Cause pressure on the nostril and can result in tissue necrosis

b. Help keep excessive pressure from building up when connected to the suction device

c. Keep the air lumen unobstructed

d. Keep the open lumen above the midline

3-27. Intracranial pressure (ICP) monitoring has multiple purposes. The most common site for placement of an ICP device is:

a. The subarachnoid space

b. The anterior horn of the lateral ventricle

c. The subdural space

d. An intraparenchymal site

3-28. When providing care for a patient status postendoscopic retrograde cholangiography, the perianesthesia nurse should monitor for and educate this patient about the potential for the occurrence of which pathology?

a. Gastritis

b. Acute pancreatitis

c. Hiatal hernia

d. Electrolyte imbalance

3-29. The perianesthesia nurse is "on call" for the Phase I PACU. The nurse is called in at 2 a.m. for a 21-year-old male patient status postlaparoscopic appendectomy. The patient has no significant preoperative health issues and comes out of the operating room awake. The correct staffing for the Phase I PACU would be:

a. A registered nurse who regularly works in the Phase I PACU and a nursing assistant who floats to units as needed

b. Two registered nurses, one of whom is competent in Phase I level of care

c. Two registered nurses, both of whom are competent in Phase I level of care

d. A registered nurse who is competent in Phase I level of care and a nursing assistant trained to assist in Phase I care

Consider this scenario for questions 3-30 and 3-31.

A 62-year-old female patient complaining of intermittent right-side numbness for three days presented to the emergency department (ED) early today. She is now brought to the Phase I PACU after craniotomy for correction of an arteriovenous malformation of the right middle cerebral artery. The patient responds to verbal stimulation, follows commands, and reports the presence of persistent numbness on the right side of her body.

3-30. The middle cerebral artery supplies blood to the:

a. Parietal lobes bilaterally

b. Pituitary gland

c. Lateral surfaces of the hemispheres

d. Temporal lobes bilaterally

3-31. A major risk associated with craniotomy is postoperative vasospasm. This risk can be decreased through controlled hypertension and:

a. Hemodilution and hypervolemia

b. Keeping intracranial pressure (ICP) less than 15

c. Low-dose anticoagulant therapy

d. Patient positioned head of bed (HOB) greater than 30 degrees

3-32. All surgical patients should be assessed for their risk, but those who have had a laparoscopic abdominal procedure are at a greater risk of deep vein thrombosis due to air insufflation, which can cause:

a. A rapid decrease in abdominal pressure after completion of the procedure, leading to a decrease in blood flow to the extremities

b. An increase in intraabdominal pressure with decreased venous blood return from the lower extremities

c. An increase in intraabdominal pressure causing an increase in blood flow to the extremities

d. A rapid decrease in abdominal pressure after completion of the procedure, leading to an increase in blood flow to the extremities

3-33. The perianesthesia nurse is admitting a 6-year-old female patient for an esophagogastroduodenoscopy (EGD). The patient weighs 12 kg. The mother states that her daughter has always been a very poor eater, and this test is part of her workup. The laboratory value present in the patient's chart that is of note is a serum albumin level of 2.5 mg/dL. The nurse is aware that the patient will receive a propofol infusion during the procedure. The nurse also is aware that her patient's weight will lead to a smaller dose of propofol than is normal for a patient her age. What other factor will have an impact on the dosage?

a. Her normal albumin level will require no further adaptations

b. Her sodium should be monitored due to potential fluid shifts during the procedure

c. Her low albumin level may affect the metabolism of the propofol in the liver

d. Her potassium level may require that she receive additional supplements

3-34. Common complications related to brachial plexus block include:

    a. Hoarse or weak voice, upper eyelid ptosis, anhidrosis

    b. Bleeding, distal pain, deltoid muscle spasm

    c. Intravascular injection, metallic taste, contraction of hand

    d. Hematoma, failure of the block, torso diaphoresis

3-35. Mr. S is a patient in Phase I PACU awaiting admission to the hospital status postcolostomy of the proximal transverse colon. The nurse is monitoring output from the colostomy and is aware that:

    a. Output from this ostomy should be more solid than from the descending colon

    b. Output from this ostomy may have a higher liquid content than that from the descending colon

    c. Output from this ostomy should be more solid than that from the sigmoid colon

    d. Output from this ostomy should have a higher liquid content than that from an ileostomy

3-36. The patient with an intracranial pressure (ICP) drain requires careful monitoring of the drainage system while in the Phase I PACU. The nurse is assessing for dampened waveform and:

    a. Quality of drainage

    b. Need to irrigate

    c. ICP above 20 mm Hg

    d. Leaks and breaks in the system

3-37. Mr. J is a 50-year-old man who presents for a screening colonoscopy. His history is remarkable for hypertension, which has been well controlled on hydrochlorothiazide. He presents to the prescreening area for admission. He has been NPO since midnight and states that he is having clear watery output after his bowel preparation. It is 11 a.m. now, and the nurse is aware that the procedure suite is running behind.

Mr. J's admission vitals are HR 80, RR 16, and BP 100/48. He states that his blood pressure is the lowest it has ever been and that he is feeling very weak. The nurse places Mr. J on a cardiac monitor, noting ST segment depression, and quickly starts an IV.

The nurse is most concerned that Mr. J may be:

    a. Hyperkalemic

    b. Hypokalemic

    c. Hyperchloremic

    d. Hypochloremic

3-38. The following type of surgery statistically increases a child's risk for postoperative nausea and vomiting (PONV):

    a. Hernia/hydrocele repair

    b. Tonsillectomy/adenoidectomy

    c. Strabismus

    d. Myingotomy and tube placement

3-39. The choroid plexus is the primary source for cerebrospinal fluid (CSF). CSF functions to:

    a. Inhibit intracerebral transport of waste products

    b. Act as a cushion for the brain

    c. Act as a cushion for the spine

    d. Transport blood to the central nervous system (CNS)

3-40. Reorientation returns in the reverse order from anesthesia, beginning with:

    a. Place

    b. Time

    c. Person

    d. Situation

Consider the following scenario for questions 3-41, 3-42, and 3-43.

John is a 7-year-old male patient weighing 25 kg who arrives in the Phase I PACU following open appendectomy for a ruptured appendix. John had presented in the emergency department (ED) after a 3-day history of vomiting, diarrhea, and abdominal pain. Appendicitis was diagnosed after ultrasound and laboratory tests showing a white blood cell (WBC) count of 18,000. He received two 20-mL/kg boluses of Lactated Ringer's in the ED along with ceftriaxone 650 mg and metronidazole 200 mg. John received sevoflurane inhalation anesthesia, acetaminophen 375 mg IV, and ketorolac 12 mg IV. John received a thorough irrigation of the surgical site during the procedure and presents in the Phase I PACU with a surgical incision at McBurney's site. John has a 22-gauge IV infusing Lactated Ringer's into his right hand at 65 mL/hr and received 500 mL of Lactated Ringer's in the operating room. Vital signs are HR 140, RR 36, BP 90/48, and temperature 36.4° C temporal. He is quietly awake.

After one half-hour in the Phase I PACU, John has not had any urine output, and a bladder scan shows minimal fluid in the bladder. His HR is 148, RR is 36, and systolic blood pressure remains 90. John states his pain is a 4 on the FACES scale. His extremities are cool, and his capillary refill is 4 seconds.

3-41. John is showing signs of:

a. Compensated hypovolemic shock

b. Decompensated hypovolemic shock

c. Compensated septic shock

d. Decompensated septic shock

3-42. The Phase I PACU nurse knows that hypotension is present if the systolic blood pressure for an 8-year-old is less than:

a. 60 mm Hg + (child's age in years × 2) mm Hg

b. 70 mm Hg + (child's age in years × 2) mm Hg

c. 75 mm Hg + (child's age in years × 2) mm Hg

d. 80 mm Hg + (child's age in years × 2) mm Hg

3-43. The operating room has called, and in addition to the 7-year-old patient, another patient will be coming into the Phase I PACU. There is one RN present caring for two stable adult patients: one who is awake but not meeting discharge criteria, and one who is unconscious with a stable airway. The appropriate number of staff needed to care for the current patients and additional new patient is:

a. One registered nurse and one nursing assistant

b. Two registered nurses

c. Three registered nurses

d. Four registered nurses

3-44. There are eight cranial bones. The strongest and thickest bone in the cranium is the:

a. Temporal bone

b. Sphenoid bone

c. Occipital bone

d. Frontal bone

3-45. The Roux-en-Y gastric bypass bypasses a portion of the stomach but also bypasses:

a. The duodenum

b. The jejunum

c. The ileum

d. The antrum

3-46. Some patients emerge from general anesthesia in a state of excitement, frequently called *emergence delirium.* This can be characterized by restlessness, inappropriate behavior, and:

a. Irrational speech

b. Cowering

c. Laughing

d. Twitching of limbs

3-47. The blood–brain barrier is located throughout the brain EXCEPT in the:

a. Endothelial cells of capillaries

b. Astrocyte projections near neurons

c. Floor of the fourth ventricle

d. Intercellular junctions between capillaries

3-48. A patient admitted to the Phase II PACU now complains of double vision, headache, and sudden dizziness. A focused neurologic assessment leads the perianesthesia nurse to suspect:

    a. Hypoxia

    b. Hypoglycemia

    c. Prolonged anesthesia

    d. Stroke

3-49. Following forced-air rewarming, the patient's temperature is 37° C (98.6° F). However, he has developed persistent hypotension with BP of 78/38 mm Hg. The cardiac monitor shows sinus tachycardia with HR of 110. Urine volume is 40 mL/hr, and 5% dextrose in 0.45% normal saline with 20 mEq of potassium chloride is infusing at 125 mL/hr. Hemoglobin is 12.5 gm/dL, and potassium is 3.5 mEq/L. What is the most likely potential explanation for the patient's hypotension?

    a. Extracellular fluid deficit from hypertonic IV infusions

    b. Fluid relocation with altered capillary permeability

    c. Perioperative myocardial infarction with shock

    d. Unrecognized preoperative gastrointestinal fluid loss

3-50. A patient with a history of postoperative nausea and vomiting (PONV) is given a dose of metoclopramide at the end of surgery. Shortly after being admitted to the Phase I PACU, the patient has facial grimacing and continual chewing movements. This is indicative of:

    a. Akathisia

    b. Tardive dyskinesia

    c. Tardive dystonia

    d. Myoclonus

3-51. The greatest priority nursing plan of care for a patient in the Phase I PACU after a subtotal gastrectomy procedure is:

    a. Monitoring recurrence of peritoneal ascites

    b. Stimulating frequent deep breaths and position shift

    c. Reporting 25mL bright-red nasogastric returns

    d. Administering prophylactic antibiotics

3-52. A patient in the Phase II PACU has jerking movements that gradually slow and then stop. This is associated with what kind of seizure activity?

    a. Tonic

    b. Petit mal

    c. Clonic

    d. Generalized tonic-clonic

3-53. Assessment of motor and sensory functioning in the immediate postoperative period is:

    a. Necessary to know when motor function returns to normal

    b. An essential part of an ongoing neurologic assessment compared with baseline function

    c. Focused on laterality changes

    d. Done to determine movement that increases pain intensity

3-54. During emergence excitement it is appropriate to keep the patient safe through:

    a. Lightly applying soft wrist restraints

    b. Having security come to the bedside

    c. Administering a muscle relaxant

    d. Encouraging the patient to calm down

3-55. The basics of care for vomiting in the Phase I PACU include giving oxygen immediately and placing the patient in:

    a. Semi-Fowler's position with head turned to one side

    b. Head-down position

    c. High Fowler's position, head forward

    d. Left lateral position

3-56. When educating an 82-year-old geriatric patient who was a former military officer about home care needed after an esophagogastroduodenoscopy (EGD), the perianesthesia nurse provides instructions verbally. The nurse sits close to the patient, with hands on the patient's arm, and calls the patient by the patient's first name. The nurse is demonstrating:

a. Person-centered care and cultural competence

b. A lack of cultural competence and person-centered care

c. An understanding of interindividual diversity

d. A lack of understanding of interindividual diversity

3-57. A patient has an epidural laceration with leak after lumbar hemilaminectomy with discectomy. It is important to:

a. Ensure a patent indwelling catheter

b. Log-roll the patient

c. Keep head of bed (HOB) at 45 degrees elevation

d. Keep the knees flexed

Consider this scenario for questions 3-58, 3-59, and 3-60.

After a motor vehicle accident, a motorcyclist was admitted to the hospital comatose with multiple injuries. A depressed skull fracture was surgically repaired 6 hours later. At 24 hours after injury, he is admitted to the Phase I PACU after an exploratory laparotomy and a splenectomy, and he has had an open reduction and internal fixation repair of a left hip fracture.

3-58. During initial assessment, the Phase I PACU nurse would be *most* concerned about which value?

a. Platelets 98,000/mm

b. Hemoglobin 8.8 g/dL

c. Urine output 35 mL/hr

d. Temperature 39.8° C (103.6° F)

3-59. During Phase I PACU admission, the patient actively shivers, blood pressure is 100/50 mm Hg, and respiratory rate is 28 breaths per minute. The bedside monitor shows sinus tachycardia; shivering artifact makes initial SpO_2 measurement difficult. The perianesthesia nurse:

a. Automatically initiates an analgesia protocol

b. Applies layers of warm blankets

c. Anticipates an order for meperidine

d. Documents skin warmth, dryness, and redness

3-60. Classic indicators of early respiratory distress in an adult with septic shock are:

a. Hyperventilation with respiratory alkalosis and elevated lactate

b. Hypoventilation with decreased pulse pressure and excess circulation of corticosteroids

c. Hyperventilation with peripheral cyanosis and acidosis

d. Hypoventilation with elevated lactate and low serum glucose

3-61. The Phase I PACU nurse is preparing to send a status postdiaphragmatic hernia repair patient to the surgical unit. The patient has a stable airway and is awake but has been vomiting and has some increasing bloody drainage noted at the surgical site that the surgeon wants to continue to closely monitor on the unit. The patient should be transported to the floor by:

a. A hospital transporter certified in basic life support (BLS)

b. A perianesthesia registered nurse

c. A hospital transporter and a medical assistant

d. A registered nurse not trained in perianesthesia care

Consider this scenario for questions 3-62, 3-63, and 3-64.

A 39-year-old male patient is having right shoulder rotator cuff repair under general anesthesia with a brachial plexus nerve block. The injury occurred on his job with a construction company, and he has been attending physical therapy for two months before approval was given for surgical intervention. He admits to smoking half a pack of cigarettes per day and using marijuana at least weekly. Before his injury he regularly ran five miles at least three times per week. He denies routine alcohol consumption but admits to "going out" with friends occasionally.

3-62. The brachial plexus block chosen is an interscalene block. The site for injection is:

a. Between the clavicle and the first rib anteriorly

b. Groove between the middle and anterior scalene muscles

c. Below the scalene muscles in the brachial plexus

d. Behind the subclavian groove in the middle scalene muscle

3-63. Physical assessment reveals diminished breath sounds on the right, and the monitor shows an SpO_2 of 94% on room air. The patient reports feeling like he cannot get enough air. A possible cause is:

a. Poor ventilation related to history of smoking

b. Lingering effects of general anesthesia

c. Phrenic nerve block causing dyspnea

d. Surgical pain limiting respiratory effort

3-64. The Phase I PACU nurse reassures the patient and calls the anesthesia provider for consultation. The patient is placed on supplemental oxygen via nasal cannula at 2 L/m. What does the nurse anticipate might be a next step?

a. Chest radiograph to rule out pneumothorax

b. Working with an incentive spirometer to improve ventilation

c. Administer a nebulizer treatment to open the airways

d. Reposition the patient with the head of the bed elevated 45 degrees

3-65. The patient begins to shiver and complains of feeling cold. The nurse understands that shivering:

a. Raises the body core temperature by increasing the metabolic rate and generating heat

b. Resolves without intervention and is a normal response to anesthesia

c. Occurs only in adult patients and older adolescents

d. Effectively raises temperature by decreasing the metabolic rate

Answers and Rationales for Chapter 3, Neurologic and Gastrointestinal Systems

3-1. *Correct answer:* **d**

Along with vital signs, the Phase I PACU nurse assesses the patient for the sensory and motor function of the lower extremities, skin color and temperature, and pedal pulses. In addition, check for the presence of muscle spasms, a frequent post–lumbar surgery finding. (Odom-Forren J. *Drain's Perianesthesia Nursing: A Critical Care Approach.* 6th ed. St. Louis, MO: Saunders; 2013:576.)

3-2. *Correct answer:* **b**

A minimum of every 15 minutes for the first 2 hours in the Phase I PACU is recommended. If the findings remain stable after 2 hours, the neurologic assessment may be extended to every 30 minutes. (Odom-Forren J. *Drain's Perianesthesia Nursing: A Critical Care Approach.* 6th ed. St. Louis, MO: Saunders; 2013:567.)

3-3. *Correct answer:* **b**

When assessing the surgical repair from the L4 microdiscectomy with hemilaminectomy, the Phase I PACU nurse must assess for intact sensation at the L4 level. This can be assessed from the lateral area above the knee through the medial anterior calf of the same side. (Schick L, Windle PE. *PeriAnesthesia Nursing Core Curriculum: Preprocedure, Phase I and Phase II PACU Nursing.* 3rd ed. St. Louis, MO: Saunders; 2016:673-674.)

3-4. *Correct answer:* **a**

Preoperatively the patient was exhibiting signs of progressive foot drop. With the release of the compression on the nerve root, the patient should now be able to dorsiflex the affected foot. Assessment of the ability to dorsiflex and the strength of the movement is important. (Schick L, Windle PE. *PeriAnesthesia Nursing Core Curriculum: Preprocedure, Phase I and Phase II PACU Nursing.* 3rd ed. St. Louis, MO: Saunders; 2016:680.)

3-5. *Correct answer:* **c**

On the strength scale, a score of 4 equates to ability to lift the extremity against gravity and to maintain the position without wavering. Zero score equals no movement, and 5 on the scale would indicate full strength with no deficit or weakness. (Schick L, Windle PE. *PeriAnesthesia Nursing Core Curriculum: Preprocedure, Phase I and Phase II PACU Nursing.* 3rd ed. St. Louis, MO: Saunders; 2016:680.)

3-6. *Correct answer:* **c**

Decreased gastric secretions and decreased gastric emptying. Though the sympathetic nervous system is mainly excitatory in function, it has an inhibitory effect on the gastrointestinal tract. (Odom-Forren J. *Drain's Perianesthesia Nursing: A Critical Care Approach.* 6th ed. St. Louis, MO: Saunders; 2013:215-216.)

3-7. *Correct answer:* **c**

Although PONV is aggravating and uncomfortable for the patient, the most correct answer is physiologic consequences. Other physiologic consequences include gastric herniation, increased ocular pressure, and dehydration. Other considerations are the increased cost of delays from discharge from the Phase I and II PACUs and the fact that the cost of treating PONV is greater than the cost of prevention. PONV frequently appears on patient surveys as an undesirable outcome of surgery. (Schick L, Windle PE. *PeriAnesthesia Nursing Core Curriculum – Preoperative, Phase I and Phase II PACU Nursing.* 3rd ed. St. Louis, MO: Saunders; 2016:422.)

3-8. *Correct answer:* **a**

Infants are sensitive to heat loss because of their large body surface area, small amount of subcutaneous fat, poor vasomotor control, and decreased ability to produce heat. Hypothermia is defined as a core body temperature less than 36° C. The Phase I PACU nurse should begin active warming measures. This is especially important for young infants who are unable to shiver, relying on brown fat thermogenesis for heat production. This requires an increase in metabolism, which can result in hypoxia, hypoglycemia, and metabolic acidosis. (Odom-Forren J. *Drain's Perianesthesia Nursing: A Critical Care Approach.* 6th ed. St. Louis, MO: Saunders; 2013:694; Schick L, Windle PE. *PeriAnesthesia Nursing Core Curriculum: Preprocedure, Phase I and Phase II, PACU Nursing.* 3rd ed. St. Louis, Mo: Elsevier; 2016:232; Urden LD, Stacy KM, Lough ME. *Critical Care Nursing: Diagnosis and Management.* 7th ed. St. Louis, Mo: Elsevier/Mosby; 2014:1111-1112.)

3-9. *Correct answer:* **b**

Alkalosis decreases the respiratory drive as the body attempts to retain CO_2 to correct the acid–base imbalance. This decrease leads to episodes of apnea, which is already at a greater risk in young infants after receiving general anesthesia. (Odom-Forren J. *Drain's Perianesthesia Nursing: A Critical Care Approach.* 6th ed. St. Louis, MO: Saunders; 2013:378.)

3-10. *Correct answer:* **b**

A maintenance IV rate for an infant of 0 to 10 kg is 4 mL/kg/hr for each kilogram of body weight, or 100 mL/kg. This demonstrates an IV rate of 14 mL/hr. The current rate infusing is over one and a half times the maintenance fluid rate for an infant weighing 3.4 kg. (Schick L, Windle PE. *PeriAnesthesia Nursing Core Curriculum: Preprocedure, Phase I and Phase II PACU Nursing.* 3rd ed. St. Louis, MO: Elsevier; 2016:1239.)

3-11. *Correct answer:* **c**

Adolescence is the period when the sense of "I" is being developed, as children gain independence from their parents. This is also the time when children identify strongly with their peers, who become very important. The patient is demonstrating difficulty adjusting to his diagnosis, which makes him different from his peer group. (Schick L, Windle PE. *PeriAnesthesia Nursing Core Curriculum: Preprocedure, Phase I and Phase II PACU Nursing.* 3rd ed. St. Louis, MO: Elsevier; 2016:254-257.)

3-12. *Correct answer:* **d**

Meals should be frequent, small (less than 30 mL), and low calorie. Fluids should be taken separately from solids. Foods that can encourage dumping syndrome include high-calorie liquids and soft foods such as ice cream; easily dissolvable foods such as cookies and bread; and foods that can obstruct such as meats, pastas, and citrus fruit membranes. (Schick L, Windle PE. *PeriAnesthesia Nursing Core Curriculum: Preprocedure, Phase I and Phase II PACU Nursing.* 3rd ed. St. Louis, MO: Elsevier; 2016:1147-1178.)

3-13. *Correct answer:* **c**

Normothermia is defined as a core temperature ranging from 36° C to 38° C. This patient's temperature is considered hypothermic and requires active warming measures, such as the application of a forced-air warming system and warmed humidified inspired oxygen. (American Society of PeriAnesthesia Nurses. *2015–2017 Perianesthesia Nursing Standards, Practice Recommendations, and Interpretive Statements.* Cherry Hill, NJ: ASPAN; 2014; Odom-Forren J. *Drain's Perianesthesia Nursing: A Critical Care Approach.* 6th ed. St. Louis, MO: Saunders; 2013:740-750.)

3-14. *Correct answer:* **c**

Postanesthesia Phase I priorities for patients having an esophagogastrectomy are pain management, usually with low thoracic epidural or patient-controlled analgesia and to maintain nasogastric tube patency and position. It is frequently ordered to have the tube set to low-pressure intermittent suction (20–80 mm Hg). Usually only low-pressure intermittent suction is used because excessive negative pressure in either the stomach or the bowel pulls the mucosa into the lumen of the tube and can cause traumatic ulcers. If the patient has had gastric, pancreatic, or esophageal surgery, the tube should not be manipulated. (Odom-Forren J. *Drain's Perianesthesia Nursing: A Critical Care Approach.* 6th ed. St Louis, MO: Elsevier; 2013:40, 582-593; Schick L, Windle PE. *PeriAnesthesia Nursing Core Curriculum: Preprocedure, Phase I and Phase II PACU Nursing.* 3rd ed. St. Louis, MO: Saunders; 2016:23, 740-767.)

3-15. *Correct answer:* **c**

The pediatric patient at this age should ride in a rear-facing car seat in the back seat. It is recommended that two adults be in the vehicle, one of whom is seated with the child. (American Society of PeriAnesthesia Nurses. *2015–2017 PeriAnesthesia Nursing Standards, Practice Recommendations and Interpretive Statements.* Cherry Hill, NJ: ASPAN; 2014:60.)

3-16. *Correct answer:* **a**

The spinal accessory nerve sends impulses to and from the voluntary muscles of the pharynx, larynx, and palate for swallowing. Motor, sensory, and autonomic messages to and from the pharynx also originate from CN X, the vagus nerve. (Odom-Forren J. *Drain's Perianesthesia Nursing: A Critical Care Approach.* 6th ed. St. Louis, MO: Saunders; 2013:112.)

3-17. *Correct answer:* **b**

The safe oral dose of midazolam is 0.25 to 0.50 mg/kg to a maximum dose of 20 mg. Onset usually occurs in 10 to 20 minutes. (Skidmore-Roth L. *Mosby's 2016 Nursing Drug Reference.* 29th ed. St. Louis, MO: Elsevier; 2016:780.)

3-18. *Correct answer:* **a**

Risk is significant for a patient for a patient to develop a DVT or embolism post–spinal surgery secondary to venous pooling and lack of movement. Use of a sequential compression device may prevent the development of a thrombus in the postoperative period. Early ambulation continues to be the best defense against developing DVT. (Odom-Forren J. *Drain's Perianesthesia Nursing: A Critical Care Approach.* 6th ed. St. Louis, MO: Saunders; 2013:543-544.)

3-19. *Correct answer:* **d**

This patient is at a 60% to 80% risk for nausea and vomiting due to her gender, being a nonsmoker, and her history of motion sickness and previous history of postoperative nausea and vomiting. The level of PONV risk increases with each risk factor noted. Her multiple risk factors place her in a severe to very severe risk depending on the assessment tool used. (American Society of PeriAnesthesia Nurses. *ASPAN's evidence-based clinical practice guideline for the prevention and/or management of PONV/PDNV.* JOPAN. 2006; 21(4):230-250; Odom-Forren J. *Drain's Perianesthesia Nursing: A Critical Care Approach.* 6th ed. St. Louis, MO: Saunders; 2013:404-405.)

3-20. *Correct answer:* **d**

Chronic subdural hematomas can mimic any of the diseases that affect the brain. Most often in the older adult it does not have a direct causative injury, but rather progressive mental or personality changes are noted. Treatment consists of evacuation of the accumulated blood through multiple burr holes or a craniotomy incision. (Schick L, Windle PE. *PeriAnesthesia Nursing Core Curriculum: Preprocedure, Phase I and Phase II PACU Nursing.* 3rd ed. St. Louis, MO: Saunders; 2016:684; Odom-Forren J. *Drain's Perianesthesia Nursing: A Critical Care Approach.* 6th ed. St. Louis, MO: Saunders; 2013:557.)

3-21. *Correct answer:* **a**

An essential element in any postoperative neurologic assessment is documentation of the preoperative baseline functioning. Basic baseline data that are readily measured postoperatively are the vital signs, LOC, pupillary response, and skin color and temperature. (Odom-Forren J. *Drain's Perianesthesia Nursing: A Critical Care Approach.* 6th ed. St. Louis, MO: Saunders; 2012:14, 374, 404.)

3-22. *Correct answer:* **c**

A patient with a severe risk of postoperative nausea and vomiting (PONV) will need a multimodal approach to PONV prophylaxis. P6 accupoint stimulation has been shown to be effective in some populations for relief of PONV. This is one additional way that the patient's potential for PONV can be addressed before arrival for surgery. Some studies have shown that drinking clear fluids up until 2 hours before surgery is helpful in preventing PONV. Five ounces of clear fluids has been found to stimulate peristalsis and facilitate gastric emptying. Thus, encouraging the patient to be NPO for at least 8 hours may not be helpful. (Peterson C. The hepatobiliary and gastrointestinal system. In: Odom-Forren J. *Drain's Perianesthesia Nursing: A Critical Care Approach.* 6th ed. St. Louis, MO: Saunders; 2013:405; American Society of PeriAnesthesia Nurses. *ASPAN's evidence-based clinical practice guideline for the prevention and/or management of PONV/PDNV.* JOPAN. 2006; 21(4):230-250; Odom-Forren J. *Drain's Perianesthesia Nursing: A Critical Care Approach.* 6th ed. St. Louis, MO: Elsevier/Saunders; 2013:404-405.)

3-23. *Correct answer:* **d**

The adjunctive reversal agent glycopyrrolate, an anticholinergic protects against the peripheral muscarinic effects (e.g., bradycardia and excessive secretions) of cholinergic agents such as neostigmine; it causes mydriasis, resulting in photophobia. (Kizior RJ, Hodgson, BB. *Saunders Nursing Drug Handbook 2015.* 1st ed. St. Louis, MO: Saunders; 2016.)

3-24. *Correct answer:* **c**

Tracheal edema may result from nerve damage or hematoma formation. Respiratory status is especially important to monitor with cervical procedures. Aside from noting the midline position of the trachea, it is important to document the rate and character of respirations. Additional assessment of the patient's ability to handle secretions can provide insight into any respiratory difficulties. (Schick L, Windle PE. *PeriAnesthesia Nursing Core Curriculum: Preprocedure, Phase I and Phase II PACU Nursing.* 3rd ed. St. Louis, MO: Saunders; 2016:714.)

3-25. *Correct answer:* **c**

The mechanism of injury to the spine or spinal cord is seen with hyperflexion as a result of a head-on collision, hyperextension from a rear-end collision or elderly who fall and strike the chin, or rotational forces from extreme twisting or flexion of the head and neck. Surgical intervention is done to decompress the spinal cord or spinal nerves to prevent further pain, loss of function, or ischemia of neural tissue. (Schick L, Windle PE. *PeriAnesthesia Nursing Core Curriculum: Preprocedure, Phase I and Phase II PACU Nursing.* 3rd ed. St. Louis, MO: Saunders; 2016:702-704; Odom-Forren J. *Drain's Perianesthesia Nursing: A Critical Care Approach.* 6th ed. St. Louis, MO: Saunders; 2013:571.)

3-26. *Correct answer:* **a**

Taping the tube to the nose and then up to the forehead can cause undue pressure on the nostril. This pressure can quickly cause tissue necrosis. The tube should be taped to prevent pressure on the naris, and to prevent further pressure the tube can be pinned or taped to the patient's gown. (Odom-Forren J. *Drain's Perianesthesia Nursing: A Critical Care Approach.* 6th ed. St. Louis, MO: Saunders; 2012:586.)

3-27. *Correct answer:* **b**

The anterior horn of the lateral ventricles, numbers 1 and 2, is the most common placement for an ICP monitoring device or drain. ICP monitoring is the standard of care for patients at risk for intracranial hypertension. A measurement of the pressure can be obtained from the lateral ventricles, subarachnoid space, or epidural or subdural spaces. (Schick L, Windle PE. *PeriAnesthesia Nursing Core Curriculum: Preprocedure, Phase I and Phase II PACU Nursing.* 3rd ed. St. Louis, MO: Saunders; 2016:687-688; Odom-Forren J. *Drain's Perianesthesia Nursing: A Critical Care Approach.* 6th ed. St. Louis, MO: Saunders; 2013:783-785.)

3-28. *Correct answer:* **b**

Pancreatitis can occur as a result of common bile duct exploration. It presents with excessive pain, vomiting, fever, and jaundice. The surgeon should be informed of the occurrence of these symptoms. (Odom-Forren J. *Drain's Perianesthesia Nursing: A Critical Care Approach.* 6th ed. St. Louis, MO: Saunders; 2013:219-220.)

3-29. *Correct answer:* **b**

The correct staffing for Phase I is "a minimum of two RNs should be present in the Phase I PACU whenever a Phase I patient is being recovered. At least one of the two RNs should be competent in Phase I level of care." Minimum standards do not vary in an "on-call" situation. Safety is the primary concern in staffing situations. (American Society of PeriAnesthesia Nurses. *2015–2017 PeriAnesthesia Nursing Standards, Practice Recommendations and Interpretive Statements.* Cherry Hill, NJ: ASPAN; 2014:35.)

3-30. *Correct answer:* **c**

The middle cerebral artery is the largest branch of the internal carotid artery. It supplies blood to two thirds of the lateral surfaces of cerebral hemispheres. This artery also sends off branches to the corpus striatum and the internal capsule. (Schick L, Windle PE. *PeriAnesthesia Nursing Core Curriculum: Preprocedure, Phase I and Phase II PACU Nursing.* 3rd ed. St. Louis, MO: Saunders; 2015:650; Odom-Forren J. *Drain's Perianesthesia Nursing: A Critical Care Approach.* 6th ed. St. Louis, MO: Saunders; 2013:118-119.)

3-31. *Correct answer:* **a**

Vasospasm postcraniotomy can lead to stroke and death. Triple-H therapy (hypertension, hemodilution, hypervolemia) postoperatively can prevent and treat cerebral vasospasm. This therapy forces constricted blood vessels to dilate and restores perfusion to an affected area. (Schick L, Windle PE. *PeriAnesthesia Nursing Core Curriculum: Preprocedure, Phase I and Phase II PACU Nursing.* 3rd ed. St. Louis, MO: Saunders; 2016:698.)

3-32. *Correct answer:* **b**

The insufflation increases pressure in the abdomen. This pressure decreases venous blood return, especially from the lower extremities. The stasis of venous blood in the extremities can contribute to the formation of thrombosis. (Schick L, Windle PE. *PeriAnesthesia Nursing Core Curriculum: Preprocedure, Phase I and Phase II PACU Nursing.* 3rd ed. St. Louis, MO: Saunders; 2016:815.)

3-33. *Correct answer:* **c**

Her low albumin level will affect the propofol dosage because propofol is protein binding and metabolized in the liver. The decreased availability of albumin to bind to the propofol will allow more drug to be available in circulation. The patient may need to be closely monitored longer than is usual because it may take longer to metabolize the propofol. (Odom-Forren J. *Drain's Perianesthesia Nursing: A Critical Care Approach,* 6th ed. St. Louis, MO: Saunders; 2013:218.)

3-34. *Correct answer:* **a**

Common complications of brachial plexus block include hoarse or weak voice, upper eyelid ptosis, and anhidrosis (inability to sweat). These experiences are distressing to the patient but self-limiting. The patient benefits from reassurance that once the blocking agent wears off, function will return to normal. (Schick L, Windle PE. *PeriAnesthesia Nursing Core Curriculum: Preprocedure, Phase I and Phase II PACU Nursing.* 3rd ed. St. Louis, MO: Saunders; 2016:354; Odom-Forren J. *Drain's Perianesthesia Nursing: A Critical Care Approach.* 6th ed. St. Louis, MO: Saunders; 2012:334-338.)

3-35. *Correct answer:* **b**

This ostomy should have a higher liquid content than that from the descending colon because it is in a more proximal location. The absorption of water and electrolytes occurs mostly in the proximal half of the colon, as opposed to the storage of fecal material, which occurs in the distal colon. (Odom-Forren J. *Drain's Perianesthesia Nursing: A Critical Care Approach.* 6th ed. St. Louis, MO: Saunders; 2013:217.)

3-36. *Correct answer:* **d**

For the patient with an intracranial pressure (ICP) drain/monitor, it is essential that the nurse observe the patient for any leaks or breaks in that system. If the patient develops a leak in the drainage system, the surgeon must be contacted immediately. An ICP drain is never irrigated, and ideally the intracranial pressure is kept below 20 mm Hg. (Schick L, Windle PE. *PeriAnesthesia Nursing Core Curriculum: Preprocedure, Phase I and Phase II PACU Nursing.* 3rd ed. St. Louis, MO: Saunders; 2016:688.)

3-37. *Correct answer:* **b**

The fact that Mr. J went through an excessive bowel prep resulting in a large loss of fluid, along with the use of hydrochlorothiazide, could contribute to hypokalemia. Thiazide diuretics act on the distal tubule of the loop of Henle and work to impair the reabsorption of sodium, chloride, and potassium, which is excreted with water. Though Mr. J may be hypochloremic, he is demonstrating many of the symptoms of hypokalemia, which is the most common negative side effect of thiazide diuretics. Some of the symptoms of hypokalemia are severe muscle weakness, hypotension, atrial and ventricular dysrhythmias, and paralytic ileus. (Odom-Forren J. *Drain's Perianesthesia Nursing: A Critical Care Approach.* 6th ed. St. Louis, MO: Saunders; 2013:184-193, 214-221.)

3-38. *Correct answer:* **c**

The Society for Ambulatory Anesthesia (SAMBA) Consensus Guidelines were established in 2014 after a Cochrane Collaboration search strategy developed an evidence-based risk assessment tool for postoperative nausea and vomiting (PONV), postoperative vomiting (POV), and postdischarge nausea and vomiting (PDNV) in pediatric patients. Guideline number one was to identify a patient's risk for PONV. In order to be able to align with this guideline, a risk factor assessment tool was developed for pediatrics using evidence-based data. The tool assesses the pediatric patient for risk factors. The risk factors include surgery greater than or equal to 30 minutes, age greater than or equal to 3 years, strabismus surgery, and a history of POV or PONV in relatives. Each factor contributes to the risk, with basic POV being 10% in pediatrics with no risk factors present. The risk remains at 10% for one factor and increases to 30%, 50%, and 70% for each additional factor. (Schick L, Windle PE. *PeriAnesthesia Nursing Core Curriculum: Preprocedure, Phase I and Phase II PACU Nursing.* 3rd ed. St. Louis, MO: Saunders; 2016:968, 978-979; Gan TJ, Diemunsch P, Habib AS, et al. Consensus Guidelines for the Management of Postoperative Nausea and Vomiting. *Anesthesia & Analgesia.* 2014;118(1):85-113.)

3-39. *Correct answer:* **b**

The primary function of the cerebrospinal fluid (CSF) is to act as a cushion for the brain. The specific gravity of both the brain and CSF is essentially the same, so the brain floats in the skull. CSF additionally serves as the medium to transport nutrients and waste products between the bloodstream and the cells of the central nervous system (CNS). The choroid plexus is a highly vascular, tufted structure with many small granular pouches that project into the ventricles of the brain and are the primary source for CSF formation. (Odom-Forren J. *Drain's Perianesthesia Nursing: A Critical Care Approach.* 6th ed. St. Louis, MO: Saunders; 2012:116.)

3-40. *Correct answer:* **c**

Reorientation after anesthesia progresses, first becoming oriented to person, then place, then time, and finally situation. If the patient was confused or disoriented preoperatively, this sequence may not hold true. (Odom-Forren J. *Drain's Perianesthesia Nursing: A Critical Care Approach.* 6th ed. St. Louis, MO: Saunders; 2013:374.)

3-41. *Correct answer:* **a**

John is showing signs of compensated hypovolemic shock. His heart and respiratory rate are above normal for his age. Due to the deficiency of his circulating blood volume, as well as extravascular fluid volume (his hypovolemia), John is demonstrating compensatory mechanisms. His tachycardia is an attempt to maintain cardiac output. The cool extremities and delayed capillary refill are the mechanisms to shunt blood to the vital organs and away from the periphery. Tachypnea is the compensatory mechanism to combat metabolic acidosis. His shock is compensated because he is still maintaining a normal blood pressure for his age. (Chameides L, Samson R, Schexnayder S. *American Heart Association Pediatric Advanced Life Support Provider Manual.* Dallas, TX: American Heart Association; 2011.)

3-42. *Correct answer:* **b**

Hypotension is present if the systolic blood pressure is less than 70 mm Hg + (child's age in years × 2) mm Hg. Hypotension is a late sign in pediatric patients, and the progression from hypotension to cardiopulmonary failure and cardiac arrest can be rapid. (Chameides L, Samson R, Schexnayder S. *American Heart Association Pediatric Advanced Life Support Provider Manual.* Dallas, TX; American Heart Association; 2011.)

3-43. *Correct answer:* **c**

The first RN is caring for two patients who meet the criteria for a one RN to two patients staffing. The RN who is caring for John has a 7-year-old patient who is without a family member or other support staff and is demonstrating signs of being hemodynamically unstable, which makes him a 1:1 class of patient. The fourth patient will require the third nurse. (American Society of PeriAnesthesia Nurses. *2015–2017 PeriAnesthesia Nursing Standards, Practice Recommendations and Interpretive Statements.* Cherry Hill, NJ: ASPAN; 2014:35.)

3-44. *Correct answer:* **c**

The occipital bone forms the back and largest portion of the base of the skull. The two temporal bones form the remaining portion. The bones at the base of the skull are both thicker and stronger than the sides and top. (Odom-Forren J. *Drain's Perianesthesia Nursing: A Critical Care Approach.* 6th ed. St. Louis, MO: Saunders; 2013:113-114.)

3-45. *Correct answer:* **a**

The Roux-en-Y creates a small pouch at the top, or antrum, of the stomach. This portion of the stomach is then connected directly to the jejunum, or middle portion of the small intestine. This serves two purposes in that it limits the volume of food taken in, as well as allowing fewer calories to be absorbed due to bypassing a portion of the intestine. (Odom-Forren J. *Drain's Perianesthesia Nursing: A Critical Care Approach.* 6th ed. St. Louis, MO: Saunders; 2013:642.)

3-46. *Correct answer:* **a**

Emergence excitement, often referred to as *emergence delirium,* is characterized by restlessness, inappropriate behavior, crying, moaning, disorientation, and irrational speech. The nurse wants to rule out hypoxemia, anxiety, medications, pain, metabolic disturbance, bladder distention, or anesthesia as a cause for the excitement. (Odom-Forren J. *Drain's Perianesthesia Nursing: A Critical Care Approach.* 6th ed. St. Louis, MO: Saunders; 2013:402-403.)

3-47. *Correct answer:* **c**

The blood–brain barrier is located throughout the brain except in the hypothalamus, pineal gland area, and floor of the fourth ventricle in the upper medulla. The site of the barrier is not on the neurons themselves, but in a network of endothelial cells (cells of capillaries) and projections from astrocytes close to the neurons. The function of the blood–brain barrier is to tightly regulate what may enter the extracellular environment of the brain from the capillaries. (Schick L, Windle PE. *PeriAnesthesia Nursing Core Curriculum: Preprocedure, Phase I and Phase II PACU Nursing.* 3rd ed. St. Louis, MO: Saunders; 2016:653-655; Odom-Forren J. *Drain's Perianesthesia Nursing: A Critical Care Approach.* 6th ed. St. Louis, MO: Saunders; 2013:116-117.)

3-48. *Correct answer:* **d**

Interruption of oxygen delivery related to decreased blood flow to the brain results in neural tissue destruction. Some warning signs may be loss of strength and/or sensation on one side of the body, decreased vision or double vision, difficulty speaking or understanding speech, severe headache, sudden dizziness, nausea and/or vomiting, and difficulty swallowing. These are symptoms that lead the nurse to suspect stroke and ask for expert consultation. (Schick L, Windle PE. *PeriAnesthesia Nursing Core Curriculum: Preprocedure, Phase I and Phase II PACU Nursing.* 3rd ed. St. Louis, MO: Saunders; 2016:690-691.)

3-49. *Correct answer:* **b**

Despite adequate overall fluid volume replacement, the patient's hypotension likely results when fluid moves from the vascular compartment into the abdominal tissues and spaces that normally contain little fluid. This sequestered volume is unavailable to support cardiac output. Extensive bowel manipulation, tissue trauma or infection, decreased serum protein, and altered capillary permeability are among forces that could allow fluids to exit the vascular compartment after a major abdominal surgical procedure. (Schick L, Windle PE. *PeriAnesthesia Nursing Core Curriculum: Preprocedure, Phase I and Phase II PACU Nursing.* 3rd ed. St. Louis, MO: Saunders; 2016:318-319; Odom-Forren J. *Drain's Perianesthesia Nursing: A Critical Care Approach.* 6th ed. St. Louis, MO: Saunders; 2013:197, 582-593.)

3-50. *Correct answer:* **b**

Tardive dyskinesia is an extrapyramidal side effect resulting from the administration of metoclopramide, a medication used to prophylactically treat postoperative nausea and vomiting in the surgical patient. It is also seen in people who have long-term use of metoclopramide for a digestive disorder. It is important that the preoperative nurse obtain a complete medication history to aid in postoperative care. (Odom-Forren J. *Drain's Perianesthesia Nursing: A Critical Care Approach.* 6th ed. St. Louis, MO: Saunders; 2013:108.)

3-51. *Correct answer:* **b**

Poor ventilation, atelectasis, and pneumonia are likely outcomes if the patient does not move, breathe deeply and often, and have adequate pain management to participate in her pulmonary care. After the high upper abdominal incision used for gastrectomy, the patient is likely to "splint" her incision and restrict her breathing to limit her pain. (Schick L, Windle PE. *Perianesthesia Nursing Core Curriculum: Preprocedure, Phase I and Phase II PACU Nursing.* 3rd ed. St. Louis, MO: Saunders; 2016:740-767.)

3-52. *Correct answer:* **c**

Clonic seizure activity is characterized by jerking movements that gradually slow and then stop. They usually last 1 to 2 minutes, and it is not unusual for the patient to stop breathing for 30 seconds to a minute. Tonic seizures are characterized by increased muscle tone and rigidity of the patient. Petit mal seizures are sometimes called *absence seizures.* These are short, 5 to 20 seconds, and may occur 30 or more times per day. Myoclonus is the jerky, spasmodic contraction of a group of muscles. (Schick L, Windle PE. *PeriAnesthesia Nursing Core Curriculum: Preprocedure, Phase I and Phase II PACU Nursing.* 3rd ed. St. Louis, MO: Saunders; 2016:689-690.)

3-53. *Correct answer:* **b**

It is essential that there is a preprocedure neurologic assessment on which to measure postoperative function. In addition to sensory and motor function after cranial procedures, it is important to assess vital signs, level of consciousness (LOC), and pupillary reaction. (Odom-Forren J. *Drain's Perianesthesia Nursing: A Critical Care Approach.* 6th ed. St. Louis, MO: Saunders; 2013:567.)

3-54. *Correct answer:* **a**

During emergence excitement it is the responsibility of the nurse to keep the patient safe from physical harm. This may require the application of soft wrist restraints while the patient is exhibiting inappropriate behavior. Additionally you want to reassure the patient that he or she is safe and that surgery is over and reorient them to person, place, time, and situation frequently. (Schick L, Windle PE. *PeriAnesthesia Nursing Core Curriculum: Preprocedure, Phase I and Phase II PACU Nursing.* 3rd ed. St. Louis, MO: Saunders; 2016:1234; Odom-Forren J. *Drain's Perianesthesia Nursing: A Critical Care Approach.* 6th ed. St. Louis, MO: Saunders; 2013:402-403.)

3-55. *Correct answer:* **b**

The purpose of the head-down position is to allow fluid to flow away from the lungs rather than into the lungs. Consequently, the patient should be placed in this position if aspiration is suspected. Fluid should be suctioned rapidly while administration of oxygen continues. (Odom-Forren J. *Drain's Perianesthesia Nursing: A Critical Care Approach.* 6th ed. St. Louis, MO: Saunders; 2013:409.)

3-56. *Correct answer:* **b**

It is critical when preparing to discharge any patient, but especially so with geriatric patients, that the nurse is aware of not only the developmental needs of the patient, but also of cultural issues that affect the care given. Although this nurse is addressing the educational needs of this patient, he or she is not demonstrating person-centered care or cultural competence.

This patient would benefit from written instructions in a large font. The area should be well lit before demonstrating care. The nurse needs to be sensitive to her patient's preferred name or title. When speaking to her patient, she or he should be aware that the patient may not be comfortable with the close proximity or touch. (Odom-Forren J. *Drain's Perianesthesia Nursing: A Critical Care Approach*, 6th ed. St. Louis, MO: Saunders; 2013:711-720.)

3-57. *Correct answer:* **b**

An epidural leak will cause a searing headache with movement, sitting, or standing, and is generally diminished by lying down. These patients need to remain on bed rest for 24 hours with administration of pain medications and possibly caffeine. Minimizing movement can limit or prevent postdural puncture headache. (Odom-Forren J. *Drain's Perianesthesia Nursing: A Critical Care Approach.* 6th ed. St. Louis, MO: Saunders; 2013:330-331, 410.)

3-58. *Correct answer:* **d**

Mortality for sepsis ranges from 20% to more than 50%. Infection results from many possible sources and can initiate a progression of events that contribute to shock, disseminated intravascular coagulation, renal failure, gastrointestinal bleeding, and pulmonary failure. Vigilant effort is directed toward finding and eradicating the infectious source. The nurse monitors the patient's currently acceptable platelets and urine output; the patient's hemoglobin level, although less than the accepted normal range of 12 to 15 g/dL, may reflect increase in the fluid content of blood, not new bleeding, after abdominal exploration. (Schick L, Windle PE. *PeriAnesthesia Nursing Core Curriculum: Preprocedure, Phase I and Phase II PACU Nursing.* 3rd ed. St. Louis, MO: Saunders; 2016:1200-1201; Urden LD, Stacy KM, Lough ME. *Critical Care Nursing: Diagnosis and Management.* 7th ed. St. Louis, MO: Elsevier; 2014:902-908.)

3-59. *Correct answer:* **c**

Shivering, a result of hypothermia or exposure to certain anesthesia agents, can have deleterious effects on patients, including increased metabolic rates and oxygen demands. Warm blankets may be helpful, but low doses of meperidine have been found to mitigate the shivering response. (Odom-Forren J. *Drain's Perianesthesia Nursing: A Critical Care Approach.* 6th ed. St. Louis, MO: Saunders; 2013:392.)

3-60. *Correct answer:* **a**

Hyperventilation and $PaCO_2$ less than 32 mm Hg (respiratory alkalosis) are hallmarks of septic shock. Alkalosis is the body's initial attempt to compensate for metabolic acidosis, indicated by a still-elevated serum lactate. Hypoxemia declares the development of acute respiratory distress syndrome. Sepsis stresses all body organ systems. Pulmonary dysfunction occurs as a result of increased pulmonary capillary membrane permeability, pulmonary microemboli, and pulmonary vasoconstriction. Ventilatory failure and acute respiratory distress syndrome (ARDS) develop. (Schick L, Windle PE. *PeriAnesthesia Nursing Core Curriculum: Preprocedure, Phase I and Phase*

II PACU Nursing. 3rd ed. St. Louis, MO: Saunders; 2016:1200-1201; Odom-Forren J. *Drain's Perianesthesia Nursing: A Critical Care Approach.* 6th ed. St. Louis, MO: Saunders; 2012:764-765, 791-794; Urden L. *Critical Care Nursing, Diagnosis and Management.* 7th ed. St. Louis, MO: Elsevier; 2014:35, 887-925.)

3-61. *Correct answer:* **b**

"A perianesthesia registered nurse should accompany patients who require evaluation, treatment or are at risk of cardiopulmonary compromise during transport . . . Patients who require evaluation during transfer include patients who have a potential for bleeding, airway compromise vomiting, etc." Because this patient has been vomiting and has a surgical site that is still being evaluated for bleeding, he should have a perianesthesia registered nurse accompany him. (American Society of PeriAnesthesia Nurses. *2015–2017 PeriAnesthesia Nursing Standards, Practice Recommendations and Interpretive Statements.* Cherry Hill, NJ: ASPAN; 2014:60.)

3-62. *Correct answer:* **b**

The interscalene block provides paresthesia to upper, middle, and lower trunks of the brachial plexus between the anterior and middle scalene muscles. This block is contraindicated in a patient with chronic obstructive pulmonary disease (COPD) secondary to the risk of pneumothorax and phrenic nerve blockade. (Schick L, Windle PE. *PeriAnesthesia Nursing Core Curriculum: Preprocedure, Phase I and Phase II PACU Nursing.* 3rd ed. St. Louis, MO: Saunders; 2016:354, 673-674; Odom-Forren J. *Drain's Perianesthesia Nursing: A Critical Care Approach.* 6th ed. St. Louis, MO: Saunders; 2013:335-337.)

3-63. *Correct answer:* **c**

Dyspnea can result from phrenic nerve blockade related to the interscalene block. Notify an anesthesia provider immediately when the patient complains of dyspnea. (Schick L, Windle PE. *PeriAnesthesia Nursing Core Curriculum: Preprocedure, Phase I and Phase II PACU Nursing.* 3rd ed. St. Louis, MO: Saunders; 2016:354; Odom-Forren J. *Drain's Perianesthesia Nursing: A Critical Care Approach.* 6th ed. St. Louis, MO: Saunders; 2013:335-337.)

3-64. *Correct answer:* **a**

Portable chest x-ray to assure that the dyspnea is not related to a pneumothorax. It is additionally beneficial to instruct the patient in the use of an incentive spirometer to promote good pulmonary function postoperatively. (Schick L, Windle PE. *PeriAnesthesia Nursing Core Curriculum: Preprocedure, Phase I and Phase II PACU Nursing.* 3rd ed.

St. Louis, MO: Saunders; 2016:354; Odom-Forren J. *Drain's Perianesthesia Nursing: A Critical Care Approach.* 6th ed. St. Louis, MO: Saunders; 2013:335-337.)

3-65. *Correct Answer:* **a**

The body initiates shivering through the hypothalamus as a response to a decrease in core temperature. The intent of shivering is to raise the core temperature; this occurs from the increase in metabolic rate with generation of heat from the act of shivering. Feeling cold and shivering were reported as the most unpleasant experiences after surgery by postoperative patients. (Stannard D, Krenzischek D, eds. *Perianesthesia Nursing Care: A Bedside Guide for Safe Recovery.* Sudbury, MA: Jones and Bartlett Learning; 2012; In: Urden LD, Stacy KM, Lough ME. *Critical Care Nursing: Diagnosis and Management.* 7th ed. St. Louis, MO: Elsevier; 2013:1111-1112.)

4

Renal and Integumentary Systems

Carolyn Kiolbasa, Theresa Clifford, Renee Smith, Charlotte West, and Susan Norris

4-1. Patients who are hypothermic after surgery require gradual rewarming in the Phase I PACU to prevent:

a. Fluid loss

b. Hypotension

c. Nausea

d. Bradycardia

4-2. The Phase I PACU nurse is caring for a male patient who underwent a revision of a total hip arthroplasty and had a reported blood loss of 900 mL. Postoperatively, the nurse notices that the patient has had low urine output for the last hour. The physician orders hetastarch. The nurse knows that hetastarch:

a. Is more expensive than blood products

b. Tends to produce allergic reactions

c. Does not cause fluid overload

d. Metabolizes slowly and remains in the vascular system

4-3. Neonates are intolerant of both dehydration and fluid overload. This is because:

a. Their larger body surface area allows for more insensible fluid loss

b. Neonates' increased metabolic rate causes more fluid shifts

c. Neonates retain sodium, rapidly clear fluid overload, and conserve fluid

d. Neonates lose sodium, slowly clear fluid overload, and have an inability to conserve fluid

4-4. The perianesthesia nurse is aware that all general anesthetic agents:

a. Increase renal blood flow and decrease urine output

b. Decrease renal blood flow and increase urine output

c. Increase renal blood flow and increase urine output

d. Decrease renal blood flow and decrease urine output

4-5. The acronym POUR denotes for:

a. Postoperative urinary release

b. Preoperative urinary review

c. Postoperative urinary retention

d. Postoperative urological reassessment

4-6. A patient has arrived in the Phase I PACU after a 4-hour laparoscopic-assisted colectomy for recurrent diverticulitis. During emergence the patient complains of spasms in the lower back and bilateral buttock pain. At this time, the most appropriate nursing intervention is to:

a. Assess for lumbar strain

b. Reposition the patient

c. Notify the surgeon of the new complaint

d. Provide sedation with multimodal analgesia

4-7. Patients at risk for an allergic reaction to latex include all of the following EXCEPT:

a. History of contact dermatitis

b. Allergies to bananas and papayas

c. Allergies to tomatoes and grass

d. Repeated bladder catheterizations

4-8. According to measures supported by the Surgical Care Improvement Project (SCIP), which of the following actions would NOT decrease the patient's risk for postoperative infection?

a. Maintaining normothermia

b. Administering an IV antibiotic before incision

c. Avoiding wide glucose swings

d. Preparing the surgical site with surgical razors

4-9. The diuretic used to treat patients with fluid overload due to cirrhosis is:

a. Triamterene

b. Hydrochlorothiazide

c. Furosemide

d. Spironolactone

4-10. A patient requires a potassium-sparing diuretic postoperatively. The nurse anticipates giving the patient:

a. Furosemide

b. Acetazolamide

c. Spironolactone

d. Hydrochlorothiazide

4-11. Electrocardiogram (ECG) monitoring is important for patients with acute renal failure with hyperkalemia. ECG tracings may show all of the following EXCEPT:

a. High-peaked T waves

b. Heart block

c. U waves

d. Depressed ST segment

4-12. The nurse is caring for a patient with extensive burns who has now been diagnosed with acute renal failure. The nurse recognizes the renal failure is probably prerenal and a result of:

a. Volume depletion

b. Volume shifts

c. Volume expansion

d. Vascular anomalies

4-13. The nurse is caring for a patient after a procedure to create an arteriovenous (AV) fistula for dialysis. The patient is complaining of pain distal to the graft site along with pallor and diminished pulses. The nurse suspects:

a. Infection

b. Aneurysm

c. Thrombosis

d. Steal syndrome

4-14. When performing an integumentary assessment of a patient with arterial insufficiency, the nurse finds the skin:

a. Thick, scaly, and scarred

b. Brawny (reddish-brown color)

c. Thin, shiny, and dry

d. Warm and mottled

4-15. A perianesthesia nurse is caring for a 6-month-old infant status postinguinal hernia repair who weighs 8.4 kilograms. He has been out of surgery for 3 hours. He has breastfed twice, with the mother reporting that he appeared to feed normally and has an IV of Lactated Ringer's now at TKO. He received a total of 320 mL of IV fluid in the operating room and an additional 30 mL since being on the unit. He is smiling and playful. During discharge teaching the nurse assesses the infant's surgical site, which is still clean, dry, and intact, and notes that his abdomen is soft. She shows the site to the baby's mother and changes the diaper. After weighing the diaper the nurse notes that the infant has had 100 mL of urine output. His HR is 112 and RR is 32. The mother states that the diaper seems pretty dry. The correct response of the nurse is:

a. I am going to call the surgeon because I, too, am concerned that his diaper is so dry

b. This is an acceptable amount of urine for your baby's body weight

c. It is normal for your baby not to urinate; he hasn't received much IV fluid

d. I am going to get an order to increase your baby's IV rate so he can produce more urine

4-16. When assessing the function of a new graft or fistula for hemodialysis, the perianesthesia nurse should monitor for the presence of:

a. Pink skin with a brisk capillary refill at the access site

b. A clean, dry, and intact pressure dressing

c. A pulse and audible bruit with a stethoscope

d. Ease when drawing blood from the site

4-17. A 63-year-old female patient had a full face resurfacing as an outpatient. The Phase II PACU nurse gives discharge instructions that include all the following EXCEPT:

a. Elevate head of bed to help minimize swelling

b. The patient may resume using glycolic acid products within 24 hours of the procedure

c. Avoid sun exposure while the skin is healing

d. Continue applying ointment to keep the facial area moist and promote healing

4-18. The trauma team has just stabilized the spine, level T5, of a young victim of a diving accident. The patient presents to the Phase I PACU complaining of severe pain, with a BP 180/110, profuse diaphoresis, and generalized vasodilation evidenced by ruddy, flushed skin. The nurse recognizes that these are symptoms of:

a. Autonomic hyperreflexia

b. Horner's syndrome

c. Sympathetic dysreflexia

d. Anaphylactic reaction

4-19. Perioperative implications of renal changes in the older adult include all of the following EXCEPT:

a. Altered thirst response

b. Increased ability to concentrate urine

c. Continued urine excretion in the face of hypovolemia

d. Decreased glomerular filtration rate

4-20. While assessing an 87-year-old postoperative patient on admission to the Phase I PACU, the nurse initiates a plan for active warming to maintain normothermia. This patient is considered to be at risk for hypothermia as a result of normal changes in the integumentary system due to aging. This increased risk of hypothermia is related to:

a. Hyperactive sweat glands

b. Decreased production of melanocytes

c. Loss of subcutaneous fat

d. Epidural atrophy

4-21. The MOST common skin injuries related to surgical positioning are:

a. Pressure injuries

b. Superficial areas of ecchymosis

c. Breaks in skin integrity from shearing

d. Multiple variegated petechiae

4-22. The surgical approach for a prostatectomy that presents the greatest risk for water intoxication and hyponatremia is:

a. Retropubic resection of prostate

b. Suprapubic resection of prostate

c. Transurethral resection of prostate

d. Simple perineal resection of prostate

4-23. The ability of a surgical wound to heal is directly related to:

a. Nutritional state

b. Presence of pulmonary disease

c. Osteoarthritis

d. Perinatal status

4-24. The prescreening nurse receives a telephone call from a mother of an 8-year-old female patient who will have an indwelling catheter after her ureteral reimplantation surgery. The mother is looking for advice regarding preparing her daughter for surgery. The nurse knows that this patient is in this stage of Piaget's cognitive development and will base her recommendations accordingly:

a. Sensorimotor

b. Preoperational

c. Concrete operations

d. Formal operations

4-25. Glomerulonephritis can contribute to the development of acute renal failure (ARF). This is an example of what type of failure?

a. Prerenal failure

b. Postrenal failure

c. Intrarenal (intrinsic) failure

d. Infectious failure

4-26. The nurse is caring for a patient after unilateral pyelolithotomy. The patient comes to the Phase I PACU with ureteral and urethral catheters in place, with pink-tinged urine draining from both catheters. Over the next hour the drainage from the ureteral catheter is less than 5 mL of darker pink drainage, and the urethral catheter has drained 75 mL. The nurse suspects this is due to:

a. Compression of the dependent side during surgery

b. Occlusion of the ureteral catheter

c. Perforation of the ureter during surgery

d. Acute renal failure due to surgery

4-27. All of the following are functions of the skin EXCEPT:

a. Protection

b. Thermoregulation

c. Communication

d. Proprioception

4-28. The nurse is caring for a young male patient who fell while straddling a bicycle. He is now scheduled for an orchiopexy. The nurse recognizes this procedure is needed to repair his:

a. Cryptorchidism

b. Varicocele

c. Hydrocele

d. Testicular torsion

4-29. Care of the patient with a surgical wound drain includes assessing that the drain is activated or maintains the proper vacuum:

a. Every 30 minutes

b. Every shift

c. At every handoff

d. Every 1 to 2 hours

4-30. Prostaglandins are produced in the renal medulla and help maintain several renal functions. Which of the following medications may block the production of prostaglandins?

a. Nonsteroidal anti-inflammatory drugs (NSAIDs)

b. Aspirin

c. Acetaminophen

d. Ketamine

4-31. The nurse reviewing the patient's medical history in the preoperative holding area sees a history of acute glomerulonephritis. Potential causes of this disorder include all of the following EXCEPT:

a. Streptococci infection

b. Staphylococci infection

c. Osteoarthritis

d. Autoimmune disease

4-32. A 28-year-old female patient arrives in the Phase I PACU with an initial temperature of 35.5° C (95.9° F) after exploratory laparotomy for lysis of adhesions. Perioperative hypothermia is defined as:

a. Patient complaint of feeling cold

b. Core temperature less than 36° C (96.8° F)

c. Patient shivering with a temperature of 36.7° C (98.1° F)

d. Skin feels cold to touch

4-33. The goal of the nursing intervention should address all of the following EXCEPT:

a. Preventing radiant heat loss

b. Improving tissue perfusion

c. Suppressing muscle activity

d. Minimizing desquamation

4-34. Comprehensive preanesthesia teaching for the patient undergoing skin grafting for extensive scar revision includes all of the following EXCEPT:

a. Aggressive prehabilitation therapy for optimal strengthening

b. Smoking cessation

c. Nutritional counseling

d. Preoperative cardiovascular screening

4-35. The perianesthesia nurse is aware that anemia in a patient with chronic kidney disease:

a. May be present in all stages of kidney disease but becomes more prevalent as the disease progresses

b. Is a sign that end-stage kidney disease has occurred

c. Is a rare occurrence that indicates other comorbidities

d. Is only seen in older adults with kidney disease

4-36. A newly graduated nurse is beginning a clinical orientation to the same-day surgery unit. On the third day of orientation, the new nurse shows her preceptor her hands. The skin is red and cracked and reportedly painful. The preceptor suspects that the new nurse MOST likely has a reaction due to:

a. Anxiety over her skill set

b. Exposure to latex

c. Prolonged keyboard work

d. Handling various policy books

4-37. The patient with diabetes mellitus is more prone to developing postoperative infections in surgical wounds. Aseptic techniques are critical during wound care to prevent exposure to pathogens. The most important activity in the prevention of disease transmission during the period of perianesthesia patient care is:

a. Hand washing

b. Preoperative use of chlorhexidine

c. Use of gloves

d. Administration of appropriate antibiotics

4-38. A patient having a prostatectomy has a decreased likelihood of nerve damage with which approach?

a. Transurethral

b. Suprapubic

c. Perineal

d. Laparoscopic robotic

4-39. A patient has had a laparoscopic nephrectomy. On examination the trocar sites are dry and intact, and the catheter is draining an adequate amount of slightly pink urine. When the nurse assesses the patient's pain, he is complaining of a feeling of facial swelling with a crackling sensation when he touches it. The nurse recognizes this subcutaneous emphysema is a result of:

a. Increased fluid retention

b. Reaction to anesthetic gases

c. Leak of CO_2 from insufflation

d. Reaction to latex products

4-40. The Phase II PACU nurse is caring for a patient status post extracorporeal shock wave lithotripsy (ESWL). She is reviewing discharge instructions when her patient begins complaining of flank pain on the treated side. The patient had one episode of hematuria but states now that he is unable to void. The most critical point the nurse is aware of is that:

    a. This can occur after ESWL due to swelling from the shock wave trauma, which will rapidly subside

    b. She will need to encourage her patient to drink more during the postoperative period

    c. The bruising from the ESWL can cause pain and hematuria

    d. Obstructions can develop after ESWL

4-41. The nurse is caring for a patient after transurethral resection of the prostate (TURP). During report the circulating nurse indicated that 6000 mL of irrigation was used. The patient is now exhibiting shortness of breath, confusion, tachycardia, and hypotension. The nurse suspects that the symptoms are related to the amount of irrigation fluid that has caused:

    a. Hypokalemia

    b. Hyponatremia

    c. Hypochloremia

    d. Hypophosphatemia

Consider this scenario for questions 4-42 to 4-45.

    Jane is a 5-year-old female patient who presents with her mother and father for a bilateral intravesicular ureteral reimplantation. The current plan for care is that Jane will stay in the extended care unit for a 23-hour admission. Jane has a history of recurrent urinary tract infections and has been diagnosed with grade IV vesicoureteral reflux. When the nurse comes to meet Jane, she hides behind her father's leg.

4-42. While admitting the patient, the perianesthesia nurse is aware that the patient is in this stage of Piaget's cognitive development:

    a. Sensorimotor

    b. Preoperational thought

    c. Concrete operations

    d. Formal operations

4-43. The admission nurse is explaining an inhalation anesthetic to Jane. Being aware of Piaget's stage of preoperational thought, the nurse introduces the mask to Jane stating "This mask will help you fall asleep." Which of the following statements would be most appropriate for a patient of Jane's age?

    a. You get to pick a fun smell for the mask!

    b. It doesn't hurt.

    c. The doctor will put it on your face for you.

    d. All the kids like it.

The scenario continues with 4-44 and 4-45.

    Jane has returned to the extended care unit status postbilateral intravesicular reimplantation. She will be staying for 23 hours. Vital signs are heart rate 84, RR 20, and BP 92/42, and weight on admission was 18.6 kg. She has an indwelling catheter in place to a leg bag, which was emptied before arrival on the unit. Jane had a total of 45 mL of urine in the Phase I PACU, reported to be pink tinged with small clots. She is alert and tolerating clear liquids. She had a caudal block for pain during the procedure and received ketorolac and ondansetron intravenously. She can move her legs and wiggle her toes. Jane is rating her pain a 2 on the FACES scale. She has an IV in her left hand of D5 1/2NS with 20 mEq (milliequivalents) KCL infusing at 58 mL/hr. Her mother is at her bedside.

4-44. Two hours after arriving on the unit, Jane is rating her pain at a 6 on the FACES scale. She runs her hand over her abdomen when asked where the pain is. The patient is very restless and complaining of nausea. Her HR is 116, RR is 28, and BP is 114/58. The nurse notes that there has been no urine evident in the leg bag since arrival on the unit. The perianesthesia nurse is aware that the patient's symptoms most likely indicate:

    a. Decreased urine production after the surgical procedure and anesthesia

    b. Bladder spasms related to surgery and potential obstruction of the urinary catheter

    c. Postoperative nausea related to anesthesia and anxiety

    d. Postoperative pain due to the surgical procedure

4-45. The kidney site for acid–base regulation, hydrogen ion secretion, and bicarbonate reabsorption is:

a. Glomerulus

b. Proximal tubule

c. Distal tubule

d. Loop of Henle

4-46. A 34-year-old truck driver is having a preanesthesia assessment in anticipation of a video-assisted thoracoscopic surgery (VATS) to evaluate and treat a lung lesion. He is reportedly a heavy smoker, and he says he has cut down but has not stopped completely. Complications associated with the use of inhaled tobacco include all of the following EXCEPT:

a. Hypertension

b. Postoperative nausea and vomiting (PONV)

c. Poor tissue healing

d. Surgical wound dehiscence

4-47. The epidermis provides a physical barrier due largely to the presence of:

a. Melanin

b. Carotene

c. Collagen

d. Keratin

4-48. During the early postoperative period, patients who have received a kidney transplant from living donors commonly experience:

a. Polyuria

b. Anuria

c. Gross hematuria

d. Agitation

4-49. The primary cause of chronic contact dermatitis among health care workers is:

a. Repeated use of hand hygiene products

b. Wrong sized gloves

c. Unsterile keyboard sharing

d. Hospital-laundered scrubs

4-50. A Jewish patient is having a skin graft. Which graft would the patient be culturally opposed to?

a. Autograft

b. Homograft

c. Bilaminate skin substitute

d. Heterograft

4-51. When a patient requires a muscle flap to repair a congenital or acquired tissue defect, the Phase I PACU nurse will monitor all of the following EXCEPT:

a. Hypocalcemia

b. Hypovolemia

c. Hypotension

d. Hypothermia

4-52. A Phase I PACU nurse receives a patient with basal cell carcinoma on the left side of the nose. The patient underwent a Mohs procedure and forehead flap. The initial assessment findings of the flap's condition would be:

a. Normal color immediately postop; the flap will be bluish in color

b. The flap would be cool to touch

c. The flap will be white or gray in color

d. Capillary refill blanching is 4 seconds

4-53. During the hand-off report after an ear-nose-throat (ENT) procedure, the certified nurse anesthetist (CRNA) mentions that the patient has a history of von Willebrand's disease. The Phase I PACU nurse creates a postoperative plan of care. The plan includes frequent assessments for:

a. Patient complaint of palpitations and shortness of breath

b. Speech difficulty and peripheral numbness

c. Dyspnea and hypotension

d. Mucosal bleeding and mild bruising

4-54. An otherwise healthy patient reports a recent diagnosis of localized shingles. The preoperative nurse is aware that herpes zoster is caused by reactivation of the varicella zoster virus. When considering precautions to implement during care of the patient, the perianesthesia nurse considers that the virus spreads via:

a. Airborne transmission

b. Direct contact with a dry, crusty lesion

c. Direct contact with a clear vesicle rash

d. Droplet transmission

4-55. A patient with a body mass index (BMI) of 52 faces a number of potential postoperative complications, including:

a. An increased risk of wound dehiscence and decreased risk of infection

b. An increased risk of wound dehiscence and increased risk of infection

c. A decreased risk of wound dehiscence and decreased risk of infection

d. A decreased risk of wound dehiscence and increased risk of infection

4-56. A 42-year-old construction worker experienced a traumatic injury while at work. He is presenting to the hospital now for surgery to treat third-degree burns sustained on his left lower extremity. A third-degree burn involves:

a. Red, dry, nonblistered skin with allodynia

b. Superficial, oozing, and painful blisters

c. Moist, painful skin that blanches

d. Leathery, dry wound with little or no pain

4-57. The nurse is caring for a patient after a kidney transplant. Vital signs are stable, and the urine output is clear yellow and greater than 30 mL on evaluation. The patient is receiving medication via patient-controlled analgesia (PCA) pump and reports good control of postoperative pain. At the next check of vital signs the nurse sees that the end-tidal carbon dioxide reading is 52 mm Hg and recognizes this is a result of:

a. Hypoperfusion

b. Hypoventilation

c. Hypovolemia

d. Hypocarbia

4-58. Creatinine is an important indicator of glomerular filtration ability because:

a. It is a large molecule that should not fit through the glomeruli

b. Creatinine is the only filtered substance not reabsorbed

c. Creatinine is reabsorbed in limited quantities along with urea and phosphate

d. It helps play a role in the secretion of hydrogen and potassium ions

Consider this scenario for questions 4-59, 4-60, and 4-61.

Matt is a 26-year-old male trauma patient with significant burns on the left leg and a partial burn on the right leg when his jeans caught on fire. It was determined that 18% of his body has been burned. He is conscious with pain level at 10 (0-10 numerical rating scale). The burn area is mostly deep red and moist, with areas of white/yellow tissue on the left with a delay in capillary refill. The left anterior lower leg had a blackish-tan, nonblanching area with no pain. BP is 98/54, HR is 138, RR is 32, SpO$_2$ is 94% on 3 L/m nasal cannula, and temperature is 36.4° C (97.5° F).

4-59. The left anterior lower leg injury is considered a:

a. Superficial injury

b. Superficial partial-thickness injury

c. Deep partial-thickness injury

d. Full-thickness injury

4-60. Matt received morphine 4 mg for pain. What is the main consideration to maintain hemostasis and renal function?

a. Providing a warming blanket

b. Infusion of isotonic crystalloid fluids

c. Draw and monitoring labs

d. Initiating antibiotics

4-61. Matt had a skin graft to his lower right leg with an autograft. The perianesthesia nurse's interventions will include all of the following EXCEPT:

a. Assess blood and fluid collection under the graft site

b. Elevate grafted extremity

c. Allow blood and fluid to collect under the graft

d. Avoid pressure or shearing

4-62. This medication should be avoided in the patient with impaired renal function:

a. Furosemide

b. Morphine

c. Acetaminophen

d. Ketorolac

4-63. In patients with multiple skin folds and redundant skin, the nurse is aware that a thorough inspection of the skin is necessary to determine if there are any excoriations or rashes. Problem areas tend to be found in the groin, perineum, axilla, and large skin folds and:

a. Between the toes

b. Behind the knees

c. Under the chin folds

d. Beneath the breasts

4-64. When assessing a bariatric patient preoperatively, the preoperative nurse knows that the presence of multiple skin folds predisposes the patient to all of the following EXCEPT:

a. Impaired hygiene

b. Highly vascularized tissue

c. Excoriations of redundant skin

d. Occult wound infections

4-65. Postoperative assessment and care of an arteriovenous (AV) fistula should include all of the following EXCEPT:

a. Gentle palpation for thrill

b. Auscultation for bruit

c. Elevation of surgical arm

d. Limb alert bracelet on surgical arm

Answers and Rationales for Chapter 4, Renal and Integumentary Systems

4-1. *Correct answer:* **b**
If the patient is warmed too rapidly, the vasodilation can result in hypotension. This can be exacerbated in the patient with a regional sympathetic block, which inhibits vasoconstriction in response to the hypotension. (Schick L, Windle PE. *PeriAnesthesia Nursing Core Curriculum: Preprocedure, Phase I and Phase II PACU Nursing.* St. Louis, MO: Saunders; 2016:488.)

4-2. *Correct answer:* **d**
Hetastarch (hydroxyethyl starch) is a synthetic colloid that is an effective plasma volume expander. It is less expensive than blood products; however, it has minimal coagulation effects, is less likely to cause allergic reactions, and metabolizes slowly and remains in the vascular system (but not as long as colloids). (Schick L, Windle PE. *PeriAnesthesia Nursing Core Curriculum: Preprocedure, Phase I and Phase II PACU Nursing.* 3rd ed. St. Louis, MO: Saunders; 2016:320-321.)

4-3. *Correct answer:* **d**
Neonate renal function is characterized by obligate sodium loss, slow clearance of fluid overload, and an inability to conserve fluid. Newborns have a low glomerular filtration rate, and dehydration is harmful to renal function. By 20 weeks of age, glomerular filtration and tubular function are nearly complete. (Odom-Forren J. *Drain's Perianesthesia Nursing: A Critical Care Approach.* 6th ed. St. Louis, MO: Saunders; 2013:692-694.)

4-4. *Correct answer:* **d**
All anesthetics decrease renal blood flow and decrease urine output. Renal blood flow is depressed due to renal vasoconstriction or systemic hypotension. Urine output can be decreased by the secretion of antidiuretic hormone (ADH) in response to the stress of surgery. Patients who have had major abdominal or thoracic surgery may have a period of diuresis in the Phase I PACU, but the stress of surgery can cause fluid volume retention for up to 48 hours postoperatively. (Odom-Forren J. *Drain's Perianesthesia Nursing: A Critical Care Approach.* 6th ed. St. Louis, MO: Saunders; 2013:190.)

4-5. *Correct answer:* **c**
Postoperative urinary retention (POUR) is defined as a urine volume greater than 500 mL upon admission with inability to void for 30 minutes or longer. Complications of POUR include damage to the detrusor muscle and ischemia, increased vulnerability to urinary tract infections from high bladder pressures, tachycardia, and hypertension. (Odom-Forren J. *Drain's Perianesthesia Nursing: A Critical Care Approach.* 6th ed. St. Louis, MO: Saunders; 2013:598.)

4-6. *Correct answer:* **b**
All surgical patients should be considered at risk for pressure injuries. The nurse repositions the patient to assess the skin and relieve pressure on the lower back. The patient's back pain and buttock tenderness are probably results of a supine position during a 4-hour surgical procedure. Skin circulation over bony prominences such as the heels, scapulae, elbows, and sacrum is easily compromised. Other methods to alleviate the risks of pressure injuries include maintaining proper body alignment, repositioning occasionally, elevating the heels from the mattress to avoid tissue trauma, and providing gentle, passive range-of-motion movement. (Schick L, Windle PE. *PeriAnesthesia Nursing Core Curriculum: Preprocedure, Phase I and Phase II PACU Nursing.* 3rd ed. St. Louis, MO: Saunders; 2016:291.)

4-7. *Correct answer:* **c**

A complete medical history is the most reliable screening examination for prediction of a reaction to latex; however, patients with the following histories should be considered at high risk for latex allergic reactions: atopic immunologic reactions; contact dermatitis; documented immunologic reactions of unknown etiology during a medical or surgical procedure; allergies to food products, including fruits, nuts, bananas, avocados, celery, figs, chestnuts, and papayas; neural tube defects (including spina bifida, myelomeningocele/meningocele, and lipomyelomeningocele); multiple operations in the past; and repeated bladder catheterizations. (Odom-Forren J. *Drain's Perianesthesia Nursing: A Critical Care Approach.* 6th ed. St. Louis, MO: Saunders; 2013:232-233.)

4-8. *Correct answer:* **d**

According to the Surgical Care Improvement Project (SCIP) measures, appropriate hair removal must be done by clipping or depilatory. Shaving by razors will cause microabrasions to the skin, predisposing the patient to infection. (Schick L, Windle PE. *PeriAnesthesia Nursing Core Curriculum: Preprocedure, Phase I and Phase II PACU Nursing.* 3rd ed. St. Louis, MO: Saunders; 2016:94.)

4-9. *Correct answer:* **d**

Spironolactone is a potassium-sparing diuretic used to treat ascites and fluid overload due to cirrhosis of the liver. When compared with furosemide, spironolactone has a greater rate of diuresis in patients with ascites. (Odom-Forren J. *Drain's Perianesthesia Nursing: A Critical Care Approach.* 6th ed. St. Louis, MO: Saunders; 2013:189-190.)

4-10. *Correct answer:* **d**

Hydrochlorothiazide acts on the distal convoluted tubules to increase urine output without the loss of potassium. (Stannard D, Krenzischek DA, eds. *Perianesthesia Nursing Care: A Bedside Guide for Safe Recovery.*

Sudbury, MA: Jones and Bartlett Learning; 2012:247; Odom-Forren J. *Drain's Perianesthesia Nursing: A Critical Care Approach.* 6th ed. St. Louis, MO: Saunders; 2013:189.)

4-11. *Correct answer:* **c**

U waves are typically seen in hypokalemia. (Stannard D, Krenzischek DA, eds. *Perianesthesia Nursing Care: A Bedside Guide for Safe Recovery.* Sudbury, MA: Jones and Bartlett Learning; 2012:247; Stillwell SB. *PDQ for Critical Care.* St. Louis, MO: Elsevier-Mosby; 2011:35; Schick L, Windle PE. *PeriAnesthesia Nursing Core Curriculum: Preprocedure, Phase I and Phase II PACU Nursing.* St. Louis, MO: Saunders; 2016:307.)

4-12. *Correct answer:* **a**

Burns can cause dehydration due to the loss of fluids from the injury. (Schick L, Windle PE. *PeriAnesthesia Nursing Core Curriculum: Preprocedure, Phase I and Phase II PACU Nursing.* St. Louis, MO: Saunders; 2016:855.)

4-13. *Correct answer:* **d**

Steal syndrome is ischemic pain that is related to vascular insufficiency due to fistula formation. This should be reported to the physician because revision or additional procedures are needed to correct the problem. (Schick L, Windle PE. *PeriAnesthesia Nursing Core Curriculum: Preprocedure, Phase I and Phase II PACU Nursing.* 3rd ed. St. Louis, MO: Saunders; 2016:858.)

4-14. *Correct answer:* **c**

The skin of patients with arterial insufficiency is pale and cyanotic and is often cool, shiny, dry, and thin, whereas the skin of patients with venous insufficiency is warm; has a reddish-brown pigmentation; and is scaly, scarred, and thick. (Schick L, Windle PE. *PeriAnesthesia Nursing Core Curriculum: Preprocedure, Phase I and Phase II PACU Nursing.* 3rd ed. St. Louis, MO: Saunders; 2016:600.)

4-15. *Correct answer:* **b**

The infant has produced approximately 5 mL/kg/hr of urine, which is above the minimum expected 2 to 3 mL/kg/hr. He is not demonstrating signs of dehydration, as his vital signs are in the normal range for his age. He is eating well and not demonstrating signs and symptoms of pain or a distended bladder. (Schick L, Windle PE. *PeriAnesthesia Nursing Core Curriculum: Preprocedure, Phase I and Phase II PACU Nursing.* 3rd ed. St. Louis, MO: Saunders; 2016:231.)

4-16. *Correct answer:* **c**

The nurse should assess for a functional graft or fistula. This would be demonstrated by a soft pulse and a bruit audible on auscultation. This demonstrates that the access is patent with good blood flow. If the site is visible due to a dressing, then a Doppler ultrasound should be used to document the presence of a pulse or bruit. (Schick L, Windle PE. *PeriAnesthesia Nursing Core Curriculum: Preprocedure, Phase I and Phase II PACU Nursing.* 3rd ed. St. Louis, MO: Saunders; 2016:858-859.)

4-17. *Correct answer:* **b**

Glycolic acid is used for chemical peels and would not be used immediately after laser resurfacing. The application of the prescribed ointment frequently promotes the skin to heal and prevent scab formation. (Schick L, Windle PE. *PeriAnesthesia Nursing Core Curriculum: Preprocedure, Phase I and Phase II PACU Nursing.* 3rd ed. St. Louis, MO: Saunders; 2016:1131.)

4-18. *Correct answer:* **a**

Autonomic hyperreflexia is an abnormal overreaction of the nervous system to stimulation and is a common finding in patients with spinal cord injuries above the level of T6. The most common symptoms of the reaction include high blood pressure, skin color changes (flushing), profuse sweating, muscle spasms, and piloerection occurring above the level of the injury. Prompt treatment includes raising the head of the bed and relieving the cause of the overstimulation. (Schick L, Windle PE. *PeriAnesthesia Nursing Core Curriculum: Preprocedure, Phase I and Phase II PACU Nursing. Approach.* 3rd ed. St. Louis, MO: Saunders; 2016:175-178.)

4-19. *Correct answer:* **b**

The older patient loses renal mass and filtering surface with a decreased glomerular filtration rate (GFR), resulting in a decreased ability to concentrate urine. (Stannard D, Krenzischek DA, eds. *Perianesthesia Nursing Care: A Bedside Guide for Safe Recovery.* Sudbury, MA: Jones and Bartlett Learning; 2012:135-136; Schick L, Windle PE. *PeriAnesthesia Nursing Core Curriculum: Preprocedure, Phase I and Phase II PACU Nursing.* 3rd ed. St. Louis, MO: Saunders; 2016:293.)

4-20. *Correct answer:* **c**

The process of aging predisposes the integumentary system to have fewer sweat glands, decreased production of melanocytes (which decreases skin pigmentation), epidural atrophy, and loss of collagen (which leads to increased risks of skin breakdown and decreased elasticity and turgor). It is the loss of subcutaneous fat that compromises thermoregulation in the older patient and exposes the patient to an increased risk of hypothermia. (Schick L, Windle PE. *PeriAnesthesia Nursing Core Curriculum: Preprocedure, Phase I and Phase II PACU Nursing.* 3rd ed. St. Louis, MO: Saunders; 2016:291.)

4-21. *Correct answer:* **a**

Pressure injuries are the most common skin injuries caused by inappropriate positioning. A lower pressure on the skin surface sustained for a prolonged time cannot be tolerated as easily as a greater pressure for a shorter time. The perianesthesia nurse should note the time surgery began to determine the possibility of the formation of pressure ulcers from lengthy surgical procedures. (Odom-Forren, J. *Drain's Perianesthesia Nursing: A Critical Care Approach.* 6th ed. St. Louis, MO: Saunders; 2013:349-350.)

4-22. *Correct answer:* **c**

The transurethral resection of the prostate (TURP) uses large volumes of fluid for irrigation which can lead to water intoxication and a decrease in serum sodium. The patient should be observed for signs of hyponatremia such as shortness of breath, hypoxemia, confusion, nausea, vomiting, muscle twitches, tachycardia, and/or hypotension. (Schick L, Windle PE. *PeriAnesthesia Nursing Core Curriculum: Preprocedure, Phase I and Phase II PACU Nursing.* 3rd ed. St. Louis, MO: Saunders; 2016:879-880.)

4-23. *Correct answer:* **a**

A state of malnourishment increases the potential for increased perioperative morbidity and compromised postoperative recovery and wound healing. (Schick L, Windle PE. *PeriAnesthesia Nursing Core Curriculum: Preprocedure, Phase I and Phase II PACU Nursing.* 3rd ed. St. Louis, MO: Saunders; 2016:293.)

4-24. *Correct answer:* **c**

The nurse is aware that the ages of 7 to 11 years are Piaget's Period 3 of concrete operations. At this time children become more logical and systematic. They can follow a step-by-step description but will need concrete objects and activities to fully understand the process. Books and pictures would be helpful to describe the anesthesia induction, with simple words and phrases used. The nurse can look for simple educational resources to send to the parent to help with the preparation. (Schick L, Windle PE. *PeriAnesthesia Nursing Core Curriculum: Preprocedure, Phase I and Phase II PACU Nursing.* 3rd ed. St. Louis, MO: Saunders; 2016:197.)

4-25. *Correct answer:* **c**

Glomerulonephritis is an example of an intrarenal, or intrinsic, failure. Intrarenal failure is caused by a dysfunction of one or more of the structural components of the kidney, such as the glomeruli, tubules, interstitium, or vessels. This dysfunction causes a sudden and rapid loss of kidney function. Pyelonephritis causes renal scarring and formation of renal lesions, which can lead to acute or chronic renal failure and hypertension. It has been found that renal scarring can occur even after a single first episode of urinary tract infection. (Schick L, Windle PE. *PeriAnesthesia Nursing Core Curriculum: Preprocedure, Phase I and Phase II PACU Nursing.* 3rd ed. St. Louis, MO: Saunders; 2016:855.)

4-26. *Correct answer:* **b**

The nurse must provide meticulous maintenance of the catheters and be aware that they may become occluded by clots or debris. (Schick L, Windle PE. *PeriAnesthesia Nursing Core Curriculum: Preprocedure, Phase I and Phase II PACU Nursing.* 3rd ed. St. Louis, MO: Saunders; 2016:872.)

4-27. *Correct answer:* **d**

As the largest organ of the body, the skin is the first line of defense against trauma and infection, and this protective barrier is its most important function. It aids in thermoregulation by way of vasoconstriction, vasodilation, and evaporation of water. The skin also serves to support reaction to environmental stimuli, including sensation and communication of pressure, pain, touch, and temperature. (Odom-Forren, J. *Drain's Perianesthesia Nursing: A Critical Care Approach.* 6th ed. St. Louis, MO: Saunders; 2013:222-224.)

4-28. *Correct answer:* **d**

Orchiopexy is a procedure to return the testicle to the correct position. It can be performed when the patient has congenital cryptorchidism, but in this case the trauma to the scrotum most likely caused torsion of the testicle that must be repaired. (Schick L, Windle PE. *PeriAnesthesia Nursing Core Curriculum: Preprocedure, Phase I and Phase II PACU Nursing.* 3rd ed. St. Louis, MO: Saunders; 2016:861)

4-29. *Correct answer:* **d**

If a drain is present, it should be checked to ensure that it is activated, or it may be connected to a vacuum blood tube. The drain is placed to minimize the bleeding into the wound and to reduce the possibility of infection. Drains should be checked every 1 or 2 hours to maintain a proper vacuum, and the output should be recorded on the intake and output records. (Odom-Forren J. *Drain's Perianesthesia Nursing: A Critical Care Approach.* 6th ed. St. Louis, MO: Saunders; 2013:546.)

4-30. *Correct answer:* **a**

NSAIDs must be used cautiously to prevent blocking production of prostaglandins that help regulate vascular resistance in arterioles of the glomerular capillaries. NSAIDs can also affect sodium and water retention, as well as cause acute renal failure in the presence of dehydration. (Schick L, Windle PE. *PeriAnesthesia Nursing Core Curriculum: Preprocedure, Phase I and Phase II PACU Nursing.* 3rd ed. St. Louis, MO: Saunders; 2016:851.)

4-31. *Correct answer:* **c**

Contributing causes of acute glomerulonephritis include streptococci, staphylococci, autoimmune diseases (e.g., lupus), polyarteritis nodosa, amyloidosis, and Alport's syndrome. (Schick L, Windle PE. *PeriAnesthesia Nursing Core Curriculum: Preprocedure, Phase I and Phase II PACU Nursing.* 3rd ed. St. Louis, MO: Saunders; 2016:853-854.)

4-32. *Correct answer:* **b**

Normothermia is defined as a core temperature ranging from 36° C to 38° C. This patient's temperature is considered hypothermic and requires active warming measures, such as the application of a forced-air warming system and warmed humidified inspired oxygen. (American Society of PeriAnesthesia Nurses. *ASPAN's Evidence-Based Clinical Practice Guideline for the Promotion of Perioperative Normothermia: Second Edition.*

Available at: http://www.aspan.org/Portals/6/docs/ClinicalPractice/Guidelines/Normothermia_Guideline_12-10_JoPAN.pdf. Accessed November 28, 2016.)

4-33. *Correct answer:* **d**

The goal is to return to normothermia while decreasing adverse effects of patient discomfort, surgical site infections, impaired wound healing, altered drug metabolism, increased adrenergic stimulation, and coagulopathy. (American Society of PeriAnesthesia Nurses. *ASPAN's Evidence-Based Clinical Practice Guideline for the Promotion of Perioperative Normothermia: Second Edition.* Available at: http://www.aspan.org/Portals/6/docs/ClinicalPractice/Guidelines/Normothermia_Guideline_12-10_JoPAN.pdf. Accessed November 28, 2016.)

4-34. *Correct answer:* **a**

Preoperative assessment for the patient undergoing skin grafting should include evaluation of smoking status and smoking cessation education; assessment for vascular concerns that may threaten the healing process, such as diabetes; identification of peripheral vascular disease or hypertension; nutritional assessment of the patient; and patient education regarding the postoperative needs. (Odom-Forren J. *Drain's Perianesthesia Nursing: A Critical Care Approach.* 6th ed. St. Louis, MO: Saunders; 2013:632.)

4-35. *Correct answer:* **a**

Anemia can be seen in patients in early chronic kidney disease, but as the disease process progresses, it becomes more pronounced. It is thought that cytokine production in the damaged kidneys leads to decreased erythropoietin production, which affects the bone marrow. (Odom-Forren J. *Drain's Perianesthesia Nursing: A Critical Care Approach.* 6th ed. St. Louis, MO: Saunders; 2013:184-193; Favero H, McMahon M. Care of the adult chronic kidney disease patient in the perianesthesia setting. *J PeriAnesth Nurs.* 2012; 25(3):162-170.)

4-36. *Correct answer:* **b**

Reactions to exposure to any latex are varied. Symptoms of contact dermatitis, a nonallergic reaction, include dry, itchy, or irritated areas that may be red and cracked and usually occur within the first 6 to 24 hours after exposure. The reaction can be caused by exposure to powders added to the gloves, repeated hand washing and drying, or the use of cleaners and sanitizers. Because this reaction is not a true allergy, it usually clears after the irritant is removed. (Odom-Forren J. *Drain's Perianesthesia Nursing: A Critical Care Approach.* 6th ed. St. Louis, MO: Saunders; 2013:232-233.)

4-37. *Correct answer:* **a**

Special precautions to reduce the introduction of opportunistic organisms should be taken with patients who are prone to infection. This group includes patients who are obese, anemic, or debilitated; those with vascular insufficiency, chronic obstructive pulmonary disease, and diabetes mellitus; and those with an immune deficiency. Good hand washing technique is the most important activity in the prevention of disease transmission. In addition, the patient's surgical wound site should be kept clean, and the dressings should remain sterile, dry, and intact. Aseptic technique in wound care for these patients should include isolation techniques, such as wearing a surgical mask and using sterile gloves and drapes. (Odom-Forren J. *Drain's Perianesthesia Nursing: A Critical Care Approach.* 6th ed. St. Louis, MO: Saunders; 2013:803.)

4-38. *Correct answer:* **d**

One of the potential advantages of the robotic approach is that it is nerve sparing. (Schick L, Windle PE. *PeriAnesthesia Nursing Core Curriculum: Preprocedure, Phase I and Phase II PACU Nursing.* 3rd ed. St. Louis, MO: Saunders; 2016:878-882.)

4-39. *Correct answer:* **c**

If a weak area in the diaphragm exists, it can allow the CO_2 used for insufflation to leak into the mediastinum. This can result in crepitus in the head, neck, chest, and conjunctiva. (Schick L, Windle PE. *PeriAnesthesia Nursing Core Curriculum: Preprocedure, Phase I and Phase II PACU Nursing.* 3rd ed. St. Louis, MO: Saunders; 2016:817.)

4-40. *Correct answer:* **d**

The shock waves from extracorporeal shock wave lithotripsy (ESWL) break the renal calculi into small fragments, which are washed out in the urine. Larger calculi can potentially form a blockage in the ureter or kidney, which then causes pain and decreased output of urine. The blockage can cause renal colic as well as urine backing up into the kidney. This must be corrected to prevent damage to the kidney. Pain, bruising, and hematuria are common occurrences after ESWL, with hematuria subsiding in 2 to 3 days. The patient should be encouraged to drink large amounts of fluids to help flush the calculi from the kidney and ureter, but if an obstruction is occurring, the extra fluids may not be helpful. (Schick L, Windle PE. *PeriAnesthesia Nursing Core Curriculum: Preprocedure, Phase I and Phase II PACU Nursing.* 3rd ed. St. Louis, MO: Saunders; 2016:871-872.)

4-41. *Correct answer:* **b**

Transurethral resection of the prostate (TURP) patients are at risk for transurethral resection syndrome with hyponatremia due to dilutional syndrome and water intoxication. (Schick L, Windle PE. *PeriAnesthesia Nursing Core Curriculum: Preprocedure, Phase I and Phase II PACU Nursing.* St. Louis, MO: Saunders; 2016:880.)

4-42. *Correct answer:* **b**

At 5 years of age Jane is in Piaget's cognitive developmental stage of preoperational thought. This is the stage where cognition is dominated by egocentrism and magical thought. Thought is dominated by perception. (Schick L, Windle PE. *PeriAnesthesia Nursing Core Curriculum: Preprocedure, Phase I and Phase II PACU Nursing.* 3rd ed. St. Louis, MO: Saunders; 2016:197.)

4-43. *Correct answer:* **a**

This statement relates to the egocentric nature of preoperational thought, informing the patient of all of the things that she will think and do, giving her the perception of being in control. The reference to fun smells will appeal to the child's magical thinking, allowing her to better process the procedure. (Schick L, Windle PE. *PeriAnesthesia Nursing Core Curriculum: Preprocedure, Phase I and Phase II PACU Nursing.* 3rd ed. St. Louis, MO: Saunders; 2016:197.)

4-44. *Correct answer:* **b**

Manipulation of the bladder during the surgical procedure, along with the catheter and potentially distended bladder, can all contribute to the occurrence of bladder spasms. The fact that there is no urine output should be concerning because clots were visible in the Phase I PACU. Bladder spasms occur more frequently in patients who have undergone intravesicular reimplantation because there is more manipulation to the bladder itself. Although nausea can cause discomfort and the change in vital signs, nausea is associated with bladder spasms, as is the characteristic of poorly localized pain. (Fleisher LA, Roizen MF, eds. Essence of Anesthesia Practice: Expert Consult- Online and Print. 3rd ed. Philadelphia, PA: Elsevier Science; 2011: 560.)

4-45. *Correct answer:* **c**

The distal tubule is made up of the distal convoluted tubule and collecting ducts. It is the site of aldosterone actions and the primary mechanism for potassium secretion. It is also the site for acid–base regulation, as well as the site of antidiuretic hormone action and water reabsorption. (Schick L, Windle PE. *PeriAnesthesia Nursing Core Curriculum: Preprocedure, Phase I and Phase II PACU Nursing.* 3rd ed. St. Louis, MO: Saunders; 2016:842.)

4-46. *Correct answer:* **b**

Smoking is associated with an increased risk of chronic obstructive pulmonary disease (COPD), heart disease, hypertension,

peripheral vascular disease, hypoxia, poor tissue healing, wound dehiscence, postoperative pulmonary complications (six times greater than that of nonsmokers), hyperreactive airway, and a higher rate of prolonged mechanical ventilation. Patients who are nonsmokers actually have a higher risk for PONV. (Schick L, Windle PE. *PeriAnesthesia Nursing Core Curriculum: Preprocedure, Phase I and Phase II PACU Nursing.* 3rd ed. St. Louis, MO: Saunders; 2016:104-105.)

4-47. *Correct answer:* **d**

Keratinocytes produce keratin, a protein that gives skin its strength and flexibility and waterproofs the skin surface. The epidermis also has keratinizing and glandular appendages. Keratinizing appendages comprise the hair and the nails. (Schick L, Windle PE. *PeriAnesthesia Nursing Core Curriculum: Preprocedure, Phase I and Phase II PACU Nursing.* 3rd ed. St Louis, MO: Saunders; 2016:1113-1116; Odom-Forren J. *Drain's Perianesthesia Nursing: A Critical Care Approach.* 6th ed. St. Louis, MO: Saunders; 2013:222-224.)

4-48. *Correct answer:* **a**

Adult renal transplant patients often receive mannitol and diuretics during the surgical procedure. Polyuria (more than 500 mL of urine output) is common in the early postoperative period. Fluids should be replaced and a careful record of output maintained. A common protocol posttransplant is to restrict fluid replacement to a maximum of 500 mL/hour. This is done to stimulate the kidney to begin concentrating the urine. (Barone C, Lightfoot M, Barone G. The postanesthesia care of an adult renal transplant recipient. *J PeriAnesth Nurs.* 2003; 18(1):32-41; Odom-Forren J. *Drain's Perianesthesia Nursing: A Critical Care Approach.* 6th ed. St. Louis, MO: Saunders; 2013:594-609; Fleisher LA, Roizen MF. *Essence of Anesthesia Practice: Expert Consult- Online and Print.* 3rd ed. Philadelphia, PA: Elsevier Science; 2011: 478.)

4-49. *Correct answer:* **a**

Frequent and repeated use of hand hygiene products, particularly soaps and other detergents, is a primary cause of chronic irritant contact dermatitis among health care workers. To minimize this condition, personnel should use hospital-approved hand lotion frequently and regularly on their hands. (Odom-Forren J. *Drain's Perianesthesia Nursing: A Critical Care Approach.* 6th ed. St. Louis, MO: Saunders; 2013:45-46.)

4-50. *Correct answer:* **d**

Heterograft is tissue from another species, usually pork. (Schick L, Windle PE. *PeriAnesthesia Nursing Core Curriculum: Preprocedure, Phase I and Phase II PACU Nursing.* 3rd ed. St Louis, MO: Saunders; 2016:1141.)

4-51. *Correct answer:* **a**

Hypocalcemia does not have an effect on the flap site. Hypothermia, hypovolemia, and hypotension could result in vasoconstriction and arterial flow compromise for the viability of the graft. (Schick L, Windle PE. *PeriAnesthesia Nursing Core Curriculum: Preprocedure, Phase I and Phase II PACU Nursing.* 3rd ed. St Louis, MO: Saunders; 2016:1138-1140.)

4-52. *Correct answer:* **c**

The normal color is white or gray immediately postoperatively. When the flap is cool to touch, there may be reduced blood flow. Bluish color indicates venous congestion, and delayed blanching indicates arterial insufficiency. All of these could cause flap failure. (Schick L, Windle PE. *PeriAnesthesia Nursing Core Curriculum: Preprocedure, Phase I and Phase II PACU Nursing.* 3rd ed. St Louis, MO: Saunders; 2016:1139.)

4-53. *Correct answer:* **d**

von Willebrand's disease is a common hematologic disorder that predisposes patients to mucosal bleeding, epistaxis, and mild bruising. Not all patients with von Willebrand's disease require treatment; however, patients scheduled for surgery should be given coagulation factors to supplement essential clotting factors.

Desmopressin acetate (DDAVP®, Ferring Pharmaceuticals, Inc., Parsippany, NJ), given intravenously in the preoperative area, is a synthetic replacement for vasopressin and for homologous factors in the blood to help minimize bleeding. (Schick L, Windle PE. *PeriAnesthesia Nursing Core Curriculum: Preprocedure, Phase I and Phase II PACU Nursing.* 3rd ed. St Louis, MO: Saunders; 2016:833.)

4-54. *Correct answer:* **c**

The virus spreads when a person has direct contact with the active herpes zoster lesions. The lesions are infectious until they dry and crust over. Standard precautions should be followed carefully, and any lesions should be completely covered. (Fleisher LA, Roizen MF, eds. *Essence of Anesthesia Practice: Expert Consult—Online and Print.* 3rd ed. Philadelphia, PA: Elsevier Science; 2011:180.)

4-55. *Correct answer:* **b**

Obesity, defined as weight greater than 20% ideal body weight, presents an increased incidence of wound dehiscence and infection. In addition, obese patients generally have poorly vascularized adipose, which increases the risk of ischemia. (Schick L, Windle PE. *PeriAnesthesia Nursing Core Curriculum: Preprocedure, Phase I and Phase II PACU Nursing.* 3rd ed. St. Louis, MO: Saunders; 2016:639-642.)

4-56. *Correct answer:* **d**

Superficial, or first-degree, burns damage only the outer layer of skin (epidermis). Partial-thickness, or second-degree, burns injure the outer layer and the layer underneath. Full-thickness, or third-degree, burns cause severe injury or destruction to the deepest layer of skin, tissues, hair follicles, and sweat glands. A fourth-degree burn involves bone, muscle, and often organs. Full-thickness burns are often the least painful because nerve endings have been destroyed, causing the absence of sensation. (Odom-Forren J. *Drain's Perianesthesia Nursing: A Critical Care Approach.* 6th ed. St. Louis, MO: Saunders; 2013:225.)

4-57. *Correct answer:* **b**

Hypoventilation as a result of residual anesthetic along with the introduction of the patient-controlled analgesia (PCA) has caused the patient to become sedated. If there are no perfusion issues, the mismatch in perfusion and ventilation will result in the increased carbon dioxide reading. (Schick L, Windle PE. *PeriAnesthesia Nursing Core Curriculum: Preprocedure, Phase I and Phase II PACU Nursing.* 3rd ed. St. Louis, MO: Saunders; 2016:474; Pfander V, Schumacher KE, eds. *ASPAN's Redi-Ref for Perianesthesia Practice.* Cherry Hill, NJ: ASPAN; 2016:24.)

4-58. *Correct answer:* **b**

Creatinine is the only filtered substance that is not reabsorbed. It is entirely secreted, which allows creatinine to serve as an indicator of glomerular filtration ability and kidney function. The National Kidney Foundation Kidney Disease Outcome Quality Initiative has created a definition and guidelines of chronic kidney disease, which are based on glomerular filtration rate. Urea and phosphate are reabsorbed in limited quantities, which is why some is apparent in the urine. (Favero H, McMahon M. Care of the adult chronic kidney disease patient in the perianesthesia setting. *J PeriAnesth Nurs.* 2012; 25(3):162-170; Odom-Forren J. Drain's *Perianesthesia Nursing: A Critical Care Approach.* 6th ed. St. Louis, MO: Saunders; 2013:184-193.)

4-59. *Correct answer:* **d**

A full-thickness burn can extend to the subcutaneous tissue, muscle, or bone with an appearance that is hard, dry, leathery, and nonblanching. Color may be black, tan, or white, and the patient has minimal to no pain. (Schick L, Windle PE. *PeriAnesthesia Nursing Core Curriculum: Preprocedure, Phase I and Phase II PACU Nursing.* 3rd ed. St. Louis, MO: Saunders; 2016:1112.)

4-60. *Correct answer:* **b**

To prevent burn shock, acute renal failure, and hypovolemia, a burn patient requires fluid resuscitation at 2 to 4 mL/kg body weight per percentage of burn. The recommended Parkland burn formula employs Lactated Ringer's alone for the first 24 hours. Fluid management of the burn patient requires attention to detail to prevent morbidity associated with either underresuscitation or overresuscitation. Overresuscitation can be a major source of morbidity by increasing pulmonary complications and wound edema. (Schick L, Windle PE. *Peri-Anesthesia Nursing Core Curriculum: Preprocedure, Phase I and Phase II PACU Nursing.* 3rd ed. St. Louis, MO: Saunders; 2016:1143.)

4-61. *Correct answer:* **c**

Allowing fluid to collect under the graft will not allow the graft to adhere to the site. Blood and fluid may be removed by rolling fluid to the edges of the graft with a cotton-tipped applicator or aspiration with a small-gauge needle. Elevating the extremity will promote venous return and minimize edema. (Schick L, Windle PE. *PeriAnesthesia Nursing Core Curriculum: Preprocedure, Phase I and Phase II PACU Nursing.* 3rd ed. St. Louis, MO: Saunders; 2016:1144-1145.)

4-62. *Correct answer:* **d**

Ketorolac should be avoided because it can be nephrotoxic. It is not recommended for use in patients with impaired renal function. (Odom-Forren J. *Drain's Perianesthesia Nursing: A Critical Care Approach.* 6th ed. St. Louis, MO: Saunders; 2013:273.)

4-63. *Correct answer:* **d**

The bariatric patient with multiple skin folds experiences issues related to impaired hygiene due to the difficulty the patient has with reaching and properly cleaning and drying skin. The larger skin folds as well as tissue around the groin, perineum, breasts, and axilla are susceptible to breakdown. (Odom-Forren J. *Drain's Perianesthesia Nursing: A Critical Care Approach.* 6th ed. St. Louis, MO: Saunders; 2013:641.)

4-64. *Correct answer:* **b**

Retained moisture on redundant skin can lead to excoriations or rashes if not kept clean and dry. Wound infections can develop and commonly include yeast and fungi. Adipose tissue is poorly vascularized and can cause delayed wound healing. (Odom-Forren J. *Drain's Perianesthesia Nursing: A Critical Care Approach.* 6th ed. St. Louis, MO: Saunders; 2013:641.)

4-65. *Correct answer:* **d**

Any circumferential dressing, including arm bands, should be avoided on the surgical arm due to potential interference with circulation. (Schick L, Windle PE. *PeriAnesthesia Nursing Core Curriculum: Preprocedure, Phase I and Phase II PACU Nursing.* 3rd ed. St. Louis, MO: Saunders; 2016:858.)

5

Genitourologic, Reproductive, and Musculoskeletal Systems

Janice Lopez, Charlotte West, and Carolyn Kiolbasa

5-1. The function of the proximal tubule in the glomerulus is to:
   a. Reabsorb 65% of filtered solute and water
   b. Reabsorb 25% of glomerular filtrate
   c. Primarily secrete potassium
   d. Secrete antidiuretic hormone (ADH), leading to water reabsorption

5-2. The preadmission nurse makes a screening phone call to a 32-year-old male patient scheduled for a varicocelectomy. A varicocele is caused by:
   a. Collection of fluid within the scrotal sac
   b. Strangulation of testicular blood supply
   c. Engorged veins of the spermatic cord
   d. Obstruction of the sperm-carrying tubular system

5-3. While monitoring the patient's vital signs, the Phase I PACU nurse may notice some of the normal physiologic changes related to pregnancy. Normal clinical findings include all of the following EXCEPT:
   a. Cola-tinged urine in the urinary catheter
   b. Mild pitting edema of the lower extremities
   c. Monitor tracing suggesting T wave inversion in lead III
   d. Elevated resting heart and respiratory rates

5-4. John Jones is a 16-year-old male patient who presents to outpatient surgery with his parents for arthroscopy with anterior cruciate ligament (ACL) repair. He is an athlete with no preexisting health problems before tearing his ACL while being tackled in football. John arrives with crutches that were used by his father.

The day-of-surgery nurse notes that the patient's father is significantly taller than his son. To assess for proper fit of his axillary crutches, the nurse must have the patient stand upright with the crutches in place and note that the central post allows:
   a. Two to three fingers to be inserted between the axilla and the pad and the hand grips allow the elbows to be bent 20 to 30 degrees
   b. The pad to fit directly under the axilla and the hand grips allow the elbows to be bent 10 to 20 degrees
   c. The pad to reach one hand width below the axilla and the hand grips allow the elbows to be bent 30 to 40 degrees
   d. One finger to be inserted between the axilla and the pad and the hand grips allow the elbows to be bent 5 to 10 degrees

5-5. The drug of choice for postoperative pain control in a patient with chronic renal failure is:
   a. Morphine
   b. Fentanyl
   c. Meperidine
   d. Hydromorphone

5-6. The preadmisson nurse makes a preoperative phone call to a 66-year-old patient scheduled for a total abdominal hysterectomy (TAH), bilateral salpingo-oophorectomy (BSO), anteroposterior (AP) repair, and cystoscopy. The patient has questions because she does not understand what an AP repair is. The nurse explains what this is because she knows an AP repair is repair of:
   a. A cystocele and rectocele
   b. A cystocele and enterocele
   c. A rectocele and enterocele
   d. An enterocele and urethrocele

5-7. The Phase I PACU nurse admits a 33-year-old patient after an emergent appendectomy. The patient is 34 weeks pregnant. Upon arrival, what is the *best* position for the patient?

a. In the right lateral recumbent position

b. In the left lateral recumbent position

c. Supine

d. In reverse Trendelenburg

5-8. The renin–angiotensin–aldosterone (RAA) system is a major renal hormonal regulator for all of the following EXCEPT:

a. Production of new red blood cells (RBCs)

b. Systemic blood pressure (BP)

c. Regional blood flow

d. Sodium and potassium balance

5-9. The Phase I PACU nurse admits an 8-year-old child after hypospadius repair. Which of the following is a postanesthesia priority for this patient?

a. Catheter care and maintenance

b. Monitoring for infection

c. Monitoring for urinary retention

d. Frequent bladder scans

5-10. A Phase II PACU nurse gives discharge instructions to a 32-year-old patient after a diagnostic laparoscopy. Her vital signs have remained stable throughout her Phase I and II course, pain is moderately controlled with a rating of 5/10, she has taken a few sips of water with her oral pain medication, and she voided when she got up to get dressed. She states she felt slightly nauseated, but it is late in the day and she wants to get home. The instructions given to the patient should include information to notify the physician if she has symptoms of unrelieved pain, nausea and vomiting, and unresolved fever due to the possible complication of a:

a. Deep vein thrombosis (DVT)

b. Pulmonary embolus

c. Surgical infection

d. Bowel injury

5-11. The Phase II PACU nurse gives discharge instructions to a 25-year-old patient who had a cervical cerclage under spinal anesthesia. The patient should be instructed that which of the following is expected after this surgery?

a. A moderate amount of bleeding

b. A minimal amount of bloody spotting

c. Low back pain

d. Uterine contractions

5-12. The Phase II PACU discharge nurse continues to give instructions to this same patient regarding her spinal. She instructs the patient to do which of the following if she develops a persistent headache?

a. Increase her activity

b. Call the surgeon for a prescription for oxycodone

c. Decrease her fluid intake

d. Drink caffeinated beverages

Consider this scenario for questions 5-13 and 5-14.
    An 88-year-old male patient is transferred to the Phase I PACU after receiving general anesthesia for a left-sided extracorporeal shock wave lithotripsy (ESWL). Report is received, and the initial assessment is completed. The patient's health history includes hypertension that is controlled with hydrochlorothiazide, 25 mg once daily, and an omega-3 fish oil supplement daily.

5-13. The patient is complaining of mild discomfort, and ketorolac 15 mg IV is ordered. It is MOST important to understand that ketorolac:

a. Is classified as a nonopioid adjunct (NOA)

b. Should be used with caution to preserve renal function

c. Must be given in higher doses to mature adults for adequate results

d. Must be used cautiously to prevent unwanted sedation

5-14. It is most important to assess this patient's urinary output because of:

a. The potential for obstruction

b. The patient's age

c. The need to collect stone fragments for testing

d. The potential for hematuria after any renal procedure

5-15. The Phase II PACU nurse is discharging a patient after insertion of a neurostimulator implant for urge incontinence. The nurse should tell the patient to avoid:

a. Computed tomography (CT) scans

b. Magnetic resonance imaging (MRI) scans

c. Ultrasounds

d. Airport scanners

5-16. The preadmission nurse is making a screening telephone call to a 90-year-old patient scheduled for a cystoscopy and fulguration bladder tumors on an outpatient basis. Her history includes hypertension, coronary artery disease, gastric reflux, and osteoarthritis. She lives alone in an assisted care facility. Regarding NPO guidelines, the preadmission nurse should instruct the patient that it is permissible to:

a. Take her beta-blocker medication before arrival to the hospital

b. Chew gum to reduce risk of gastric reflux

c. Use throat lozenges or cough drops

d. Suck on a piece of hard candy

5-17. The Phase I PACU nurse is preparing to transfer a patient who is status post–anterior cruciate ligament (ACL) repair and has an indwelling nerve catheter of 0.1% ropivacaine in 100 mL of normal saline infusing at 8 mL/hr. He quickly becomes increasingly agitated, stating that he has a metallic taste in his mouth and his lips are numb. The nurse's first response after calling for help should be:

a. Attempt to calm the patient down, offer him some juice, and clamp the nerve catheter

b. Clamp the nerve catheter, reapply monitors to the patient, and continue to assess

c. Clamp the nerve catheter, begin oxygen at 100% by nonrebreather, and reapply monitors

d. Call a code, reapply the monitors, and begin oxygen

5-18. While obtaining a patient's preoperative history, the preadmission nurse learns that the patient has symptoms of urgency and frequency. Urinary urgency is:

a. The urge to urinate at frequent intervals

b. Caused by residual urine

c. A strong sensation of the need to void immediately

d. Caused by inadequate bladder capacity

5-19. For a patient exhibiting symptoms of local anesthetic systemic toxicity (LAST), the recommended initial dose of intralipids is:

a. 1 mL/kg of 20% lipid emulsion

b. 1.5 mL/kg of 20% lipid emulsion

c. 1.5 mL/kg of 10% lipid emulsion

d. 2.5 mL/kg of 10% lipid emulsion

5-20. A 50-year-old female patient is admitted to the preoperative unit in preparation for a triple arthrodesis on the right foot. Pertinent baseline assessments for this surgery include:

a. Color and temperature of the right foot and toes

b. Range of motion of the right foot and toes

c. Sensation in right and left feet and toes

d. Capillary refill time in right toes

5-21. The Phase II PACU nurse has initiated discharge teaching to a patient who is going home with an indwelling femoral nerve catheter. The instructions will include reminding the patient that after removing the catheter, it is critical to immediately check:

a. For lower leg sensation

b. For sensation behind the knee joint

c. That the fluid chamber connected to the catheter is empty

d. That the catheter tip is intact

5-22. The nurse knows that the patient who is being treated with chlorothiazide for high blood pressure may present with a potassium deficiency. This deficiency may affect the function of neuromuscular blocking agents by:

a. Preventing depolarization

b. Enhancing depolarization

c. Decreasing circulating potassium

d. Increasing circulating potassium

5-23. The Phase I PACU nurse is caring for Mrs. Smith after surgical reduction of a displaced femoral fracture requiring pinning. She was struck by a car while crossing the street. The report indicated the patient had no preexisting health problems. No loss of consciousness occurred during the event, and the patient was alert, verbal, and oriented before surgery. The patient arrived in the Phase I PACU awake and responsive to verbal stimuli.

While assessing the patient, the nurse notes a petechial rash evident on the patient's head, neck, and chest. The patient's SpO_2 is 85%, and crackles are evident bilaterally to auscultation of her lungs. She does not respond to verbal stimuli. The perianesthesia nurse is concerned the patient is exhibiting symptoms of:

a. Hypovolemic shock

b. Bleeding to the brain

c. Fat embolism syndrome

d. Heart failure

5-24. The most common complication after lower extremity joint arthroplasty is:

a. Hypovolemia

b. Compartment syndrome

c. Fat embolism

d. Deep vein thrombosis (DVT)

5-25. A patient demonstrating weak or absent dorsiflexion of the foot and ankle and numbness of the lateral aspect of the great toe and medial aspect of the second toe is demonstrating what complication of hip arthroplasty?

a. Femoral head displacement

b. Femoral nerve impingement

c. Femoral nerve palsy

d. Peroneal nerve palsy

5-26. The Phase I PACU nurse receives a 10-year-old patient who fell skateboarding and suffered a comminuted fracture of his humerus. This type of fracture is defined as:

a. A fracture line that runs at a 90-degree angle to the longitudinal axis of the bone

b. A fracture line that twists around the bone shaft

c. Multiple fracture lines that divide the bone into multiple fragments

d. A fracture line that runs at a 45-degree angle to the axis of the bone

5-27. The Phase I PACU nurse receives a 57-year-old female patient after placement of an arteriovenous (AV) graft in her right upper extremity for hemodialysis. Besides her chronic renal failure, her history includes diabetes, hypertension, systemic lupus erythematosus (SLE), stroke, myocardial infarction (MI), cataracts, fibromyalgia, morbid obesity, and polycystic kidney disease. Which of the following is a primary cause of chronic renal failure?

a. Diabetes

b. Hypertension

c. Systemic lupus erythematosus (SLE)

d. Polycystic kidney disease

5-28. A preadmission nurse makes a screening phone call to a 75-year-old female patient scheduled for outpatient surgery to repair a right radial Colles's fracture that she sustained when she fell getting out of bed. The patient's history includes hypertension, coronary artery disease (CAD), Type I diabetes, and stroke with slight left arm weakness. The patient uses a walker or cane and lives alone. The patient states she is worried because she does not have any family to help her at home when she is discharged. There is a neighbor who will bring her to the hospital and take her home, but no one to stay with her. Based on this information, the preadmission nurse should:

 a. Cancel the patient's surgery

 b. Suggest regional anesthesia to the anesthesia provider

 c. Instruct the patient to find a neighbor or friend who can stay with her

 d. Collaborate with the surgeon on a plan for postoperative care

5-29. The broad ligaments of the uterus:

 a. Attach the uterus to either side of the pelvic cavity

 b. Are fibrous sheets that extend to the lateral pelvic wall from the cervix and vagina

 c. Connect the uterus to the sacrum

 d. Are located in front of and below the uterine tubes

5-30. The Phase I nurse admits a 45-year-old patient who had a repair of a vesicovaginal fistula. Which of the following is correct regarding this fistula?

 a. It is an abnormal passage between the rectum and vagina

 b. It develops after previous surgery or trauma

 c. It is an occlusion in the duct system of the Bartholin's gland leading to a fluid-filled sac

 d. It can be a congenital abnormality

5-31. The union of the vas deferens with the duct from the seminal vesical forms the:

 a. Ejaculatory duct

 b. Ejaculatory vesicle

 c. Prostate gland

 d. Cowper's gland

5-32. The Phase I PACU nurse performs a neurologic assessment on a patient who had an L4–5 laminectomy. The patient is asked to move his foot by bending the toes and foot forward. This movement is called:

 a. Plantar flexion

 b. Dorsiflexion

 c. Hyperextension

 d. Supination

5-33. Aldosterone is released from the:

 a. Pituitary gland

 b. Adrenal cortex

 c. Bowman's capsule

 d. Hypothalamus

5-34. A strain injury is most likely a result of:

 a. A ligamentous injury to a joint

 b. Forcible hyperextension of a joint

 c. Rupture of the body of the ligament

 d. A musculotendinous injury

5-35. The preadmission nurse calls a 35-year-old patient at 30 weeks' gestation scheduled for a fractured ankle repair after falling on ice. During the interview the patient mentions some symptoms that she has been having that she did not experience with prior pregnancies. Which of the following cardiovascular changes during pregnancy that mimic cardiac disease would need further investigation?

 a. Fatigue

 b. Orthopnea

 c. Peripheral edema

 d. Chest pain with exertion

5-36. A 25-year-old male patient arrives to the Phase I PACU after repair of a left tibial plateau fracture after a motor vehicle crash. The nurse assesses the patient frequently for signs of compartment syndrome, which include all of the following EXCEPT:

a. Unrelieved intense pain

b. Paresthesia

c. Painless passive stretching of the left great toe

d. Decreased capillary refill

5-37. In the preoperative unit, the nurse is called to assist with placement of an interscalene block on a 40-year-old patient scheduled for shoulder arthroscopy. Anesthesia has ordered midazolam 1 mg IV and fentanyl 50 mcg IV to be given for the procedure. Which of the following statements is correct regarding assisting with this procedure?

a. The unit maintains a two patient–to–one nurse staffing ratio, so the nurse will help with the procedure as able while getting another patient ready for surgery

b. The nurse took vital signs on admission, so vitals do not need to be done again

c. The nursing assistant can assist anesthesia with the procedure and monitor the patient

d. The patient may need pulse oximetry, sedation assessments, and frequent vital signs

5-38. A 45-year-old male patient who works in a warehouse is admitted to the Phase I PACU after a rotator cuff repair. His history includes previous shoulder injuries, including subluxations. A subluxation injury is:

a. Displacement of bone from its normal joint position

b. Partial disruption of a joint

c. A break or disruption of normal continuity of a bone

d. A first-degree strain

5-39. The Phase I PACU nurse performs frequent neurovascular assessments on a patient's postoperative hand. Which of the following is done to test radial nerve sensation?

a. Touch the web space between the thumb and index finger

b. Touch the tip of the index finger

c. Touch the tip of the small finger

d. Touch the tip of the thumb with the small finger

5-40. A patient was diagnosed with pyelonephritis. Which laboratory value supports this diagnosis?

a. Myoglobinuria

b. Ketonuria

c. Pyuria

d. Leukopenia

5-41. A late-stage compartment syndrome symptom is:

a. Pain

b. Pulselessness

c. Paresthesia

d. Pallor

5-42. A patient has arrived from the operating room with a urinary catheter in place. Which of the following findings is AGAINST standard practice?

a. The catheter is anchored with the tubing under the thigh

b. The catheter is anchored with the tubing over the leg

c. The tubing has no proximal loops and is free of kinks

d. The urine collection system is kept below the level of the mattress

5-43. The Phase II PACU is providing discharge teaching to a 65-year-old male patient going home after a shoulder arthroscopy. The patient received preoperative medications, including midazolam 2 mg IV, acetaminophen 1000 mg PO, oxycodone 10 mg PO, and gabapentin 600 mg PO. In the operating room, he received general anesthesia, and the surgeon placed a disposable pump device for postoperative pain control. The bulb is filled with 400 mL of 0.5% bupivacaine and will infuse at 5 mL/hr with an additional PRN demand dose of 5 mL/hr. The nurse provided discharge instructions regarding diet, wound care, showering, pain management, follow-up appointment, and care/removal of the pump infusion line. For what issue should the nurse instruct the patient to call the surgeon?

   a. The bulb is empty on the third postop day

   b. A temperature of 99.5° F

   c. Generalized sore muscles

   d. Difficulty urinating

5-44. The preadmission nurse is making a screening phone call to a 65-year-old patient scheduled for a cystoscopy and retrograde pyelogram (RPG). The nurse explains that the RPG provides:

   a. Fluoroscopic views of the ureters and kidneys

   b. Evaluation of the retroperitoneal lymph nodes

   c. Evaluation of renal blood flow and function

   d. Visualization of the entire urinary system through IV administration of contrast dye

5-45. The Phase I PACU nurse receives a 63-year-old patient following a total abdominal hysterectomy (TAH), bilateral salpingo-oophorectomy (BSO), and omentectomy.

She has a history of hypertension, heart failure, hypothyroidism, and chronic pain. She received 1500 mL Lactated Ringer's in the operating room and had a 300 mL blood loss. After 3 hours in the Phase I PACU, the patient's urine output is averaging 10 mL/hr, BP is 99/60, and HR is 110. The surgeon orders a complete blood count (CBC) and basic metabolic panel (BMP). The patient's creatinine was 1.6 preop and is now 3.0. This is a sign of:

   a. Acute renal failure

   b. Chronic renal failure

   c. Renal insufficiency

   d. Uremia

5-46. The Phase I PACU nurse admits a 23-year-old patient after a diagnostic laparoscopy and excision of an ovarian cyst. The patient presents to the Phase I PACU restless and complaining of abdominal pain, nausea, and right shoulder pain. The patient's BP is 140/88, HR is 120, RR is 26, and SpO_2 is 99%. These symptoms are likely related to:

   a. A pulmonary embolus

   b. Retained gas from the pneumoperitoneum

   c. Pulmonary edema

   d. Perforated bowel

5-47. The nurse in the Phase I PACU is caring for a 58-year-old male patient after receiving general anesthesia during a 4-hour procedure. He repeatedly attempts to get out of bed, removes his oxygen mask, and picks at his abdominal dressing. The perianesthesia nurse attempts to reorient the patient and reassure him while assessing for likely causes of his restlessness, including hypoxia, pain, and:

   a. Distended bladder

   b. Sepsis

   c. Electrolyte imbalance

   d. Emergence delirium

5-48. A 59-year-old, 100-kg female patient is in the Phase II PACU preparing for discharge after ankle surgery. The nurse has given discharge instructions to the patient and family member. Physical therapy provided crutch-walking instructions for non–weight bearing, and the patient demonstrated correct use of the crutches. In order to decrease the risk of postoperative deep vein thrombosis (DVT), the nurse should instruct the patient to do which of the following?

    a. Limit fluid intake to decrease having to get up frequently to go to the bathroom

    b. Stay in bed or a recliner with her leg elevated

    c. Do range-of-motion exercises once daily

    d. Take the anticoagulant prescribed by her surgeon

5-49. While caring for a patient with a posterior hip arthroplasty, which measure should be taken to prevent the risk of hip dislocation?

    a. Elevate the foot of the bed

    b. Avoid hip abduction

    c. Avoid hip flexion greater than 90 degrees

    d. Avoid external rotation

5-50. A 33-year-old male patient has had a percutaneous lithotripsy. The Phase II PACU nurse should instruct the patient to:

    a. Limit oral fluid intake for 1 to 2 weeks

    b. Report the passing of sandlike particles through the nephrostomy tube

    c. Notify the physician if urine becomes cloudy or foul smelling

    d. Report bright pink urine lasting up to 24 hours postprocedure

5-51. A patient is being discharged from the Phase II PACU after knee arthroscopy. Anesthesia placed a regional nerve block, and the patient is going home with a disposable pump device. The patient should be instructed to be alert for which of the following signs and symptoms of local anesthetic toxicity?

    a. Dry mouth

    b. Nausea and vomiting

    c. Numbness or tingling in the toes

    d. Numbness around the mouth

5-52. The Phase I PACU nurse admits a 30-week-gestation pregnant patient after undergoing surgery for an emergency exploratory laparotomy and splenectomy after a motor vehicle crash. The patient is on a ventilator, and blood gases are ordered by the anesthesiologist. Which of the following blood gas interpretations is normal in pregnancy?

    a. Compensated respiratory alkalosis

    b. Respiratory acidosis

    c. Compensated metabolic alkalosis

    d. Metabolic acidosis

5-53. A preoperative nurse is preparing a 45-year-old patient for removal of a peritoneal dialysis catheter. He had a successful kidney transplant 2 months ago. He expresses concern regarding signs of rejection of his cadaveric transplant. The patient is instructed to watch for which of the following signs and symptoms of allograft rejection?

    a. Increased urine output

    b. Weight loss

    c. Increased appetite

    d. Low-grade fever

Consider this scenario for questions 5-54 and 5-55.
    A 44-year-old female patient presents to the Phase I PACU after robotic-assisted hysterectomy due to cancer. Health history includes hypertension controlled by lisinopril 10 mg daily. Preoperative vital signs include BP 128/82 mm Hg, HR 77, RR 16, and SpO$_2$ 99%. A urinary catheter is secure and draining yellow urine.

5-54. The patient is awake and talking. She complains of pain increasing from level 4 to 8 despite being medicated with hydromorphone 2 mg. There is no vaginal bleeding, but the abdomen is distended. BP is now 144/88, HR is 126, RR is 18, and SpO$_2$ saturation is 98 on 3 L nasal cannula. The perianesthesia nurse should be concerned about:

    a. Hypoxia

    b. Dehydration

    c. Abdominal hemorrhage

    d. Low pain tolerance

5-55. A urinary catheter was placed in surgery and will remain in place secondary to:

a. Temporary paralysis of the puborectalis muscle

b. Urethral edema from the surgical procedure

c. Patient need for overnight rest

d. Surgeon's preference

5-56. Patient education priorities after extracorporeal shock wave lithotripsy (ESWL) focus primarily on:

a. Antibiotic effect

b. Scheduled analgesia

c. Hematuria

d. Forced hydration

5-57. Following an orchiopexy, the Phase I PACU nurse's observations and interventions include all of the following EXCEPT:

a. Providing scrotal support

b. Applying heat to the surgical area

c. Conducting frequent checks for edema and bleeding

d. Titrating small doses of pain medicine

5-58. Signs of bladder distention include all of the following EXCEPT:

a. Restlessness

b. Hypertension

c. Hypotension

d. Tachycardia

5-59. Which of the following laboratory results are components of the triad of HELLP syndrome?

a. Hemolysis and elevated leukocytes

b. Elevated leukocytes and low protein

c. Hemolysis and low platelets

d. Hematuria and elevated liver enzymes

5-60. The micturition reflex is stimulated by all of the following EXCEPT:

a. Higher centers in the brainstem

b. Increased pressure in the bladder

c. Irritation of the bladder or urethra

d. Absence of bladder contractions

5-61. Surgical management of urinary incontinence includes all of the following EXCEPT:

a. Tension-free vaginal tape (TVT) sling

b. Modified Burch's procedure

c. Culdoscopy

d. Bladder neck suspension

5-62. A 38-year-old male patient is admitted to the Phase I PACU after an exploratory laparotomy for lower abdominal pain. Preoperative history includes type II diabetes. He had several days of nausea and vomiting before the emergency department visit. Preoperative laboratory test results include blood urea nitrogen (BUN) at 29, creatinine at 1.9, and blood sugar at 290. He is diagnosed with acute renal failure (ARF). What could be the cause for this patient's ARF?

a. Dehydration

b. Diverticulitis

c. Occult peritonitis

d. Ketogenesis

Consider this scenario for questions 5-63 and 5-64.
The Phase II PACU nurse receives a patient after a prolonged stay in the PACU. Mr. J is status post–inguinal hernia repair and required a bolus of 1.5 mg/kg of succinylcholine for a laryngospasm that did not respond to positive pressure ventilation. He was monitored closely and discharged from the Phase I PACU after demonstrating full recovery from the neuromuscular blocking agent.

5-63. Mr. J states that he has a very sore throat and neck pain. The nurse realizes this pain may be due to the endotracheal tube used during surgery. Another likely cause could be:

a. Positioning during the surgical procedure

b. The extra pressure used during airway support during laryngospasm

c. Myalgia occurring from succinylcholine administration

d. Early signs of a viral upper airway infection

5-64. During the postoperative follow-up call to Mr. J on day one after surgery, the nurse determines that Mr. J is having generalized muscle pain. He was ambulating in the surgery center before discharge and denies any fever, wound drainage, nausea, vomiting, or difficulty breathing. She knows that:

a. This pain can occur in 60% to 70% of ambulatory patients after succinylcholine administration

b. The myalgia usually does not last 2 days, and the surgeon should be notified immediately

c. This pain occurs more often in patients who are not ambulatory, so this is unusual

d. This patient may require additional pain medication to help his recovery and relieve the myalgia

5-65. After surgery to repair a humerus fracture, the Phase I PACU nurse assesses the color of the patient's fingers. Cyanosis indicates:

a. Arterial obstruction

b. Venous obstruction

c. Lymphatic obstruction

d. Hyperventilation

Answers and Rationales for Chapter 5, Genitourologic, Reproductive, and Musculoskeletal Systems

5-1. *Correct answer:* **a**
Each kidney contains approximately 1.2 million nephrons, the functional units of the kidney. Each nephron contains a glomerulus, the vascular segment enclosed in Bowman's capsule. The proximal tubule is the site of 65% of resorption of filtered solutes and water. The loop of Henle reabsorbs 25% of the glomerular filtrate and is a mechanism for sodium and water reabsorption, which controls urine concentration and conservation, such as seen in dehydration and hemorrhage. The distal tubule is the site for aldosterone action and is the primary site for potassium secretion, acid–base regulation, and the action of ADH leading to water reabsorption. (Schick L, Windle PE. *PeriAnesthesia Nursing Core Curriculum: Preprocedure, Phase I and Phase II Nursing.* 3rd ed. St. Louis, MO: Saunders; 2016:839-842.)

5-2. *Correct answer:* **c**
A hydrocele is the collection of fluid within the scrotal sac, which may compromise testicular blood supply. Torsion of the testis is the strangulation of the testicular blood supply, usually caused by trauma, resulting in extreme pain and requiring immediate surgery. In a varicocele, the veins of the spermatic cord become engorged because of venous backflow. This is often painful and, if uncorrected, can affect fertility. A spermatocele is an intrascrotal cystic mass caused by obstruction of the sperm-carrying tubular system. (Schick L, Windle PE. *PeriAnesthesia Nursing Core Curriculum: Preprocedure, Phase I and Phase II Nursing.* 3rd ed. St. Louis, MO: Saunders; 2016:861.)

5-3. *Correct answer:* **a**
The body undergoes many physiologic changes to accommodate a pregnancy, in particular, in the cardiovascular, hematologic, metabolic, renal, and respiratory systems. Increases in blood glucose, breathing, and cardiac output all are required. The renal system experiences increased dilation within the kidneys secondary to mechanical compression by the pregnant uterus, and urinary tract infections can be more frequent. Urine should remain normal in color and consistency. (Udom-Forren J. *Drain's Perianesthesia Nursing: A Critical Care Approach.* 6th ed. St. Louis, MO: Saunders; 2013:721-725.)

5-4. *Correct answer:* **a**
The proper fit of axillary crutches is critical to prevent damage to the brachial plexus. Adequate space needs to be present between the axilla and the pad, with sufficient elbow flexion to keep the patient from placing full body weight directly on the axillary region when standing upright. The elbow flexion of 20 to 30 degrees also allows the elbow to straighten when the arms move forward with the crutches. (Schick L, Windle PE. *PeriAnesthesia Nursing Core Curriculum: Preprocedure, Phase I and Phase II Nursing.* 3rd ed. St. Louis, MO: Saunders; 2016:1014.)

5-5. *Correct answer:* **b**
Fentanyl appears safe for renal patients, especially for short-term use. The metabolites from fentanyl are also inactive. Do not use morphine, meperidine, or hydromorphone because the metabolites can accumulate and their adverse effects (e.g., sedation, nausea) can be prolonged. In general, consider decreased doses of medications eliminated through the kidneys. (Schick L, Windle PE. *PeriAnesthesia Nursing Core Curriculum: Preprocedure, Phase I and Phase II PACU Nursing.* 3rd ed. St. Louis, MO: Saunders; 2016:105-107.)

5-6. *Correct answer:* **a**

A cystocele is a herniation of the bladder that causes the anterior vaginal wall to bulge downward. A rectocele is formed by protrusion of the anterior rectal wall (posterior vaginal wall) into the vagina. An enterocele is a herniation of the cul-de-sac of Douglas, containing loops of small intestine. A urethrocele is a pouchlike protrusion of the urethral wall. (Schick L, Windle PE. *PeriAnesthesia Nursing Core Curriculum: Preprocedure, Phase I and Phase II Nursing.* 3rd ed. St. Louis, MO: Saunders; 2016:895.)

5-7. *Correct answer:* **b**

Cardiac output is profoundly affected by maternal position. It is highest in the lateral or semi-Fowler's position with uterine displacement. Cardiac output is lowest in the supine and standing positions. Turning from the left lateral recumbent to supine position at term can decrease cardiac output by 25% to 30% as a result of vena cava compression by the gravid uterus. (Schick L, Windle PE. *PeriAnesthesia Nursing Core Curriculum: Preprocedure, Phase I and Phase II Nursing.* 3rd ed. St. Louis, MO: Saunders; 2016:898-899.)

5-8. *Correct answer:* **a**

The renin-angiotensin-aldosterone (RAA) system, along with prostaglandin, erythropoietin, antidiuretic hormone (ADH), and vitamin D, controls renal endocrine function. The RAA is a hormonal regulator for systemic BP, regional blood flow, and sodium and potassium balance. Erythropoietin is secreted by the kidney in response to a decrease in tissue oxygen tension (PaO_2) and stimulates production of new RBCs by exerting its effect directly on the bone marrow. (Schick L, Windle PE. *PeriAnesthesia Nursing Core Curriculum: Preoprocedure, Phase I and Phase II Nursing.* 3rd ed. St. Louis, MO: Saunders; 2016:850-852.)

5-9. *Correct answer:* **a**

This procedure is a urethral or meatal reconstruction and repositioning. It is often a staged procedure and performed most frequently in pediatric populations. The postanesthesia priorities of care are catheter care and maintenance, monitoring urine output, fluid and electrolyte balance, body temperature, assessment of dressing, and changes if needed. Psychosocial concerns are reuniting the child and parents to reduce anxiety and stress. Complications of this procedure include infection, urethral stricture, scarring, and urinary retention. (Schick L, Windle PE. *PeriAnesthesia Nursing Core Curriculum: Preprocedure, Phase I and Phase II Nursing.* 3rd ed. St. Louis, MO: Saunders; 2016:883.)

5-10. *Correct answer:* **d**

Patients undergoing outpatient laparoscopic procedures should be taught to report early signs of bowel injuries. While relatively rare, bowel injuries are a potential complication. Typically the injury involves perforation of the small intestines which are micro in nature. These can go unrecognized while in the operating room and eventually develop into peritonitis and subsequent sepsis. Patients must be educated to report unrelieved pain, prolonged nausea and vomiting and unanticipated fevers to the surgeon. (Odom-Forren J. *Drain's Perianesthesia Nursing: A Critical Care Approach.* 6th ed. St. Louis, MO: Saunders; 2013:671.)

5-11. *Correct answer:* **b**

After a cervical cerclage, the patient should expect a minimal amount of bleeding or spotting. Larger amounts of bleeding should be reported to the surgeon. Low back pain and uterine contractions are signs of labor. (Schick L, Windle PE. *PeriAnesthesia Nursing Core Curriculum: Preprocedure, Phase I and Phase II Nursing.* 3rd ed. St. Louis, MO: Saunders; 2016:905, 939.)

5-12. *Correct answer:* **d**

Postdural puncture headache (PDPH) typically develops 24 to 48 hours after lumbar puncture from spinal needle placement. The headache is caused by leakage of cerebrospinal fluid. The incidence rate of PDPH is greater in younger patients and women, especially during pregnancy. Treatment is initially conservative; recommendations include mild analgesics, bed rest, caffeinated beverages, and increased fluid intake. If the symptoms continue, definitive treatment is an epidural blood patch in which fresh autologous blood is injected into the epidural space to seal the leak. Epidural blood patches are effective in greater than 95% of symptomatic patients. (Odom-Forren J. *Drain's Perianesthesia Nursing: A Critical Care Approach.* 6th ed. St. Louis, MO: Saunders; 2013:410.)

5-13. *Correct answer:* **b**

The goal of patient care includes being aware of nephrotoxic medications and preserving renal function. This patient should be watched for oliguria as a sign of reduced glomerular function or obstruction from the renal calculi moving in the kidney and passing into the ureters. Renal effects of ketorolac have been attributed to long-term use. The lowest possible dose of ketorolac should be used to minimize risk. (Odom-Forren J. *Drain's Perianesthesia Nursing: A Critical Care Approach.* St. Louis, MO: Saunders; 2013:184-193.)

5-14. *Correct answer:* **a**

After extracorporeal shock wave lithotripsy (ESWL), small fragments of calculi are washed out of the kidney and passed through the ureter. If any of the fragments are large enough, there could be obstruction. This obstruction would be noted with a decrease in renal output and pain to the operative side from renal colic and backing up of urine into that kidney. (Odom-Forren J. *Drain's Perianesthesia Nursing: A Critical Care Approach.* St. Louis, MO: Saunders; 2013:600.)

5-15. *Correct answer:* **b**

A neurostimulator implant is a type of neuromodulation device used to treat voiding dysfunctions such as urinary frequency, urgency, or incontinence. It provides pacemaker-type stimulation of the sacral nerves. A pocket is created for the pacemaker below the waist and adjacent to the pelvic bone. Thin wires are tunneled from the sacral foramen to the pacemaker. MRI scans are contraindicated with this implant. (Schick L, Windle PE. *PeriAnesthesia Nursing Core Curriculum: Preprocedure, Phase I and Phase II Nursing.* 3rd ed. St. Louis, MO: Saunders; 2016:877.)

5-16. *Correct answer:* **a**

Patients should be educated about the specifics of the fasting period. They should know that in addition to food and beverages, they are to avoid water, gum, candy, coffee, and cough drops immediately before surgery. Even though candy and gum are not swallowed, they stimulate the stomach to produce acids that can be harmful if aspirated. Patients should be informed about the seriousness of breaking the fasting period and of accurate reporting of nonadherence. Beta blockers should be continued in the perioperative period, and patients are allowed to take them preoperatively with a sip of water. (Odom-Forren J. *Drain's Perianesthesia Nursing: A Critical Care Approach.* 6th ed. St. Louis, MO: Saunders; 2013:652-653.)

5-17. *Correct answer:* **c**

The patient is exhibiting signs of local anesthetic systemic toxicity (LAST). The early symptoms of central nervous excitement, such as agitation, metallic taste in mouth, and circumoral numbness, can rapidly progress to seizures and central nervous system depression and eventual respiratory and cardiac arrest. The infusion of local anesthetic must be stopped to prevent further toxicity. Hypoxia and acidosis potentiate LAST, thus airway management and oxygenation are critical. Additional help will be needed to provide further treatment and assistance with beginning intralipid infusions. (Odom-Forren J. *Drain's Perianesthesia Nursing: A Critical Care Approach.* St. Louis, MO: Saunders; 2013: 321-322; Noble K. *Local anesthesia toxicity and lipid rescue.* J PeriAnesth Nurs. 2015; 30(4):321-335.)

5-18. *Correct answer:* **c**

Urinary frequency is characterized by the urge to urinate at frequent intervals that is caused by residual urine volume, inflamed bladder mucosa, interstitial cystitis, bladder infection, or inadequate bladder capacity. Urgency is the strong sensation of having to void immediately caused by cystitis or bladder instability. (Schick L, Windle PE. *PeriAnesthesia Nursing Core Curriculum: Preprocedure, Phase I and Phase II Nursing.* 3rd ed. St. Louis, MO: Saunders; 2016:862-864.)

5-19. *Correct answer:* **b**

The recommended initial dose of lipid for the treatment of local anesthetic systemic toxicity (LAST) is 1.5 mL/kg of the 20% lipid emulsion bolus. The initial bolus is followed by a continuous infusion at 0.25 mL/kg/min. Two additional boluses may be given if the patient continues to have cardiac instability, and the continuous infusion may be increased to 0.5 mL/kg/min. A lipid infusion should be continued for at least 10 minutes after the patient has stabilized. The maximum recommended dose of lipids within a 30-minute time period is 10 mL/kg. (Odom-Forren J. *Drain's Perianesthesia Nursing: A Critical Care Approach.* 6th ed. St. Louis, MO: Saunders; 2013:321-322; Noble K. *Local anesthesia toxicity and lipid rescue.* J PeriAnesth Nurs. 2015; 30(4):321-335.)

5-20. *Correct answer:* **c**

Preoperative assessment should provide a baseline for postoperative assessments. Both lower extremities should be assessed for pain, color, mobility, temperature, pulses, sensation, swelling, and capillary refill. Assessments are done on both lower extremities for comparisons. (Odom-Forren J. *Drain's Perianesthesia Nursing: A Critical Care Approach.* 6th ed. St. Louis, MO: Saunders; 2013:542-543. American Society of PeriAnesthesia Nurses. *2015–2017 Perianesthesia Nursing Standards, Practice Recommendations and Interpretive Statements.* Cherry Hill, NJ: ASPAN; 2014:43.)

5-21. *Correct answer:* **d**

Because the effects of the local anesthetic may last for 36 hours after the catheter is removed, sensation may not be present in the lower leg. Due to the location of the sciatic nerve, sensation may be present behind the knee even while the catheter is in place. Ideally all of the anesthetic agent in the device will have infused into the patient prior to removal of the catheter, but this does not always happen. It is critical that the catheter tip be intact, demonstrating that the entire catheter has been removed from the body. A broken catheter requires the family to notify their anesthesia provider immediately. (Odom-Forren J. *Drain's Perianesthesia Nursing: A Critical Care Approach.* 6th ed. St. Louis, MO: Saunders; 2013:335; Pasero C, McCaffery M. *Pain Assessment and Pharmacological Management,* Elsevier Health Sciences, 2011:696-704.)

5-22. *Correct answer:* **a**

A potassium deficiency appears to stabilize muscle end plates, causing less movement of ions across the cell membrane. This can lead to an increase in the blocking action of the nondepolarizing neuromuscular blocking agents, as well as cause an increase in the amount of depolarizing neuromuscular blocking agents needed to have an effect on the muscle. (Odom-Forren J. *Drain's Perianesthesia Nursing: A Critical Care Approach.* 6th ed. St. Louis, MO: Saunders; 2013:301.)

5-23. *Correct answer:* **c**

The patient is exhibiting signs and symptoms of fat embolism, which can occur as a result of fractures to the long bones. The fractures release fat droplets into circulation from the bone marrow, which eventually travel to the pulmonary vasculature, causing pulmonary congestion. The classic triad of symptoms includes petechial rash, respiratory symptoms, and neurologic changes. (Odom-Forren J. *Drain's Perianesthesia Nursing: A Critical Care Approach.* 6th ed. St. Louis, MO: Saunders; 2013:544-545; Mamaril M, Childs S, Sortman S. Care of the orthopedic trauma patient. *J PeriAnesth Nurs.* 2006; 22(3):184-194.)

5-24. *Correct answer:* **d**

Deep vein thrombosis (DVT) is the most common complication after lower extremity joint replacement. Sequential compression devices are one common form of prophylaxis that is implemented. Encouraging the patient to contract and relax the calf muscles while in bed and early ambulation is recommended for most joint replacement patients. (Schick L, Windle PE. *ASPAN's PeriAnesthesia Nursing Core Curriculum: Preprocedure, Phase I and Phase II PACU Nursing.* 3rd ed. St. Louis, MO: Saunders; 2016:1016-1017, 1032.)

5-25. *Correct answer:* **d**

The peroneal nerve has the potential of being stretched during hip arthroplasty by intraoperative hip dislocation, limb lengthening, or hematoma formation. (Schick L, Windle PE. *ASPAN's PeriAnesthesia Nursing Core Curriculum: Preprocedure, Phase I and Phase II PACU Nursing.* 3rd ed. St. Louis, MO: Saunders; 2016:1033.)

5-26. *Correct answer:* **c**

A longitudinal or linear fracture line runs parallel to the axis of the bone. An oblique fracture line runs at a 45-degree angle to the axis of the bone. A spiral fracture line twists around the bone shaft. A transverse fracture line runs at a 90-degree angle to the longitudinal axis of the bone. A comminuted fracture is multiple fracture lines that divide the bone into multiple fragments. External fixation devices such as splints and casts are usually inadequate in treating this type of fracture. Repairing a comminuted fracture often requires open surgery to restructure the bone to normal position. (Schick L, Windle PE. *PeriAnesthesia Nursing Core Curriculum: Preprocedure, Phase I and Phase II Nursing.* 3rd ed. St. Louis, MO: Saunders; 2016:1007-1009.)

5-27. *Correct answer:* **d**

Primary causes of chronic renal failure include glomerulonephritis, pyelonephritis, and polycystic kidney disease. Secondary causes are diabetes, hypertension, systemic lupus erythematosus (SLE), Alport's syndrome, and amyloidosis. (Schick L, Windle PE. *PeriAnesthesia Nursing Core Curriculum: Preprocedure, Phase I and Phase II Nursing.* 3rd ed. St. Louis, MO: Saunders; 2016:855-856.)

5-28. *Correct answer:* **d**

The surgery should not be canceled without discussing with the surgeon. Giving regional anesthesia will not solve the problem. The patient already has weakness in the left arm, and she will not be able to use her right arm due to the surgery. The patient stated she does not have a responsible adult to stay with her at home to provide assistance. The nurse should call the surgeon to discuss the situation and make a plan for safe care for the patient, which may necessitate admission to the hospital and a care management consult for assistance with home care once discharged. (American Society of PeriAnesthesia Nurses. *2015–2017 Perianesthesia Nursing Standards, Practice Recommendations and Interpretive Statements.* Cherry Hill, NJ: ASPAN; 2014:41-42.)

5-29. *Correct answer:* **a**

There are eight ligaments of the uterus. The fibrous sheets that extend to the lateral pelvic wall from the cervix and vagina are the two cardinal ligaments. They help prevent prolapse of the uterus. Two lateral or broad ligaments attach the uterus to either side of the pelvic cavity. They divide the cavity into two portions; the anterior part is the bladder, and the posterior part is the rectum. They also keep the uterus in position. Two uterosacral ligaments lie on either side of the rectum and connect the uterus to the sacrum. The two round ligaments are situated between layers of the broad ligaments in front of and below the uterine tubes. (Schick L, Windle PE. *PeriAnesthesia Nursing Core Curriculum: Preprocedure, Phase I and Phase II Nursing.* 3rd ed. St. Louis, MO: Saunders; 2016:893.)

5-30. *Correct answer:* **b**

A urethrovaginal (vesicovaginal) fistula is an abnormal passageway between the urethra and vagina that develops after trauma such as a pelvic fracture, surgery, or radiotherapy. A vaginal urethroplasty is performed to correct the fistula. A urethral diverticulum can be a congenital abnormality that requires excision and plastic repair. A Bartholin's gland cyst and abscess is an occlusion in the duct system of the gland that leads to a fluid-filled sac. An abscess can result if the cyst becomes infected. A rectovaginal fistula is an abnormal passage between the rectum and vagina. (Schick L, Windle PE. *PeriAnesthesia Nursing Core Curriculum: Preprocedure, Phase I and Phase II Nursing.* 3rd ed. St. Louis, MO: Saunders; 2016:861-862.)

5-31. *Correct answer:* **a**

The epididymis leads to the vas deferens, which converge into the ejaculatory duct. Once sperm cells are produced in the testis and accumulate in the epididymis, they rely on the ductus (vas) deferens and ejaculatory duct to propel them into the urethra and out of the penis during ejaculation. The ejaculatory duct delivers sperm into the urethra, adding secretions and additives from the prostate necessary for sperm function, while providing an interface between the reproductive and urinary systems in men (Schick L, Windle PE. *ASPAN's PeriAnesthesia Nursing Core Curriculum: Preprocedure, Phase I and Phase II PACU Nursing.* 3rd ed. St. Louis, MO: Saunders; 2016:845-846.)

5-32. *Correct answer:* **a**

Plantar flexion increases the angle between the foot and front of the leg by bending the foot and toes down and back. Dorsiflexion decreases the angle between the foot and front of the leg by bending the toes and foot upward. Hyperextension is stretching a part beyond its normal anatomical limits. Supination describes the palm of the hand turned upward while the forearm rotates outward. Assessment of motor and sensory function is part of an ongoing neurologic assessment and is performed to note changes from the baseline assessment. It can provide clues to bleeding, edema, or nerve injury. (Schick L, Windle PE. *PeriAnesthesia Nursing Core Curriculum: Preprocedure, Phase I and Phase II Nursing.* 3rd ed. St. Louis, MO: Saunders; 2016:999; Odom-Forren J. *Drain's Perianesthesia Nursing: A Critical Care Approach.* 6th ed. St. Louis, MO: Saunders; 2013:568.)

5-33. *Correct answer:* **b**

Aldosterone is released from the adrenal cortex, which is stimulated by decreased sodium levels or increased potassium levels. This prompts the kidney to absorb more sodium in the distal tubule and conserve sodium and water. The pituitary gland and hypothalamus work in a feedback system controlling adrenocorticotropic hormone (ACTH), antidiuretic hormone (ADH), and oxytocin. Bowman's capsule houses the glomeruli in the nephrons of the kidney. (Schick L, Windle PE. *PeriAnesthesia Nursing Core Curriculum: Preprocedure, Phase I and Phase II Nursing.* 3rd ed. St. Louis, MO: Saunders; 2016:314-315, 841-842; Odom-Forren J. *Drain's Perianesthesia Nursing: A Critical Care Approach.* 6th ed. St. Louis, MO: Saunders; 2013:208-209.)

5-34. *Correct answer:* **d**

A strain is a musculotendinous injury caused by overstretching, repetitive stress, or misuse. Tendons connect muscles to bones. A sprain is a ligamentous injury to a joint that is caused by forcible hyperextension of a joint, and it can lead to rupture of the body of the ligament. Ligaments connect bones to bones. (Schick L, Windle PE. *PeriAnesthesia Nursing Core Curriculum: Preprocedure, Phase I and Phase II Nursing.* 3rd ed. St. Louis, MO: Saunders; 2016:1007.)

5-35. *Correct answer:* **d**

Normal physiologic adaptations of the cardiopulmonary system during pregnancy may mimic cardiac disease. These include dyspnea, decreased exercise tolerance, fatigue, orthopnea, syncope, and chest discomfort. Clinical findings that warrant further investigation to rule out underlying cardiac disease include hemoptysis, syncope or chest pain with exertion, progressive orthopnea, and paroxysmal nocturnal dyspnea. Normal findings that may mimic cardiac disease include peripheral edema, mild tachycardia, jugular distention after midpregnancy, and lateral displacement of the left ventricular apex. (Schick L, Windle PE. *PeriAnesthesia Nursing Core Curriculum: Preprocedure, Phase I and Phase II Nursing.* 3rd ed. St. Louis, MO: Saunders; 2016:900.)

5-36. *Correct answer:* **c**

The hallmark symptoms of compartment syndrome include intense pain unrelieved with conventional methods, paresthesia, and sharp pain on passive stretching of the middle finger of the affected arm or the large toe of the affected leg. Progressive symptoms include decreased capillary refill; peripheral pulses are not generally compromised. A serious complication of a tibial plateau fracture is compartment syndrome. (Odom-Forren J. *Drain's Perianesthesia Nursing: A Critical Care Approach.* 6th ed. St. Louis, MO: Saunders; 2013:545.)

5-37. *Correct answer:* **d**

The nurse caring for a patient receiving sedation for an invasive procedure should not have any other assignment that would call the nurse away from monitoring the patient. An RN needs to be monitoring and assessing the patient. This patient will probably need pulse oximetry, telemetry monitoring, frequent vital signs, and sedation assessments, as well as monitoring for signs and symptoms of local anesthetic toxicity. (American Society of PeriAnesthesia Nurses. *2015–2017 Perianesthesia Nursing Standards, Practice Recommendations and Interpretive Statements.* Cherry Hill, NJ: ASPAN; 2014:43, 62-65.)

5-38. *Correct answer:* **b**

A dislocation is displacement of bone from its normal position; articulating surfaces lose contact. Subluxation is a partial disruption of a joint; there is partial loss of contact. Dislocations and subluxation injuries are more common in the shoulder joint, followed by the elbow, and may be accompanied by soft tissue injury, including nerve palsy. Recurrent dislocation may necessitate surgical repair or reconstruction of the joint. A break or disruption of normal continuity of a bone is a fracture. A first-degree strain is a mild stretching injury in a joint. (Schick L, Windle PE. *PeriAnesthesia Nursing Core Curriculum: Preprocedure, Phase I and Phase II Nursing.* 3rd ed. St. Louis, MO: Saunders; 2016:1007.)

5-39. *Correct answer:* **a**

To test sensory function of the radial nerve, touch the web space between the thumb and index finger. To test motor function, have the patient extend the wrist and hyperextend the thumb. To test sensory function of the median nerve, touch the tip of the index finger. To test motor function, have the patient pinch, abduct, and oppose the thumb to the small finger. To test sensory function of the ulnar nerve, touch the tip of the small finger. To test motor function, have the patient abduct all fingers. (Schick L, Windle PE. *PeriAnesthesia Nursing Core Curriculum: Preprocedure, Phase I and Phase II Nursing.* 3rd ed. St. Louis, MO: Saunders; 2016:1016.)

5-40. *Correct answer:* **c**

Pyelonephritis is diagnosed by the presence of leukocytosis, hematuria, pyuria, and bacteriuria. The patient exhibits fever, chills, and flank pain. Pyuria is the presence of white blood cells in the urine. Ketonuria indicates a diabetic state. Myoglobinuria is the presence of myoglobin in the urine, usually associated with rhabdomyolysis or muscle destruction. (Fleisher LA, Roizen MF. *Essence of Anesthesia Practice: Expert Consult- Online and Print.* 3rd ed. Philadelphia, PA: Elsevier Science; 2011:703.)

5-41. *Correct answer:* **b**

Pain is the most universal symptom related to muscle ischemia. It is extreme, unrelieved, aggravated by passive flexion or extension of the digit or limb, and not well localized—it involves the entire compartment. Pallor is seen in the early stage and is related to compression of an artery. Later it may be seen as cyanosis. Paresthesias are commonly seen changes related to compression of a sensory nerve and described as burning, searing, or electric sensations. In the early stage, a pulse with decreased strength is found. Later, the pulse is non-palpable but present by Doppler. In later stages, no pulse is found by Doppler. Muscle and nerve ischemia can be occurring without occluding an artery. (Schick L, Windle PE. *PeriAnesthesia Nursing Core Curriculum: Preprocedure, Phase I and Phase II Nursing.* 3rd ed. St. Louis, MO: Saunders; 2016:1021.)

5-42. *Correct answer:* **a**

Urinary catheters should be properly secured by a leg strap or a locking device to the patient's thigh. Care must be taken that the tubing is not beneath the patient. This will help reduce irritation and allow for adequate bladder drainage. The connecting tubing should be arranged to allow free flowing urine without proximal loops of tubing or kinks lying below the distal tubing. The urine receptacle should always be kept below the bladder level to prevent urine reflux up the tubing. (Odom-Forren J. *Drain's Perianesthesia Nursing: A Critical Care Approach.* St. Louis, MO: Saunders; 2013:596-597.)

5-43. *Correct answer:* **d**

Discharge instructions should be given to the patient and responsible home care provider. They should include written information about diet, hygiene, wound care, ambulation, return physician visit, telephone numbers for assistance, care of equipment/devices, and what symptoms may be usual and what should be reported to the physician. Knowledge that a slight sore throat or generalized sore muscles may follow general anesthesia helps patients avoid worry. Following the instructions with suggestions for alleviating possible minor symptoms, the patient has an even greater chance of recuperating comfortably. If the pump is infusing at 5 mL/hr, after 72 hours, 360 mL would have infused, allowing 40 mL for PRN demand doses. If it is empty on postop day 3, this is expected, and the patient should be able to remove the device following the instructions that were given. A temperature of 99.5° F is considered low grade and is generally not a concern. Temperatures over 100.4° F are more alarming. Generalized sore muscles are not unusual. If the patient is having difficulty urinating or has minimal urine output, this is a symptom that should be checked into further. The patient may have underlying benign prostatic hypertrophy (BPH) or is not taking in enough oral fluids. (Odom-Forren J. *Drain's Perianesthesia Nursing: A Critical Care Approach.* 6th ed. St. Louis, MO: Saunders; 2013:657.)

5-44. *Correct answer:* **a**

A computed tomography (CT) scan can evaluate the retroperitoneal lymph nodes. A renal scan evaluates renal blood flow and function. An intravenous pyelogram (IVP) involves the administration of contrast dye. Retrograde pyelograms (RPGs) are done with cystoscopy using radiopaque dye. The ureters are catheterized, and the surgeon can have direct vision and fluoroscopic views of the ureters and kidneys. (Schick L, Windle PE. *PeriAnesthesia Nursing Core Curriculum: Preprocedure, Phase I and Phase II Nursing.* 3rd ed. St. Louis, MO: Saunders; 2016:867-868.)

5-45. *Correct answer:* **a**

Acute renal failure arises from a decrease in glomerular filtration rate that results in a decrease in clearance of metabolites excreted by the kidney. An abnormally high creatinine level is the best serum indicator of renal failure. (Schick L, Windle PE. *PeriAnesthesia Nursing Core Curriculum: Preprocedure, Phase I and Phase II Nursing.* 3rd ed. St. Louis, MO: Saunders; 2016:854-855.)

5-46. *Correct answer:* **b**

Right shoulder pain is quite common following laparoscopic procedures due to the trapping of insufflation gases in the peritoneal cavity. This residual gas irritates the surfaces of the peritoneum and manifests as shoulder pain. It is not uncommon for this type of discomfort to persist for several days following a laparoscopic procedure. (Odom-Forren J. *Drain's Perianesthesia Nursing: A Critical Care Approach.* 6th ed. St. Louis, MO: Saunders; 2013:670.)

5-47. *Correct answer:* **a**

Bladder distension can contribute to postoperative hypertension, tachycardia, and restlessness. Emergence delirium may also be a cause of restlessness, but the stem of this question leads one to consider the length of surgery in terms of bladder requirements. (Schick L, Windle PE. *PeriAnesthesia Nursing Core Curriculum: Preprocedure, Phase I and Phase II Nursing.* 3rd ed. St. Louis, MO: Saunders; 2016:1241-1242.)

5-48. *Correct answer:* **d**

In order to decrease the risk of postoperative risk for deep vein thrombosis (DVT) patients should be taught to maintain adequate hydration, participate in physical activity as often as possible within the restrictions of surgery, and actively engage in rehabilitation and postoperative exercises. This is especially true for this patient with multiple risk factors for DVT. Generally risk factors include advanced age, pelvis, hip, femur, or tibia fractures; prolonged immobility, prior venous thromboembolic disease, surgery on the abdomen, pelvis, or lower extremities, obesity, heart failure, myocardial infarction (MI), and stroke. (Odom-Forren J. *Drain's Perianesthesia Nursing: A Critical Care Approach.* 6th ed. St. Louis, MO: Saunders; 2013:544.)

5-49. *Correct answer:* **c**

In caring for a patient after a posterior hip arthroplasty, position the lower extremity to reduce the risk of dislocation. Maintain the operative extremity in neutral alignment. Avoid hip adduction by placing a pillow or abduction device between the legs at all times. Turn the patient carefully to the unaffected side, maintaining abduction, if allowed. Avoid hip flexion greater than 90 degrees. Avoid raising the head of the bed and foot of the bed at the same time. Avoid extremes in hip rotation. Avoid internal rotation if a posterior approach was used. Avoid external rotation if an anterolateral approach was used. (Schick L, Windle PE. *PeriAnesthesia Nursing Core Curriculum: Preprocedure, Phase I and Phase II Nursing.* 3rd ed. St. Louis, MO: Saunders; 2016:1033.)

5-50. *Correct answer:* **c**

Foul-smelling urine indicates a urinary infection, which can lead to sepsis. The nephrostomy tube is placed to drain the upper urinary tract when obstructed. The obstruction can be acute or chronic from a variety of reasons, such as tumors, renal calculi, or gravid uterus. The placement of the nephrostomy tube is essential to preserve renal function and prevent urosepsis. (Schick L, Windle PE. *PeriAnesthesia Nursing Core Curriculum: Preprocedure, Phase I and Phase II Nursing.* 3rd ed. St. Louis, MO: Saunders; 2016:1208.)

5-51. *Correct answer:* **d**

Some of the early central nervous system signs and symptoms of local anesthetic toxicity are dizziness, tinnitus, drowsiness, and circumoral numbness. Confusion, dysphoria, and agitation can also occur. This can progress to seizures and coma. The most common regional anesthetic techniques that result in local anesthetic toxicity are epidural, axillary, and interscalene blocks. Most signs and symptoms of local anesthetic toxicity occur within 5 minutes, but up to 25% may occur later, from hours to days later. Numbness or tingling in fingertips is a symptom of hypocalcemia. (Odom-Forren J. *Drain's Perianesthesia Nursing: A Critical Care Approach.* 6th ed. St. Louis, MO: Saunders; 2013:322.)

5-52. *Correct answer:* **a**
Pregnancy is a state of compensated respiratory alkalosis. Chronic mild hyperventilation results in a lowered $PaCO_2$. The lowered $PaCO_2$ is critical to ensure CO_2 transfer at the placental level between the fetus and mother. (Schick L, Windle PE. *PeriAnesthesia Nursing Core Curriculum: Preprocedure, Phase I and Phase II Nursing*. 3rd ed. St. Louis, MO: Saunders; 2016:902.)

5-53. *Correct answer:* **d**
Signs and symptoms of allograft rejection include irritability, anxiousness, restlessness, lethargy, swollen and tender kidney, decreased urine output, fever that may be low grade, increased blood pressure, weight gain, and anorexia. (Odom-Forren J. *Drain's Perianesthesia Nursing: A Critical Care Approach*. 6th ed. St. Louis, MO: Saunders; 2013:603.)

5-54. *Correct answer:* **c**
With the distended abdomen, increased heart rate, and uncontrolled postoperative pain, the nurse should question hemorrhage. Although it is important to assess a patient for respiratory depression after doses of opioid analgesics such as fentanyl, this patient is not showing signs of respiratory depression. It is stated in the assessment that the nurse observed increased abdominal distention. The most common complication of any obstetric or gynecologic procedure is excessive hemorrhage and shock. The patient should be assessed frequently for circulatory status; this should include checking dressings for drainage. (Odom-Forren J. *Drain's Perianesthesia Nursing: A Critical Care Approach*. 6th ed. St. Louis, MO: Saunders; 2013:618.)

5-55. *Correct answer:* **b**
The area around the urethra can become edematous, causing a temporary stricture and bladder distension, especially after a vaginal hysterectomy. The urinary catheter is needed to keep from overdistending the bladder, causing temporary paralysis of the detrusor muscle. If this paralysis occurs, it can take several days to resolve. (Schick L, Windle PE. *PeriAnesthesia Nursing Core Curriculum: Preprocedure, Phase I and Phase II Nursing*. 3rd ed. St. Louis, MO: Saunders; 2016:951.)

5-56. *Correct answer:* **d**
After extracorporeal shock wave lithotripsy (ESWL), patients often are discharged home and must understand that high-volume fluid intake and straining urine are essential. ESWL directs multiple high-frequency shocks through the skin to pulverize renal calculi. The patient must excrete the stone fragments through the urine. Copious fluid intake is expected to promote an increase in urine output to flush the stone fragments out through the renal system. The patient should also be encouraged to maintain an active ambulatory status to facilitate stone passage. Pain is usually minimal after ESWL, although flank tenderness and slight skin redness can occur. (Schick L, Windle PE. *PeriAnesthesia Nursing Core Curriculum: Preprocedure, Phase I and Phase II PACU Nursing*. 3rd ed. St. Louis, MO: Saunders; 2016:871-872.)

5-57. *Correct answer:* **b**
An ice pack can be used to decrease swelling and comfort. If a compression dressing is used on the scrotum, it should be maintained but monitored for excessive swelling and cyanosis. The scrotum needs to be supported to decrease pain and edema. Continue to observe for increased edema and hemorrhage. (Schick L, Windle PE. *PeriAnesthesia Nursing Core Curriculum; Preprocedure, Phase I and Phase II PACU Nursing*. 3rd ed. St. Louis, MO: Saunders; 2016:884.)

5-58. *Correct answer:* **c**
Signs and symptoms of bladder distention include restlessness, hypertension, and tachycardia. (Schick L, Windle PE. *PeriAnesthesia Nursing Core Curriculum: Preprocedure, Phase I and Phase II PACU Nursing*. 3rd ed. St. Louis, MO: Saunders; 2016:1241-1242.)

5-59. *Correct answer:* **c**

The triad of HELLP syndrome is hemolysis, elevated liver enzymes, and low platelets. Hemolysis results from vasospasm, which causes endothelial damage, leading to platelet aggregation and fibrin network formation. Red blood cells (RBCs) are forced through the fibrin network at increased pressure, causing the hemolysis. Hematocrit is decreased; bilirubin and lactate dehydrogenase (LDH) levels are increased. Elevated liver enzymes occur when microemboli form in the hepatic vasculature, and hepatic blood flow decreases, resulting in ischemia. LDH is the first liver enzyme to elevate. Low platelets occur because of platelet consumption. Coagulopathies are associated with platelet counts less than 50,000. (Schick L, Windle PE. *PeriAnesthesia Nursing Core Curriculum: Preprocedure, Phase I and Phase II Nursing.* 3rd ed. St. Louis, MO: Saunders; 2016:912.)

5-60. *Correct answer:* **d**

The micturition reflex can be stimulated or inhibited by higher brain centers and is stimulated by increased pressure by irritation of the bladder or urethra. The stretch receptors in the bladder wall convey afferent impulses through the pelvic nerve to the spinal cord, which stimulates the sympathetic efferent nerves. These nerves convey impulses back to the bladder through the hypogastric nerves, which activate the internal sphincter to maintain continence and allow bladder filling. When the bladder is sufficiently distended, nerve impulses are then transmitted to the brain. (Schick L, Windle PE. *PeriAnesthesia Nursing Core Curriculum; Preprocedure, Phase I and Phase II PACU Nursing.* 3rd ed. St. Louis, MO: Saunders; 2016:844.)

5-61. *Correct answer:* **c**

Quality-of-life challenges are significant in patients with incontinence. Bladder neck suspensions in a variety of techniques are performed to correct urinary stress incontinence. These include the Raz sling, Stamey endoscopic suspension, tension-free vaginal tape (TVT), and modified Burch's procedure, to name a few. Postoperative complications for all techniques include urinary retention, wound infection, urinary tract infection, continued incontinence, retroperitoneal hemorrhage, and organ perforation. Culdoscopy is a diagnostic procedure allowing for endoscopic visualization of the pelvic structures. (Odom-Forren J. Drain's *PeriAnesthesia Nursing: A Critical Care Approach.* St. Louis, MO: Saunders; 2013:603-604; Schick L, Windle PE. *PeriAnesthesia Nursing Core Curriculum: Preprocedure, Phase I and Phase II, PACU Nursing.* 3rd ed. St. Louis, MO: Saunders; 2016:876.)

5-62. *Correct answer:* **a**

Hypovolemia, hypotension, and vasoconstriction can cause reduced renal perfusion, which is generally reversible upon correction of the underlying cause. Fluid resuscitation is required while taking care not to cause fluid overload. (Schick L, Windle PE. *PeriAnesthesia Nursing Core Curriculum: Preprocedure, Phase I and Phase II PACU Nursing.* St. Louis, MO: Saunders; 2016:105-106.)

5-63. *Correct answer:* **c**

A single injection of succinylcholine can cause fasciculation of muscles due to the initial rapid depolarization of the skeletal muscle. These contractions frequently cause myalgias, which may be apparent as early as Phase I PACU. (Odom-Forren J. *Drain's Perianesthesia Nursing: A Critical Care Approach.* 6th ed. St. Louis, MO: Saunders; 2013:300.)

5-64. *Correct answer:* **a**

The myalgia that can occur after succinylcholine administration is more common in patients who are ambulatory right after surgery. It may occur in 60% to 70% of ambulatory patients and decreases to 10% in those patients confined to bed. The pain usually does not require analgesics and subsides in 1 to 2 days. (Odom-Forren J. *Drain's Perianesthesia Nursing: A Critical Care Approach.* 6th ed. St. Louis, MO: Saunders; 2013:300.)

5-65. *Correct answer:* **b**

Neurovascular checks following any orthopedic procedures are essential to help with early detection of circulatory adverse events. Assessments should include the characteristics of pain, the color of the skin, mobility of the limb, temperature, pulse presence and quality, capillary filling times and edema. Cyanotic, or bluish color, suggests venous obstruction. (Odom-Forren J. *Drain's Perianesthesia Nursing: A Critical Care Approach.* 6th ed. St. Louis, MO: Saunders; 2013:542.)

6

Endocrine System, Fluids, and Electrolytes

Renee Smith, Marie A. Evans, and Theresa Clifford

6-1. A 62-year-old male patient has had a transurethral resection of the prostate. He arrives in the Phase I PACU with initial vital signs of BP 165/90, HR 58, RR 31, and SpO$_2$ 96%. Oxygen is placed on the patient, and the nurse receives the handover report. The patient received adequate fluid replacement in surgery and had minimal blood loss. The patient has continuous bladder irrigation at this time. On initial assessment of the patient, the nurse finds that he is complaining of feeling nauseated, short of breath, and restless. Based on the initial assessment, what would be the optimal nursing intervention for this patient?

a. Treat the patient for nausea with antiemetics

b. Adjust the oxygen and obtain an arterial blood gas

c. Notify the surgeon and obtain orders to draw serum sodium levels

d. Treat the patient for pain with analgesics

6-2. The perianesthesia nurse is providing discharge instructions for the patient who has just had a subtotal thyroidectomy. The nurse is aware that the patient could experience hypocalcemia and includes all of the following symptoms in the instructions EXCEPT:

a. Muscle cramps

b. Circumoral paresthesia

c. Numbness of feet

d. Excessive sleepiness

6-3. A 68-year-old male patient arrives in the Phase I PACU after a pancreaticoduodenectomy (Whipple procedure). There were multiple complications intraoperatively, and a pulmonary artery catheter was inserted. The nurse assesses the vital signs of the patient and reviews the first set of readings from the pulmonary artery catheter. The readings are as follows: central venous pressure (CVP) is 6, pulmonary artery pressure systolic/pulmonary artery pressure diastolic (PAS/PAD) is 16/10, pulmonary artery wedge pressure (PAWP) is 10. Vital signs are BP 107/64, HR 87, RR 19, and SpO$_2$ 98%. Reviewing the readings, the nurse recognizes that the patient is:

a. Hypervolemic

b. Normovolemic

c. Hypovolemic

d. Euvolemic

6-4. A 23-year-old male patient had spinal anesthesia for his bone marrow donation procedure. On arrival to the Phase I PACU, his vital signs are BP 80/60, HR 48, RR 20, T 96.8° F (36° C), and SpO$_2$ 97%. The nurse recognizes that the patient is experiencing:

a. Blood loss requiring immediate transfusion

b. A predictable effect of the spinal anesthesia

c. Cardiogenic shock

d. Septic shock

Consider this scenario for questions 6-5 and 6-6.

A 25-year-old male patient with type I diabetes arrives for surgery. In the preoperative interview he is complaining of nausea and thirst. His skin is warm and dry. He seems lethargic when the nurse is speaking to him. The nurse checks his glucose level with the bedside glucose meter and results are 642 mg/dL He also reports that he has been urinating every 30 minutes.

6-5. Based on the presenting symptoms, the nurse suspects that the patient has:

a. Urinary tract infection

b. Diabetic ketoacidosis

c. Hyperglycemic hyperosmolar syndrome

d. Diabetes insipidus

6-6. All of the following may have precipitated this disorder EXCEPT:

a. Presence of a soft tissue infection

b. Recent trauma

c. Doubling insulin dose

d. Normal surgical stress

6-7. A healthy 46-year-old patient arrives in the Phase I PACU after a total parathyroidectomy and will be staying in the Phase I PACU overnight. Twenty-four hours later as the nurse assists the patient with ambulation to the bathroom, he stumbles and apologizes, saying that he has numbness in his toes and has been experiencing muscle spasms. He also reports a tingling sensation around his mouth. What is the MOST likely complication that the nurse is concerned about at this time?

a. Hypokalemia

b. Hyponatremia

c. Hypocalcemia

d. Hypomagnesemia

6-8. The nurse caring for a patient with Addison's disease is aware that perioperative steroid administration can increase the risk of:

a. Hypotension

b. Stress ulcers

c. Improved wound healing

d. Increased glucose tolerance

6-9. Pheochromocytoma is a benign tumor of the adrenal medulla with release of catecholamine. Symptoms include all of the following EXCEPT:

a. Hyperglycemia

b. Severe hypertension

c. Hypermetabolism

d. Decreased epinephrine

6-10. Which of the following patients all undergoing the same procedure is most at risk for dehydration postoperatively?

a. 18-year-old male

b. 24-year-old female

c. 73-year-old male

d. 73-year-old female

6-11. The patient arrives in the Phase I PACU after a liver biopsy to rule out malignancy. His vital signs on admission are BP 96/67, HR 126, RR 27, and SpO_2 96%. The nurse places the patient on nasal cannula at 4 L/min oxygen and medicates the patient for abdominal pain with intravenous opioids. He states his pain level is 6 (numerical rating scale 0–10). After 15 minutes the patient's vital signs are BP 90/68, HR 130, RR 27, and SpO_2 95%. The patient reports a pain level of 8/10. Preoperatively the patient's vital signs were BP 134/72, HR 90, RR 18, and SpO_2 98% on room air. What would be the MOST likely course of action for the nurse to consider first?

a. Offer a combination of analgesic medications

b. Obtain ordered laboratory blood samples and anticipate physician orders for a fluid bolus

c. Obtain ordered laboratory blood samples and anticipate physician orders for a transfusion

d. Notify the physician that the patient needs different analgesic medications

6-12. The perianesthesia nurse is caring for a patient after partial thyroidectomy. While assessing the patient for potential nerve damage, the nurse will ask the patient to say:

a. "a"

b. "e"

c. "i"

d. "o"

6-13. A 37-year-old female patient arrives in the Phase I PACU after cardiac arrest in the operating room. During the arrest, it was noted that the patient was having peaked T waves and widening QRS complexes on the cardiac monitor. When reviewing potential electrolyte causes of cardiac arrest, what electrolytes would the nurse consider FIRST to be a potential cause of the arrest?

a. Calcium

b. Magnesium

c. Potassium

d. Chloride

6-14. A 53-year-old male patient has suffered a cardiac arrest, and during the code his rhythm shows that he has torsades de pointes. What is the medication of choice for terminating this rhythm?

a. Amiodarone 600 mg IV push

b. Adenosine 12 mg IV push

c. Magnesium sulfate 1-2 g IV push

d. Procainamide 250 mg IV push

6-15. The perianesthesia nurse caring for a hyperthyroidism patient with exophthalmos recognizes that in the perioperative period, the patient may be at increased risk for:

a. Dacryostenosis

b. Corneal abrasions

c. Inability to open eyelids

d. Blepharitis

6-16. A patient was diagnosed with intestinal ileus after 2 days of vomiting. In the emergency department, the patient had a nasogastric (NG) tube placed and attached to suction. The patient arrives in the Phase I PACU after colon resection and the NG tube is reattached to wall suction. As a result of this the nurse recognizes that the patient is at risk for which acid–base imbalance?

a. Metabolic acidosis

b. Metabolic alkalosis

c. Respiratory acidosis

d. Respiratory alkalosis

6-17. Thyrotoxic crisis (thyroid storm) can mimic malignant hyperthermia. Which of the following symptoms can help differentiate that the patient is experiencing thyrotoxic crisis?

a. Rapid development of hyperthermia

b. Obvious onset of tachycardia

c. Discernable hypercarbia

d. Lack of muscle rigidity

Consider this scenario for questions 6-18 and 6-19.

A patient comes to the Phase I PACU after a transsphenoidal resection of a pituitary tumor. It is reported there were no complications during surgery, vital signs were stable, 1500 mL of IV fluid were infused, urine output was 200 mL, and there was minimal blood loss.

6-18. The patient has been in the PACU for 1 hour and the nurse empties the catheter drainage bag of 2000 mL of light yellow urine. The patient is slightly tachycardic and hypotensive. IV fluids for the hour were 100 mL. The patient did not receive any diuretic medications intraoperatively or in the PACU. The nurse suspects that the patient may be exhibiting symptoms of:

a. Diabetes mellitus

b. Syndrome of inappropriate antidiuretic hormone

c. Diabetes insipidus

d. Cushing syndrome

6-19. The nurse anticipates that the patient will be treated with:

a. Adrenocorticotropin hormone (ACTH)

b. Antidiuretic hormone (ADH)

c. Thyroid-stimulating hormone (TSH)

d. Luteinizing hormone (LH)

6-20. A 57-year-old male patient underwent a transurethral resection of the prostate (TURP) and is experiencing symptoms of TURP syndrome. The patient's serum sodium level is 118 mEq/L. Due to the decreased sodium level, the nurse would anticipate an order for what fluid?

    a. Dextrose 5% with 0.45% normal saline

    b. 3% normal saline

    c. 0.9% normal saline

    d. Lactated Ringer's

6-21. What is the dosage of sodium bicarbonate for a child in arrest who has severe metabolic acidosis or hyperkalemia?

    a. 1 mEq/kg IV/IO

    b. 1.5 mEq/kg IV/IO

    c. 2 mEq/kg IV/IO

    d. 2.5 mEq/kg IV/IO

6-22. A child with poor skin turgor, sunken fontanel, marked oliguria, and tachycardia may be exhibiting the signs of what physiologic state?

    a. Dehydration

    b. Hypervolemia

    c. Normovolemia

    d. Euvolemia

6-23. A 43-year-old patient with von Willebrand disease has undergone colon resection for removal of a tumor. The patient experienced a large blood loss, and transfusion would be optimal to support the patient's fluid status; however, the patient is a devout Jehovah's Witness who will not allow blood transfusion. Which of the following colloids would be the MOST likely to be acceptable to this patient?

    a. Platelets

    b. Fresh frozen plasma

    c. Hydroxyethyl starch

    d. Autologous whole blood

6-24. The preadmission nurse is listening to the anesthesiologist explain to a hypothyroid patient that a fiber-optic scope will be used to facilitate intubation. The nurse recognizes that the patient with hypothyroidism is at risk for a difficult intubation due to:

    a. Decreased thyromental distance

    b. Muscular atrophy

    c. Enlarged tongue

    d. Lymphadenopathy

6-25. A 32-year-old female patient with Addison's disease arrives in the Phase I PACU after repair of the right tibia–fibula fracture. What electrolytes would the nurse look for that might indicate the patient was experiencing an Addisonian crisis?

    a. Increased sodium, increased potassium

    b. Increased sodium, decreased potassium

    c. Decreased sodium, decreased potassium

    d. Decreased sodium, increased potassium

6-26. What is the amount of an initial fluid bolus to be given to a child who is suspected of being in cardiogenic shock?

    a. 5 to 10 mL/kg

    b. 10 to 15 mL/kg

    c. 10 to 20 mL/kg

    d. 15 to 20 mL/kg

6-27. A patient is in cardiac arrest after surgery for an adrenal tumor. Capnography is in use, and the nurse recognizes return of spontaneous circulation with an end tidal carbon dioxide level of:

    a. 8 mm Hg

    b. 16 mm Hg

    c. 25 mm Hg

    d. 35 mm Hg

6-28. Which of the following patients has the highest risk for dehydration or fluid overload postoperatively?

    a. 35-year-old female

    b. 25-year-old male

    c. 15-year-old male

    d. 8-month-old female

6-29. A patient arrives in the Phase I PACU after a craniotomy, and mannitol is ordered to be administered. The nurse caring for the patient recognizes that the mannitol will affect intracranial pressure (ICP) by acting as:

a. A loop diuretic to decrease it

b. An osmotic diuretic to decrease it

c. A thiazide diuretic to decrease it

d. An osmotic diuretic to increase it

6-30. Postoperative nausea and vomiting is MOST likely to significantly affect which patient?

a. 18-year-old female patient having an open appendectomy

b. 45-year-old male patient having a total knee replacement

c. 73-year-old female patient having a laparoscopic hysterectomy

d. 8-year-old female patient having a tonsillectomy and adenoidectomy

6-31. After surgery for total thyroidectomy, the nurse is alert for signs of hypocalcemia that include all of the following EXCEPT:

a. Positive Chvostek sign

b. Laryngeal spasm

c. Tingling in the mouth

d. Positive Horner sign

6-32. The perianesthesia nurse is aware that in the perioperative period the most common cause of morbidity in a patient with diabetes is:

a. Surgical site infection

b. Ischemic heart disease

c. Coagulopathy

d. Respiratory insufficiency

6-33. A patient is scheduled for surgery to repair a fractured radius and ulna after a fall at home. During the preadmission interview the patient describes symptoms of increased thirst, decreased urine output, nausea, and headache. The nurse checks for edema of the lower extremities and finds none. A review of the preprocedure laboratory values shows hyponatremia. The nurse suspects that the patient may have:

a. Syndrome of inappropriate antidiuretic hormone (SIADH)

b. Diabetes insipidus (DI)

c. Acute renal failure (ARF)

d. Early congestive heart failure (CHF)

6-34. What is the impact of anesthetic agents on extracellular fluid (ECF)?

a. Decreases ECF capacity

b. Has no impact on ECF capacity

c. Increases ECF capacity

d. Reduces ECF capacity

6-35. The perianesthesia nurse caring for a patient with Cushing syndrome recognizes that the corticosteroid hypersecretion by the adrenal glands can cause:

a. Poor wound healing

b. Hypoglycemia

c. Osteoneogenesis

d. Hypercoagulopathy

6-36. A 46-year-old patient arrives in the pre-anesthesia holding area before his scheduled procedure for removal of renal calculi. The preanesthesia nurse reviews the patient's history, which includes congenital central diabetes insipidus. For treatment, the patient's medications would include:

a. Insulin glargine

b. Desmopressin

c. Paroxetine

d. Hydrochlorothiazide

6-37. A 27-year-old patient with diabetes and asthma arrives in the Phase I PACU after a total knee replacement. His surgery was delayed until late in the day. He arrives with stable vital signs, but he is drowsy, vomiting and complaining of abdominal pain, polyuria, and polydipsia. As the nurse, what would be the **first** priority for this patient?

 a. Treat the patient for the vomiting with antiemetic medication

 b. Administer analgesic medication

 c. Obtain a blood glucose measurement and laboratory work

 d. Anticipate a glucose bolus order

6-38. The nurse caring for the patient with Graves disease knows that it is most commonly a result of:

 a. Hyperaldosteronism

 b. Hyperthyroidism

 c. Hyperparathyroidism

 d. Hypersplenism

6-39. The nurse is reviewing the home medication list of a patient with diabetes. Which of the following medications may contribute to hypoglycemia?

 a. Phenytoin sodium, extended release capsules

 b. Thiazide diuretics

 c. Angiotensin-converting enzyme (ACE) inhibitors

 d. Calcium channel blockers

6-40. When the nurse in the preoperative area is preparing the patient with chronic renal failure for surgery, which set of laboratory blood work is most likely ordered other than a blood urea nitrogen (BUN) and creatinine?

 a. Magnesium and calcium

 b. Calcium and potassium

 c. Potassium and magnesium

 d. Magnesium, calcium, and potassium

6-41. Patients with diabetes who are scheduled for interventional radiology procedures with contrast should be instructed to hold which medication?

 a. Insulin

 b. Steroid inhaler

 c. Metformin

 d. Omeprazole

6-42. A patient's arterial blood gas (ABG) results are the following: pH 7.38, $PaCO_2$ 40, HCO_3 24, and PaO_2 95%. What does the nurse interpret these results to be?

 a. Respiratory alkalosis

 b. Normal ABG

 c. Respiratory acidosis

 d. Metabolic acidosis

6-43. The perianesthesia nurse is caring for a patient with diabetes in the preoperative area. The nurse recognizes that surgical stress may precipitate all of the following in this patient EXCEPT:

 a. Decreased peripheral insulin resistance

 b. Increased glucose production

 c. Impaired insulin secretion

 d. Breakdown of protein and fat

6-44. What is the dosage of magnesium to be given to a child younger than 8 years old whose electrocardiogram rhythm is identified as torsades de pointes?

 a. 5 to 10 mg/kg IV/IO

 b. 15 to 20 mg/kg IV/IO

 c. 25 to 50 mg/kg IV/IO

 d. 55 to 70 mg/kg IV/IO

6-45. The nurse has received orders to give potassium supplements to her patient who has a low potassium level. Which order would the nurse want to clarify?

a. Give 10 mEq potassium chloride intravenous over 1 hr via peripheral IV

b. Give 10 mEq potassium chloride intravenous over 1 hr via central line

c. Give 20 mEq potassium chloride intravenous over 1 hr via central line

d. Give 20 mEq potassium chloride intravenous push via central line

6-46. A 58-year-old male patient presented to the emergency department with increasing abdominal distention and nausea and vomiting for the past week. He arrived in the preoperative bay with an indwelling urinary catheter, a nasogastric tube to suction, and continuing abdominal pain controlled with intermittent opioid analgesics. The patient is attached to the physiologic monitors, and his vital signs are BP 90/46, HR 50, and RR 22. On the ECG monitor the nurse notes the QRS interval is .24 seconds and the patient is experiencing frequent premature ventricular contractions (PVCs). What electrolyte imbalance might the nurse suspect that the patient is experiencing?

a. Low calcium level

b. Low magnesium level

c. Low potassium level

d. Low phosphorous level

6-47. The perianesthesia nurse caring for the patient with hypothyroidism recognizes that the patient is predisposed to all the following EXCEPT:

a. Hyperthermia

b. Cardiac failure

c. Delayed gastric emptying

d. Delayed medication metabolism

6-48. A patient who just had surgery to remove one lobe of the thyroid gland comes to the Phase I PACU restless and thrashing. The perianesthesia nurse is assessing the surgical dressing and drain. There is no drainage in the drain, and the dressing is dry and intact. A short time later the patient is again restless, and the nurse observes that the drain has a large amount of bloody drainage and the dressing now shows bloody drainage. After calling anesthesia and the surgeon, the most important nursing task is to:

a. Control the bleeding

b. Administer sedation

c. Maintain airway patency

d. Increase IV fluids

6-49. A pregnant woman arrives in the preoperative area for the nurse to ready her for a caesarean section. The patient has been diagnosed with pregnancy-induced hypertension and is being treated with a magnesium infusion at this time. What symptoms would the nurse assess for if she was concerned that the patient was experiencing hypermagnesemia?

a. Decreased reflexes, decreased blood pressure, decreased heart rate

b. Normal reflexes, normal blood pressure, increased heart rate

c. Increased reflexes, decreased blood pressure, decreased heart rate

d. Decreased reflexes, increased blood pressure, increased heart rate

6-50. A pregnant patient comes to the Phase I PACU after an appendectomy. She is on a magnesium infusion for preeclampsia symptoms. Vital signs are currently stable. Anticipating the potential for magnesium sulfate toxicity, what preferred medication should the nurse be prepared to administer?

a. Calcium chloride

b. Calcium gluconate

c. Calcium carbonate

d. Calcium bicarbonate

6-51. The perianesthesia nurse is caring for an elderly patient with hyperparathyroidism. The nurse recognizes that the patient is at risk for which of the following?

a. Hypotension

b. Insomnia

c. Osteoporosis

d. Diarrhea

6-52. The perianesthesia nurse caring for a patient scheduled for a transsphenoidal hypophysectomy recognizes that this approach for surgery has which of the following benefits?

a. Decreased blood loss

b. Decreased incidence of cerebrospinal fluid (CSF) leak

c. Decreased chance of diabetes insipidus (DI)

d. Decreased chance of syndrome of inappropriate antidiuretic hormone secretion (SIADH)

6-53. A patient with syndrome of inappropriate antidiuretic hormone secretion (SIADH) is at risk for reparalysis after the administration of muscle relaxants due to:

a. Hyperkalemia

b. Hypercalcemia

c. Hypochloremia

d. Hyponatremia

6-54. The perianesthesia nurse is caring for a patient who is suspected to be in diabetic ketoacidosis. The nurse sees a prominent U wave on the patient's electrocardiogram (ECG). What laboratory value will the nurse need to check before instituting an insulin drip?

a. Calcium

b. Potassium

c. Sodium

d. Magnesium

6-55. A patient arrives in the Phase I PACU after a total abdominal hysterectomy. Her vital signs are BP 100/60, HR 130, RR 15, T 36.4° C, and SpO_2 97%. The patient reports a pain level of 5/10 on a numerical rating scale of 0 to 10. Intraoperatively the patient had a blood loss of 200 mL and was given 400 mL of crystalloids. The patient's vital signs preoperatively were BP 132/64, HR 85, RR 16, and SpO_2 98% on room air. The nurse has medicated the patient for pain, and the pain is now reported to be 2/10. There is no significant change on the patient's vital signs. What would be the MOST likely cause of the increased HR of the patient?

a. The patient is continuing to experience pain and needs more pain relief

b. The patient is hypovolemic

c. The patient is septic

d. The patient is continuing to respond to surgical stimulation

6-56. The nurse caring for a patient with Addison's disease anticipates giving preoperative medications to include:

a. Insulin

b. Vasopressin

c. Corticosteroid

d. Epinephrine

6-57. A 49-year-old male patient has had a carotid stent placed. He arrives in the Phase I PACU with a BP 84/64, HR 52, RR 23, and SpO_2 97%. Preoperatively he had vital signs of BP 167/76, HR 78, RR 20, and SpO_2 98%. He had blood loss of 100 mL and intravenous fluid replacement of 100 mL. He has a history of diabetes and a total hip replacement. He denies any complaints. What initial intervention may the nurse anticipate that the physician may order?

a. Blood transfusion

b. Atropine

c. Fluid bolus

d. Continue to observe the patient

6-58. According to the American Diabetic Association's SUGAR-NICE study, the goal for glucose levels of medical-surgical patients should be less than:

a. 100 mg/dL

b. 130 mg/dL

c. 150 mg/dL

d. 180 mg/dL

6-59. The Phase I PACU nurse is caring for a patient after a transsphenoidal hypophysectomy. The nurse observes the patient swallowing and wiping his nose frequently and recognizes that the patient may be experiencing:

a. Pruritus from opioids

b. Oral dryness from NPO status

c. Cerebrospinal fluid (CSF) leak

d. Medication reaction

6-60. A 64-year-old male patient arrives in the Phase I PACU after a right lung lobectomy. His estimated blood loss (EBL) is 80 mL, and intravenous fluids of 800 mL were given intraoperatively. His vital signs are BP 134/68, HR 71, RR 28, and SpO_2 92%. The patient is placed on nasal cannula at 4 L/min of oxygen, and SpO_2 is now 93%. On auscultation of lung fields the nurse hears crackles or rales. What is the first course of action for the nurse?

a. Continue to observe the patient

b. Call the physician in anticipation of diuretic orders

c. Obtain arterial blood gases (ABGs) and report the results

d. Initiate endotracheal suctioning

6-61. A 56-year-old male patient arrives in day surgery for a laparoscopic-assisted hernia repair. His vital signs on arrival are BP 168/98, HR 68 and irregular, RR 18, T 36.8° C via temporal artery thermometer, and room air SpO_2 92%. He has a history of intermittent atrial fibrillation, essential hypertension, pseudocholinesterase deficiency, and morbid obesity (body mass index [BMI] 42). Which

of the following conditions will increase his risk for pulmonary aspiration?

a. Atrial fibrillation

b. Hypertension

c. Pseudocholinesterase deficiency

d. Morbid obesity

6-62. The perianesthesia nurse is reviewing the home medications for a patient with diabetes having a hernia repair. The nurse recognizes that duloxetine may be used to treat the patient's:

a. Gastroparesis

b. Hyperglycemia

c. Diabetic neuropathy

d. Stress incontinence

6-63. The nurse transferring care after surgery knows that "handoff" communication has been shown to do all of the following EXCEPT:

a. Reduce the rate of errors

b. Reduce omission of information

c. Increase redundancy

d. Increase effectiveness of communication

6-64. Shivering in a postoperative patient puts the patient at risk for hypoxemia and which of the following?

a. Metabolic acidosis

b. Metabolic alkalosis

c. Respiratory acidosis

d. Respiratory alkalosis

6-65. Lactated Ringer's (LR) is BEST described as:

a. An isotonic colloid with the electrolyte composition of blood serum

b. A hypertonic crystalloid with the electrolyte composition of blood serum

c. A hypotonic colloid with the electrolyte composition of blood serum

d. An isotonic crystalloid with the electrolyte composition of blood serum

Answers and Rationales for Chapter 6, Endocrine System, Fluids, and Electrolytes

6-1. *Correct answer:* **c**
The patient may be experiencing transurethral resection of the prostrate (TURP) syndrome (or dilutional hyponatremia) due to irrigation that is absorbed into the vascular system during surgery. This absorption leads to hyponatremia, or decreased serum sodium, as a result of excessive fluids. Blood samples for laboratory testing should be obtained to check for low sodium serum levels and treated accordingly. (Odom-Forren J. *Drain's Perianesthesia Nursing: A Critical Care Approach.* 6th ed. St. Louis, MO: Saunders; 2013:411.)

6-2. *Correct answer:* **d**
The patient experiencing a state of hypocalcemia will exhibit nervousness in addition to muscle cramps, circumoral paresthesia (as well as paresthesias of the fingers and toes), and tingling and numbness of the feet. Other symptoms include abnormal facial muscle spasms when the facial nerve is tapped (Chvostek's sign) and carpal tunnel spasms (Trousseau's sign) due to ischemia. (Schick L, Windle PE. *PeriAnesthesia Nursing Core Curriculum: Preprocedure, Phase I and Phase II PACU Nursing.* 3rd ed. St. Louis, MO: Saunders; 2016:308t.)

6-3. *Correct answer:* **b**
The readings are normal for the patient. Normal readings are central venous pressure (CVP) 0 to 8 mm Hg, right ventricular systolic/diastolic (RVS/RVD) 15 to 25/0 to 8 mm Hg, pulmonary artery systolic/diastolic (PAS/PAD) 15 to 25/8 to 12 mm Hg, and pulmonary artery wedge pressure (PAWP) 6 to 12 mm Hg. (Odom-Forren J. *Drain's Perianesthesia Nursing: A Critical Care Approach.* 6th ed. St. Louis, MO: Saunders; 2013:368-373.)

6-4. *Correct answer:* **b**
Spinal anesthesia causes dilation of peripheral vasculature and blocks sympathetic tone, which expands the extracellular fluid (ECF). Fluid volume expansion and vasopressor administration will be needed until the impact of the anesthesia abates. (Odom-Forren J. *Drain's Perianesthesia Nursing: A Critical Care Approach.* 6th ed. St Louis, MO: Saunders; 2013:330.)

6-5. *Correct answer:* **b**
Patients with diabetic ketoacidosis exhibit symptoms of polydipsia, polyuria, polyphagia, warm dry skin, decreased level of consciousness, hypotension, tachycardia, ECG changes, nausea and vomiting, Kussmaul respirations (late sign), and fruity breath odor. (Schick L, Windle PE. *PeriAnesthesia Nursing Core Curriculum: Preprocedure, Phase I and Phase II PACU Nursing.* 3rd ed. St. Louis, MO: Saunders; 2016:735.)

6-6. *Correct answer:* **c**
Probable causes of diabetic ketoacidosis include infection, poor diabetes control, surgical stress, medication interference with medication metabolism, and trauma. A missed insulin dose (as opposed to an extra dose or too much insulin) is a possible cause of diabetic ketoacidosis. (Schick L, Windle PE. *PeriAnesthesia Nursing Core Curriculum: Preprocedure, Phase I and Phase II PACU Nursing.* 3rd ed. St. Louis, MO: Saunders; 2016:735.)

6-7. *Correct answer:* **c**
A low calcium level can be a result of the removal of the parathyroid. Symptoms of low calcium include circumoral numbness and tingling, numbness and tingling of the digits, muscle cramps, and spasms. A normal calcium level for a man is 9 to 10.3 mg/dL and for a woman is 8.9 to 10.2 mg/dL. (Odom-Forren J. *Drain's Perianesthesia Nursing: A Critical Care Approach.* 6th ed. St. Louis, MO: Saunders; 2013:210.)

6-8. *Correct answer:* **b**
The perioperative steroids may cause decreased wound healing, increase infection, increase glucose intolerance, increase blood pressure, and increase stress ulcers in patients with Addison's disease. (Schick L, Windle PE. *PeriAnesthesia Nursing Core Curriculum: Preprocedure, Phase I and Phase II PACU Nursing.* 3rd ed. St. Louis, MO: Saunders; 2016:114.)

6-9. *Correct answer:* **d**
Patients with pheochromocytoma will exhibit elevated levels of epinephrine and norepinephrine resulting in symptoms of sympathetic nervous system hyperactivity. (Schick L, Windle PE. *PeriAnesthesia Nursing Core Curriculum: Preprocedure, Phase I and Phase II PACU Nursing.* 3rd ed. St. Louis, MO: Saunders; 2016:730t-731t.)

6-10. *Correct answer:* **d**
Females have a higher fat content in their body than men. Due to the fact that there is minimal water in fat, women tend to have lower water concentrations. In addition, older adults are also known to have a lower proportion of water in their body, putting them more at risk for dehydration postop. (Odom-Forren J. *Drain's Perianesthesia Nursing: A Critical Care Approach.* 6th ed. St. Louis, MO: Saunders; 2013:194-195.)

6-11. *Correct answer:* **c**
A potential complication of liver biopsies is internal bleeding. Increasing abdominal pain and signs of hypovolemia may be indications of internal bleeding and impending shock. (American Society of PeriAnesthesia Nurses. *2015-2017 Perianesthesia Nursing Standards, Practice Recommendations and Interpretive Statements.* Cherry Hill, NJ: ASPAN; 2014:144.)

6-12. *Correct answer:* **b**
The nurse asks the patient to phonate the letter "e" to assess for nerve damage that may have occurred with retraction and stretching of the recurrent laryngeal nerve. (Schick L, Windle PE. *PeriAnesthesia Nursing Core Curriculum: Preprocedure, Phase I and Phase II PACU Nursing.* 3rd ed. St. Louis, MO: Saunders; 2016:798.)

6-13. *Correct answer:* **c**
Hyperkalemia, a serum level greater than 5 mEq/L, can precipitate cardiac arrhythmias and be represented on an electrocardiogram strip by peaked T waves and a widening QRS complex. (American Heart Association. *Advanced Cardiovascular Life Support. Provider Manual.* Dallas, TX: American Heart Association; 2016:73.)

6-14. *Correct answer:* **c**
One to two grams of magnesium sulfate is given as the initial treatment in the case of cardiac arrest due to torsades de pointes. Amiodarone is initially given as a 300 mg dose, following by 150 mg for ventricular tachycardia. Adenosine is NOT indicated for ventricular arrhythmias but for narrow-complex tachycardia. Procainamide, if used, should be considered for refractory ventricular fibrillation (VF) and in doses of 20 mg/min or 100 mg boluses up to 17 mg/kg. (American Heart Association. *Advanced Cardiovascular Life Support Provider Manual.* Dallas, TX: American Heart Association; 2016:167.)

6-15. *Correct answer:* **b**
Due to the dryness of the eyes and the inability to close the lids completely, the patient with exophthalmos is at risk for corneal abrasions. (Schick L, Windle PE. *PeriAnesthesia Nursing Core Curriculum: Preprocedure, Phase I and Phase II PACU Nursing.* 3rd ed. St. Louis, MO: Saunders; 2016:720-721.)

6-16. *Correct answer:* **b**

Metabolic alkalosis results from the loss of gastric acids or an increase in bases. In this case, the loss of gastric contents due to the presence of the nasogastric (NG) tube results in a lack of acids in the stomach. (Odom-Forren J. *Drain's Perianesthesia Nursing: A Critical Care Approach.* 6th ed. St. Louis, MO: Saunders; 2013:171.)

6-17. *Correct answer:* **d**

Both disorders exhibit hyperthermia tachycardia and hypercarbia, but malignant hyperthermia exhibits muscle rigidity, whereas thyrotoxic crisis does not. (Schick L, Windle PE. *PeriAnesthesia Nursing Core Curriculum: Preprocedure, Phase I and Phase II PACU Nursing.* 3rd ed. St. Louis, MO: Saunders; 2016:722; Odom-Forren J. *Drain's Perianesthesia Nursing: A Critical Care Approach.* 6th ed. St. Louis, MO: Saunders; 2013:580.)

6-18. *Correct answer:* **c**

Diabetes insipidus (DI) is caused by a hyposecretion of antidiuretic hormone (vasopressin). Signs of DI include dilute, sugar-free, unconcentrated urine, dehydration, and complaints of thirst. This can be due to head trauma, tumors, or surgery. (Schick L, Windle PE. *PeriAnesthesia Nursing Core Curriculum: Preprocedure, Phase I and Phase II PACU Nursing.* 3rd ed. St. Louis, MO: Saunders; 2016:726, 728.)

6-19. *Correct answer:* **b**

ADH (antidiuretic hormone), or vasopressin, will be used to treat the patient with diabetes insipidus (DI). Although there may be a decrease in adrenocorticotropin (ACTH) as well, ADH is the first treatment. (Schick L, Windle PE. *PeriAnesthesia Nursing Core Curriculum: Preprocedure, Phase I and Phase II PACU Nursing.* 3rd ed. St. Louis, MO: Saunders; 2016:726, 728.)

6-20. *Correct answer:* **b**

The patient has dilutional hyponatremia, and for serum sodium less than 120 mEq/L, 3% or 5% saline solution is generally ordered. (Odom-Forren J. *Drain's Perianesthesia*

Nursing: A Critical Care Approach. 6th ed. St. Louis, MO: Saunders; 2013:411.)

6-21. *Correct answer:* **a**

While routine use of sodium bicarbonate during cardiac arrest is not recommended, it can be used in the event of hyperkalemia and overdoses of either tricyclic antidepressants or other sodium channel blocking agents. The usual dose is 1 mEq/kg IV/IO given as a slow bolus. (Chameides L, Samson R, Schexnayder S, Hazinski MF. American Heart Association Pediatric *Advanced Life Support Provider Manual. Dallas, TX: Amercian Heart Association;* 2011:230.)

6-22. *Correct answer:* **a**

All of these are symptoms of moderate dehydration in an infant. More serious symptoms include significant tachycardia, weak or absent distal pulses, tachypnea, hypotension, and decreasing levels of consciousness. (Chameides L, Samson R, Schexnayder S, Hazinski MF. *American Heart Association Pediatric Advanced Life Support Provider Manual.* Dallas, TX: Amercian Heart Association; 2011:96-97.)

6-23. *Correct answer:* **c**

Hydroxyethel starch (also known as hetastarch) is a colloid that Jehovah's Witness practitioners often allow. Most Jehovah's Witnesses refuse transfusions of whole blood (including autologous donations), believing that once blood has left the body it must be left alone. Some Witnesses will accept transfusions of primary blood components such as albumin, cryoprecipitates, clotting factors, and immunoglobulins. (Schick L, Windle PE. *PeriAnesthesia Nursing Core Curriculum: Preprocedure, Phase I and Phase II PACU Nursing.* 3rd ed. St. Louis, MO: Saunders; 2016:320t.)

6-24. *Correct answer:* **c**
The patient with hypothyroidism has an enlarged tongue that may make intubation potentially more difficult. In addition, patients with hypothyroidism tend to have slower metabolism of medications, some airway incompetence due to neurological weakness, and overall decreased metabolic states. (Schick L, Windle PE. *PeriAnesthesia Nursing Core Curriculum: Preprocedure, Phase I and Phase II PACU Nursing.* 3rd ed. St. Louis, MO: Saunders; 2016:721.)

6-25. *Correct answer:* **d**
Addison's disease is a state of adrenocortical insufficiency requiring steroid therapy. Addisonian crisis is marked by muscle weakness, fever, dehydration, nausea, vomiting, and hypotension followed by hyponatremia and hyperkalemia. (Odom-Forren J. *Drain's Perianesthesia Nursing: A Critical Care Approach.* 6th ed. St. Louis, MO: Saunders; 2013:212.)

6-26. *Correct answer:* **a**
Many children in cardiogenic shock do not require fluid therapy; however, a child suspected to be in cardiogenic shock is best treated with a conservative fluid bolus of 5 to 10 mL/kg over 10 to 20 min to avoid fluid overload. (Chameides L, Samson R, Schexnayder S, Hazinski MF. *American Heart Association Pediatric Advanced Life Support Provider Manual.* Dallas, TX: Amercian Heart Association; 2011:104-105.)

6-27. *Correct answer:* **d**
With a return of spontaneous circulation, the capnography reading abruptly rises to 35 to 45 mm Hg. The effectiveness of chest compressions can also be evaluated with the use of capnography during cardiopulmonary resuscitation. (Lough ME. *Hemodynamic Monitoring: Evolving Technologies and Clinical Practice.* St. Louis, MO: Elsevier-Mosby; 2016:250; Odom-Forren J. *Drain's Perianesthesia Nursing: A Critical Care Approach.* 6th ed. St. Louis, MO: Saunders; 2013:358-361.)

6-28. *Correct answer:* **d**
The 8-month-old child has a higher percentage of body water to body surface area (BSA), placing her at the greatest risk for dehydration or fluid overload. Renal function is not considered mature until 2 to 3 years of age. (Odom-Forren J. *Drain's Perianesthesia Nursing: A Critical Care Approach.* 6th ed. St. Louis, MO: Saunders; 2013:692-694.)

6-29. *Correct answer:* **b**
The mannitol acts as an osmotic diuretic to pull fluid into the bloodstream from the brain cells and decrease intracranial pressure (ICP). (Odom-Forren J. *Drain's Perianesthesia Nursing: A Critical Care Approach.* 6th ed. St. Louis, MO: Saunders; 2013:563.)

6-30. *Correct answer:* **c**
Patients more at risk for postoperative nausea and vomiting are infants, children, and the elderly, as well as persons with a previous history of nausea and vomiting after surgery and laparoscopic, strabismus correction, and ear procedures. Other risk factors include length of surgery, nonsmoking, postoperative opioid use, and female gender. (Odom-Forren J. *Drain's Perianesthesia Nursing: A Critical Care Approach.* 6th ed. St. Louis, MO: Saunders: 2013: 404; Schick L, Windle PE. *PeriAnesthesia Nursing Core Curriculum: Preprocedure, Phase I and Phase II, PACU Nursing.* 3rd ed. St. Louis, MO.: Saunders; 2016: 424-426.)

6-31. *Correct answer:* **d**
The signs of hypocalcemia are a result of removal of the parathyroid glands along with the thyroid. The signs of hypocalcemia (e.g., tingling, weakness, twitching, hypotension) are usually manifested later in the recovery period, but the nurse should observe for these signs and communicate these symptoms to the nurse on the inpatient unit. Horner's syndrome is evidenced by a drooping eyelid, pupillary constriction, anhidrosis, ipsilateral nasal congestion, skin flushing, and ipsilateral temperature increases. (Schick L, Windle PE. *PeriAnesthesia Nursing Core Curriculum: Preprocedure, Phase I and Phase II PACU Nursing.* 3rd ed. St. Louis, MO: Saunders; 2016:355, 722, 725.)

6-32. *Correct answer:* **b**

Patients with diabetes are at risk for macroangiopathy disorders affecting blood vessels throughout the body (e.g., coronary artery disease, peripheral vascular disease, cerebrovascular disease). (Schick L, Windle PE. *PeriAnesthesia Nursing Core Curriculum: Preprocedure, Phase I and Phase II PACU Nursing.* 3rd ed. St. Louis, MO: Saunders; 2016:114; Odom-Forren J. *Drain's Perianesthesia Nursing: A Critical Care Approach.* 6th ed. St. Louis, MO: Saunders; 2013:684.)

6-33. *Correct answer:* **a**

The syndrome of inappropriate antidiuretic hormone (SIADH) is a disorder of the posterior pituitary that manifests with a fluid overload. This fluid overload causes a dilutional hyponatremia. Symptoms of SIADH include thirst, headache, decreased level of consciousness, decreased urine output, elevated BP and HR, nausea, vomiting, diarrhea, seizures, and heart failure. (Schick L, Windle PE. *PeriAnesthesia Nursing Core Curriculum: Preprocedure, Phase I and Phase II PACU Nursing.* 3rd ed. St. Louis, MO: Saunders; 2016:728.)

6-34. *Correct answer:* **c**

Anesthetic medications cause vascular dilation and expand the extracellular fluid (ECF) capacity. This is important for easing fluid overload and improving cardiovascular function. When the ECF volume is too low, hypotension ensues. (Schick L, Windle PE. *PeriAnesthesia Nursing Core Curriculum: Preprocedure, Phase I and Phase II PACU Nursing.* 3rd ed. St. Louis, MO: Saunders; 2016:309.)

6-35. *Correct answer:* **a**

The increase in the endogenous corticosteroids can cause poor wound healing. The nurse should observe these patients for any signs of infections and monitor white blood cell counts. (Schick L, Windle PE. *PeriAnesthesia Nursing Core Curriculum: Preprocedure, Phase I and Phase II PACU Nursing.* 3rd ed. St. Louis, MO: Saunders; 2016:731-732.)

6-36. *Correct answer:* **b**

A patient with central diabetes insipidus (DI) of either congenital or acquired origin requires hormone replacement to prevent and control polydipsia and polyuria associated with DI. A patient with a diagnosis of nephrogenic DI may be treated with thiazide diuretics; a patient with psychogenic DI may benefit from the use of anxiolytics or anti-compulsive disorder medications. (Urden LD, Stacy KM, Lough ME. *Critical Care Nursing Diagnosis and Management.* 7th ed. St. Louis, MO: Elsevier; 2013:832-835.)

6-37. *Correct answer:* **c**

The patient may be experiencing diabetic ketoacidosis (DKA) due to his fasting for surgery, leading to dehydration. Inadequate fluid resuscitation during surgery may also affect this patient. Once baseline labs are determined, the patient may receive additional insulin and rehydration. (Odom-Forren J. *Drain's Perianesthesia Nursing: A Critical Care Approach.* 6th ed. St. Louis, MO: Saunders; 2013:683.)

6-38. *Correct answer:* **b**

Graves disease is most commonly caused by an autoimmune form of hyperthyroidism. Treatments include those used for hyperthyroidism: radioactive iodine, antithyroid drugs, surgery, or a combination. (Stannard D, Krenzischek DA. *Perianesthesia Nursing Care: A Bedside Guide for Safe Recovery.* Sudbury, MA: Jones and Bartlett Learning; 2012:227; Schick L, Windle PE. *PeriAnesthesia Nursing Core Curriculum: Preprocedure, Phase I and Phase II PACU Nursing.* 3rd ed. St. Louis, MO: Saunders; 2016:719-722, 726.)

6-39. *Correct answer:* **c**

Angiotensin-converting enzyme (ACE) inhibitors can contribute to hypoglycemia, whereas the other medications listed contribute to hyperglycemia. (Schick L, Windle PE. *PeriAnesthesia Nursing Core Curriculum: Preprocedure, Phase I and Phase II PACU Nursing.* 3rd ed. St. Louis, MO: Saunders; 2016:733.)

6-40. *Correct answer:* **d**
A baseline electrolyte panel can check for dangerous electrolyte levels and can provide a baseline for comparison of kidney function postoperatively. (Odom-Forren J. *Drain's Perianesthesia Nursing: A Critical Care Approach.* 6th ed. St. Louis, MO: Saunders; 2013:192.)

6-41. *Correct answer:* **c**
Metformin is a biguanide antihyperglycemic that may not be excreted if there is decreased renal function after administration of contrast media for a procedure. Though rare, this may lead to lactic acidosis, which carries a 50% mortality rate. (Stannard D, Krenzischek DA. *Perianesthesia Nursing Care: A Bedside Guide for Safe Recovery.* Sudbury, MA: Jones and Bartlett Learning; 2012:330; Urden LD, Stacy KM, Lough ME. *Critical Care Nursing Diagnosis and Management.* 7th ed. St. Louis: Elsevier Mosby; 2013:714.)

6-42. *Correct answer:* **b**
Normal ranges for aterial blood gases (ABGs) are pH 7.35 to 7.45, $PaCO_2$ 35 to 45 mm Hg, HCO_3 22 to 26 mEq/L, and PaO_2 80 to 100 mm Hg. (Odom-Forren J. *Drain's Perianesthesia Nursing: A Critical Care Approach.* 6th ed. St. Louis, MO: Saunders; 2013:479.)

6-43. *Correct answer:* **a**
The stress response causes an increase in peripheral insulin resistance along with all the other responses listed. (Stannard D, Krenzischek DA. *Perianesthesia Nursing Care: A Bedside Guide for Safe Recovery.* Sudbury, MA: Jones and Bartlett Learning; 2012:108; Urden LD, Stacy KM, Lough ME. *Critical Care Nursing Diagnosis and Management.* 7th ed. St. Louis: Elsevier; 2013:810.)

6-44. *Correct answer:* **c**
Magnesium sulfate, 25 to 50 mg/kg IV/IO, is given when the patient's rhythm is identified as torsades de pointes. It is also recommended for treatment of hypomagnesemia. (Chameides L, Samson R, Schexnayder S,

Hazinski MF. *American Heart Association Pediatric Advanced Life Support Provider Manual.* Dallas, TX: Amercian Heart Association; 2011:132.)

6-45. *Correct answer:* **d**
Potassium is never given as an IV push because it can cause cardiac arrest. (Odom-Forren J. *Drain's Perianesthesia Nursing: A Critical Care Approach.* 6th ed. St. Louis, MO: Saunders; 2012:199.)

6-46. *Correct answer:* **c**
Low potassium can be due to losses from vomiting, diarrhea, and the presence of a nasogastric tube. Symptoms of low potassium include widened QRS interval, hypotension, bradycardia, slowed deep tendon reflexes, confusion, and arrhythmias. Left untreated, hypokalemia may result in cardiac arrest and death. The normal range for a potassium level is 3.5 to 5.3 mEq/L. (Odom-Forren J. *Drain's Perianesthesia Nursing: A Critical Care Approach.* 6th ed. St. Louis, MO: Saunders; 2013:199.)

6-47. *Correct answer:* **a**
Patients with hypothyroidism are prone to hypothermia due to their lowered metabolism. Special measures need to be taken to warm these patients to prevent complications. (Schick L, Windle PE. *PeriAnesthesia Nursing Core Curriculum: Preprocedure, Phase I and Phase II PACU Nursing.* 3rd ed. St. Louis, MO: Saunders; 2016:727.)

6-48. *Correct answer:* **c**
Due to the proximity of the surgical site to the airway, the addition of pressure from bleeding to any other swelling at the surgical site can compromise the airway. (Schick L, Windle PE. *PeriAnesthesia Nursing Core Curriculum: Preprocedure, Phase I and Phase II PACU Nursing.* St. Louis, MO: Saunders; 2016:720-722; Stannard D, Krenzischek DA. *Perianesthesia Nursing Care: A Bedside Guide for Safe Recovery.* Sudbury, MA: Jones and Bartlett Learning; 2012:224.)

6-49. *Correct answer:* **a**
Magnesium levels greater than 2.5 mEq/L may result in decreased reflexes, decreased blood pressure and decreased heart rate. (Odom-Forren J. *Drain's Perianesthesia Nursing: A Critical Care Approach.* 6th ed. St. Louis, MO: Saunders; 2013:200.)

6-50. *Correct answer:* **b**
Signs of magnesium sulfate toxicity include sedation, myocardial depression, muscular weakness with diminished reflexes, and respiratory difficulty. Calcium gluconate, 1 g given intravenously, should be readily available and followed by a diuretic and fluid bolusing. (Odom-Forren J. *Drain's Perianesthesia Nursing: A Critical Care Approach.* 6th ed. St. Louis, MO: Saunders; 2013:200.)

6-51. *Correct answer:* **c**
Signs and symptoms of hyperparathyroidism include, but are not limited to, hypertension, dysrhythmias, somnolence and lethargy, polyuria, polydipsia, osteoporosis, general muscle weakness, myalgias, and constipation. The excessive secretion of parathyroid hormone (PTH) will result in hypercalcemia that can deplete the bones of calcium and increase the risk of osteoporosis. (Schick L, Windle PE. *PeriAnesthesia Nursing Core Curriculum: Preprocedure, Phase I and Phase II PACU Nursing.* 3rd ed. St. Louis, MO: Saunders; 2016:723.)

6-52. *Correct answer:* **a.**
There is less chance of blood loss using this approach, as well as a lower infection rate. Excessive swallowing, coughing, or complaints about postnasal drainage are potential indications of cerebrospinal fluid (CSF) leaks. (Stannard D, Krenzischek DA. *Perianesthesia Nursing Care: A Bedside Guide for Safe Recovery.* Sudbury, MA: Jones and Bartlett Learning; 2012:225; Schick L, Windle PE. *PeriAnesthesia Nursing Core Curriculum: Preprocedure, Phase I and Phase II PACU Nursing.* 3rd ed. St. Louis, MO: Saunders; 2016:729.)

6-53. *Correct answer:* **d**
Patients with syndrome of inappropriate antidiuretic hormone (SIADH) are prone to dilutional hyponatremia, which is a risk factor in reparalysis when muscle relaxants are administered. (Schick L, Windle PE. *PeriAnesthesia Nursing Core Curriculum: Preprocedure, Phase I and Phase II PACU Nursing.* 3rd ed. St. Louis, MO: Saunders; 2016:386.)

6-54. *Correct answer:* **b**
U waves are typically associated with hypokalemia. Insulin will push potassium back into the cell and exacerbate the hypokalemia. Insulin is used in certain disorders with hyperkalemia (e.g., malignant hyperthermia) to push potassium back into the cell and bring potassium levels back to normal ranges. (Schick L, Windle PE. *PeriAnesthesia Nursing Core Curriculum: Preprocedure, Phase I and Phase II PACU Nursing.* 3rd ed. St. Louis, MO: Saunders; 2016:307t.)

6-55. *Correct answer:* **b**
The patient was not adequately hydrated during the operative procedure, considering the length of the procedure, fluid replacement, and her estimated blood loss. Her HR is at least 20% higher and her BP lower than her preoperative baseline values. (Schick L, Windle PE. *PeriAnesthesia Nursing Core Curriculum: Preprocedure, Phase I and Phase II PACU Nursing.* 3rd ed. St. Louis, MO: Saunders; 2016:231.)

6-56. *Correct answer:* **c**
Patients with Addison's disease do not have the ability to make cortisol and aldosterone due to a nonfunctioning adrenal cortex. These patients require a "stress dose" of corticosteroid, in addition to their baseline steroid needs, during the perioperative period. (Schick L, Windle PE. *PeriAnesthesia Nursing Core Curriculum: Preprocedure, Phase I and Phase II PACU Nursing.* 3rd ed. St. Louis, MO: Saunders; 2016:114, 730t-731t.)

6-57. *Correct answer:* **c**

One of the potential complications of this surgery is hypotension and/or bradycardia. Treat first with a fluid challenge if appropriate. The patient is asymptomatic at this time. (American Society of PeriAnesthesia Nurses. *2015-2017 Perianesthesia Nursing Standards, Practice Recommendations and Interpretive Statements.* Cherry Hill, NJ: ASPAN; 2014:144.)

6-58. *Correct answer:* **d**

Earlier studies directed tighter glycemic control for patients. Although it reduced morbidity and mortality in critically ill patients, it increased morbidity and mortality in the medical-surgical population. Striving for a glucose level below 180 mg/dL improves outcomes. (Schick L, Windle PE. *PeriAnesthesia Nursing Core Curriculum: Preprocedure, Phase I and Phase II PACU Nursing.* 3rd ed. St. Louis, MO: Saunders; 2016:734.)

6-59. *Correct answer:* **c**

One of the potential complications of this approach for surgery is a cerebrospinal fluid (CSF) leak. This is manifested by leaking of clear fluid from the nose or frequent coughing or swallowing. (Schick L, Windle PE. *PeriAnesthesia Nursing Core Curriculum: Preprocedure, Phase I and Phase II PACU Nursing.* St. Louis, MO: Saunders; 2016:729. Stannard D, Krenzischek DA. *Perianesthesia Nursing Care: A Bedside Guide for Safe Recovery.* Sudbury, MA: Jones and Bartlett Learning; 2012:225-226.)

6-60. *Correct answer:* **b**

Symptoms of pulmonary edema include fine to coarse crackles, mild tachypnea, and lower SpO_2. The patient is most likely experiencing mild pulmonary edema and may benefit most by being diuresed. (Odom-Forren J. *Drain's Perianesthesia Nursing: A Critical Care Approach.* 6th ed. St. Louis, MO: Saunders; 2013:165.)

6-61. *Correct answer:* **d**

The following patient conditions increase the risk for aspiration: morbid obesity, renal or hepatic failure, ascites, brain injury or increased intracranial pressure (ICP), decreased level of consciousness, delayed gastric emptying, difficulty swallowing, cerebral palsy, trauma, pain, drug overdose, difficult airway, gastrointestinal obstruction, anorexia, esophageal disorders, and diabetes. (Odom-Forren J. *Drain's Perianesthesia Nursing: A Critical Care Approach.* 6th ed. St. Louis, MO: Saunders; 2013:196.)

6-62. *Correct answer:* **c**

Although generally used to treat depression and anxiety, several studies have found duloxetine to be very effective in the treatment of diabetic neuropathy. (Pasero C, McCaffery M. *Pain Assessment and Pharmacologic Management,* St. Louis, MO: Elsevier-Mosby; 2011:639.)

6-63. *Correct answer:* **c**

Handoff communication can reduce errors, reduce omission of information, eliminate redundancy, improve inclusion of details, increase effective transfer of care, and decrease length of stay and costs associated with communication errors. (American Society of PeriAnesthesia Nurses. *2015-2017 Perianesthesia Nursing Standards, Practice Recommendations and Interpretive Statements.* Cherry Hill, NJ: ASPAN; 2014:59.)

6-64. *Correct answer:* **a**

Hypothermia can cause shivering, leading to metabolic acidosis and other electrolyte shifts. (Odom-Forren J. *Drain's Perianesthesia Nursing: A Critical Care Approach.* 6th ed. St. Louis, MO: Saunders; 2013:171, 742-743.)

6-65. *Correct answer:* **d**

Lactated Ringer's (LR) is an electrolyte isotonic crystalloid solution that closely resembles the electrolyte composition of blood serum. (Schick L, Windle PE. *PeriAnesthesia Nursing Core Curriculum: Preprocedure, Phase I and Phase II PACU Nursing.* 3rd ed. St. Louis, MO: Saunders; 2016:320; Odom-Forren J. *Drain's Perianesthesia Nursing: A Critical Care Approach.* 6th ed. St. Louis, MO: Saunders; 2013:201-203.)

7

Maintenance of Normothermia, Physiologic Comfort, and the Therapeutic Environment

Nancy Strzyzewski, Tanya LeCompte Hofmann, Vallire D. Hooper, and Theresa Clifford

7-1. Warming intravenous (IV) fluids helps to prevent heat loss resulting from the following mechanism:

a. Radiation

b. Conduction

c. Convection

d. Evaporation

7-2. Examples of active warming measures include all of the following EXCEPT:

a. Forced-air convection system

b. Circulating-water mattresses

c. Application of warmed blankets

d. Radiant warmers

7-3. A patient is in the Phase I PACU after surgery to remove a benign pituitary tumor. The nurse will monitor the patient's temperature carefully during this phase of recovery. The nurse is aware that a consequence of this surgery includes hyperthermia (a result of hypothalamic influence) and hypothermia, which is a result of:

a. Decreased thyroid-stimulating hormones

b. Increased thyroid-stimulating hormones

c. Impaired metabolism

d. Impaired glucose regulation

7-4. Which of the following statements is true?

a. Near-core measures of oral temperatures best approximate core

b. Near-core measures of rectal temperatures best approximate core

c. Near-core measures of tympanic temperatures best approximate core

d. Near-core measures of temporal temperatures best approximate core

Consider this scenario for questions 7-5 and 7-6.
   A nurse relieving another nurse for break asks for a report on the patient. The second nurse states, "Why should I give you a report? You won't understand it anyway." Then she rolls her eyes and walks away from the patient and relief nurse.

7-5. What term best describes this interaction?

a. Immature behavior

b. Nurse fatigue

c. Female relationships

d. Horizontal violence

7-6. This type of behavior threatens patient safety because it:

a. Forces nurses who don't like each other to work together

b. Creates barriers to effective communication

c. Distracts and entertains the rest of the staff

d. Makes nurses look unprofessional

Consider this scenario for questions 7-7 and 7-9.
   A 42-year-old male patient is in the Phase I PACU after a hernia repair under spinal anesthesia. Preoperatively his BP was 130/60 and HR was 70.

7-7. After 90 minutes, his BP is 160/90 and HR is 110. He denies any pain. Based on knowledge of evidence-based practice, the nurse suspects the patient may be at risk for:

    a. Pulmonary hypertension (PHTN)

    b. Postoperative urinary retention (POUR)

    c. Postoperative nausea and vomiting (PONV)

    d. Posttraumatic stress disorder (PTSD)

7-8. What intervention should the nurse consider as the first action?

    a. Notify the physician

    b. Treat hypertension

    c. Scan the bladder

    d. Use distraction

7-9. Loss of body heat due to transfer to the surrounding cooler air is an example of:

    a. Radiation

    b. Conduction

    c. Convection

    d. Evaporation

7-10. Mrs. Jones presents to the Phase I PACU after undergoing a right knee arthroscopy. Her surgeon has ordered ketorolac 30 mg to be given for pain. During handoff, the anesthesia provider reports that ketorolac 15 mg was administered intraoperatively. While reading Mrs. Jones's health history, the nurse has learned that this 70-year-old patient has previously been treated for acute kidney injury. The nurse should consider all of the following EXCEPT:

    a. Question the order of ketorolac 30 mg in a patient over the age of 60

    b. Limit IV fluids because she has a history of renal impairment

    c. Request an order for IV acetaminophen 1000 mg instead of ketorolac

    d. Monitor Mrs. Jones's urinary output

7-11. On arrival to the Phase I PACU, a 9-month-old child is alert and moving all extremities, with a BP of 75/40 and HR of 180. Twenty minutes after arrival, the patient's HR is 230, a strong brachial pulse is present, and her cardiac rhythm is a narrow complex tachycardia. The perianesthesia nurse immediately prepares for:

    a. Defibrillation

    b. Carotid massage

    c. Adenosine

    d. An ice pack

7-12. Potential causes of hypothermia during a pediatric surgery include all of the following EXCEPT:

    a. Neuromuscular blocking agents

    b. Opioid analgesic agents

    c. Volatile inhalation agents

    d. Intravenous fluids

7-13. Which of the following would place the patient at the highest risk of postoperative nausea and vomiting (PONV)?

    a. Stapedectomy

    b. Abdominal surgery

    c. History of seasickness

    d. Obesity

7-14. Which of the following drugs would be preferred for the management of nausea and vomiting due to motion sickness?

    a. Dexamethasone

    b. Dronabinol

    c. Haloperidol

    d. Scopolamine

7-15. A Phase I PACU nurse routinely works "double shifts" caring for patients 16 hours a day, 3 or 4 days within a 5-day work week. Understanding current evidence regarding nursing fatigue, a colleague is concerned because this work schedule can:

    a. Triple the medical error rate

    b. Double the medical error rate

    c. Increase patient length of stay

    d. Decrease patient satisfaction

7-16. Each of the following drugs could be appropriately prescribed for the management of postoperative nausea and vomiting EXCEPT:

   a. Granisetron

   b. Haloperidol

   c. Lorazepam

   d. Dolasetron

7-17. A 42-year-old female patient is admitted to the Phase I PACU after a laparoscopic cholecystectomy. The patient's BP is 130/60, HR is 84, RR is 20, and SpO_2 is 88%. The perianesthesia nurse understands this patient is at risk for:

   a. Increased lung volume

   b. Decreased lung volume

   c. Decreased dead space

   d. Increased minute volume

7-18. Normothermia is defined as a core temperature between:

   a. 34° C and 36° C

   b. 35° C and 37° C

   c. 36° C and 38° C

   d. 37° C and 39° C

7-19. Which of the following agents is likely to produce confusion, motor incoordination, and hallucinations?

   a. Scopolamine

   b. Ondansetron

   c. Granisetron

   d. Dexamethasone

Consider this scenario for questions 7-20 and 7-21.

   While monitoring an intubated patient using capnography, the nurse recognizes a sudden decrease in end-tidal CO_2 ($ETCO_2$) to near 0.

7-20. What is the first action the nurse immediately takes?

   a. Call the anesthesiologist

   b. Reset the ventilator alarm

   c. Simulate the patient

   d. Auscultate the lungs

7-21. A sudden increase in end-tidal CO_2 may be an indication of:

   a. Inadvertent narcotization

   b. Malignant hyperthermia

   c. Dislodged endotracheal (ET) tube

   d. Pulmonary embolism

7-22. Family presence in the PACU:

   a. Should be discouraged to prevent infection

   b. Should be encouraged to decrease anxiety

   c. Is a Health Insurance Portability and Accountability Act (HIPAA) violation

   d. Should be open to improve Hospital Consumer Assessment of Healthcare Providers and Systems (HCAHP) scores

7-23. Signs of pain in patients with intellectual disabilities can include all of the following EXCEPT:

   a. Fidgeting

   b. Guarding

   c. Grimacing

   d. Vital signs

7-24. When providing discharge instructions, the perianesthesia nurse in the Phase II PACU reiterates the need to call a physician when there is pain not relieved by the prescribed pain management protocol, bleeding beyond the expected volume, symptoms of urinary retention, and a fever with a temperature above:

   a. 37.8° C

   b. 38° C

   c. 38.3° C

   d. 39° C

7-25. During a busy evening in the Phase I PACU, the charge nurse decides to combine Preoperative, Phase I, and Phase II patients in one area. Patients are carefully moved so that:

  a. Preanesthesia patients are separated from recovering patients

  b. Phase I postanesthesia patients are closer to the operating room (OR) doors

  c. Phase II postanesthesia patients are nearest to the door

  d. Patients are mixed together, regardless of the level of care, as long as there are competent staff

7-26. Which of the following agents reduces nausea and vomiting by increasing gastric emptying?

  a. Diazepam

  b. Granisetron

  c. Diphenhydramine

  d. Metoclopramide

7-27. Hyperalgesia is defined as:

  a. Extreme physical or mental pain

  b. Altering or adaptation according to circumstances

  c. Increased sensitivity to pain

  d. A lessening of pain without loss of consciousness

7-28. Pain tolerance is defined as the:

  a. Decreased sensitivity to painful stimuli

  b. Point at which a person does not feel pain

  c. Maximum level of pain a person accepts

  d. Disturbance of neural pain processes

7-29. A 25-year-old female trauma patient presents from the emergency surgery under general anesthesia following a motor vehicle accident. The family indicates a possible history of malignant hyperthermia. The best course of action would be to:

  a. Conduct emergency genetic testing

  b. Pretreat with 2.5 mg/kg of dantrolene before anesthesia induction

  c. Conduct an emergency muscle biopsy

  d. Avoid exposure to malignant hyperthermia–triggering agents

7-30. A patient appears upset and tearful but denies pain and refuses pain medication because "my sibling is a drug addict and I am afraid of getting hooked." What is the priority intervention for this patient?

  a. Encourage expression of fears of past experiences

  b. Provide accurate information about the use of pain medication

  c. Explain that addiction is unlikely among acute care patients

  d. Seek family assistance in resolving this problem

7-31. A perianesthesia nurse caring for a patient in Phase I is assigned a second patient. While receiving a report for the second patient, the nurse learns this patient is classified as an ASA IV, hemodynamically unstable, and has an extensive cardiac history. The nurse immediately contacts the charge nurse because the nurse understands that safe staffing should reflect:

  a. Nurse competency

  b. Number of nurses

  c. Patient comorbidities

  d. Patient acuity

7-32. While searching for the most comprehensive evidence-based statement regarding a clinical practice issue, the perianesthesia nurse seeks out a/an:

  a. Systematic integrative study

  b. Randomized control trial

  c. ASPAN position statement

  d. Clinical practice guideline

7-33. The most common clinical symptom of malignant hyperthermia is:

a. Masseter jaw spasm

b. Unstable blood pressure

c. Hypercarbia

d. Hypoxia

7-34. To reduce the noise level in the Phase I PACU, several of the nurses have decreased the volume of the pulse oximeter alarms. The prudent perianesthesia nurse is concerned because:

a. Noise volume in the unit still remains too loud

b. PACU patient satisfaction scores are still low

c. The Joint Commission National Patient Safety Goal is not being met

d. Patients complain they cannot sleep comfortably

7-35. When caring for a young child with pain, which assessment tool is the most useful?

a. Simple description pain intensity scale

b. 0-10 numerical rating scale (NRS)

c. FACES pain-rating scale

d. McGill-Melzack pain questionnaire

7-36. When the patient develops malignant hyperthermia in the operating room, the first action that should be taken is:

a. Reconstitute dantrolene

b. Ventilate with high-flow oxygen

c. Discontinue all triggering agents

d. Initiate cooling measures

7-37. A patient with chronic low back pain who took hydromorphone around the clock for the past year was told to stop the medication preoperatively by a provider. The preoperative nurse recognizes that this patient may experience symptoms of:

a. Addiction

b. Tolerance

c. Pseudoaddiction

d. Physical dependence

7-38. Infants are at higher risk for hypothermia due to the lack of a shiver response between birth and:

a. Age 12 months

b. Age 9 months

c. Age 6 months

d. Age 3 months

7-39. A 75-year-old, frail, elderly female patient presents to the preoperative area on the day of surgery with an oral temperature of 36° C. The best intervention to prevent unplanned perioperative hypothermia in this patient would be:

a. Infuse 1 L of intravenous fluid

b. Increase the room temperature

c. Apply socks and gloves

d. Apply forced-air warming

7-40. When applying the principles of pain management, what is the first consideration?

a. Treatment is based on the patient's and family's goal

b. A multidisciplinary approach is needed

c. The patient must be believed about perceptions of their own pain

d. Medication side effects must be prevented and managed

7-41. _____ results in compulsive use of a drug despite harmful effects.

a. Addiction

b. Tolerance

c. Physical dependence

d. Addiction and physical dependence

7-42. Intravenous insulin and glucose are administered during a malignant hyperthermia episode to treat:

a. Hyperkalemia

b. Hypothyroidism

c. Hypokalemia

d. Hyperthyroidism

7-43. An elderly woman with a history of a stroke that left her confused and unable to communicate returns from the procedure area after a gastrostomy tube placement. The provider has addressed pain management with an order that reads as follows: oxycodone 2.5 mg (1/2 tab), per tube, q 4 hours, prn. Which action by the nurse is most appropriate?

a. No action is required by the nurse because the order is appropriate

b. Request to have the order changed to around-the-clock (ATC) for the first 48 hours

c. Ask for a change of medication to hydromorphone 0.2 mg IVP, q 3 hours, prn

d. Begin the oxycodone when the patient shows nonverbal symptoms of pain

7-44. An example of a preemptive intervention for postoperative pain management include all of the following EXCEPT:

a. Administration of oral acetaminophen for 24 hours preoperatively

b. Injection of local anesthetic into the tissues prior to incision

c. The provision of a peripheral nerve block in the Phase I PACU

d. A single dose of a short acting opioid just prior to entering the operating room

Consider this scenario for questions 7-45 and 7-46.

An 8-year-old child is admitted to the Phase I PACU after an appendectomy.

7-45. Considering that the child was exposed to chickenpox the day before surgery, what action does the charge nurse take?

a. Send him directly to an inpatient room

b. Place him on contact precautions in the PACU

c. Place him on airborne precautions in the PACU

d. Assign him to a nurse who was also exposed

7-46. During transport of this patient, what does the nurse advocate for?

a. No special considerations during travel

b. Transport personnel wear N-95 masks

c. Transport personnel wear goggles

d. Patient wears a face mask

7-47. When administering an analgesic to manage pain, what is the priority goal?

a. Administer the smallest dose that provides relief with the fewest side effects

b. Titrate upward until the patient is pain free

c. Titrate downwards to prevent toxicity

d. Ensure that the drug is adequate to meet the client's subjective needs

7-48. The patient who is susceptible to malignant hyperthermia (MH) should be monitored for symptoms for _____ hours postoperatively.

a. 6 to 12

b. 12 to 24

c. 24 to 48

d. 48 to 72

7-49. While checking a self-inflating ventilation bag to ensure it is properly functioning, the nurse realizes the bag will not inflate when it is connected to a flow of oxygen. What should the nurse recheck?

a. Gas flow valves are closed

b. Gas flow valves are open

c. Oxygen flow is set at 4 L

d. Oxygen flow is set at 2 L

7-50. Safe staffing in the perianesthesia area is based on:

a. Patient acuity and nursing involvement

b. Patient acuity and nursing interventions

c. Number of patients on the schedule

d. Number of beds/slots in the unit

7-51. Risk factors for postoperative nausea and vomiting (PONV) include all of the following EXCEPT:

a. Gender

b. Thermoregulation

c. Smoking status

d. Family history of PONV

7-52. Which of the following patients is at the greatest risk for developing unplanned perioperative hypothermia?

a. A 25-year-old male patient with a body mass index (BMI) of 26 undergoing a laparoscopic appendectomy under general anesthesia

b. An 80-year-old female patient with a BMI of 18 undergoing a spinal fusion under general anesthesia

c. A 60-year-old male patient with a BMI of 25 undergoing a cardiac catheterization under moderate sedation

d. A 47-year-old female patient with a BMI of 24 undergoing a total abdominal hysterectomy under general anesthesia

7-53. A 17-year-old patient has been in the Phase I PACU for 60 minutes after extensive burn debridement and scar release of his right thigh requiring general anesthesia. After several pharmacologic interventions, his pain score has decreased from 10 to 7 on a numerical rating scale. What other evidence-based intervention could the nurse use to help the patient?

a. Continuous passive motion (CPM) machine

b. Family visitation

c. Therapy dog

d. Reduce stimuli

7-54. Which of the following agents is associated with an increased risk of developing extrapyramidal effects?

a. Ondansetron

b. Diphenhydramine

c. Metoclopramide

d. Dexamethasone

7-55. In addition to volatile general inhalation agents, the other most common trigger for malignant hyperthermia with general anesthesia is:

a. Propofol

b. Midazolam

c. Fentanyl

d. Succinylcholine

7-56. Temperature should be assessed at least every _____ minutes in the hypothermic patient.

a. 10

b. 15

c. 30

d. 60

7-57. Complications of the pneumoperitoneum needed for laparoscopic abdominal surgery are exacerbated by which surgical position?

a. Supine

b. Prone

c. Lithotomy

d. Trendelenburg

7-58. The most accurate measure of core temperature is obtained via a/an:

a. Pulmonary artery catheter

b. Nasal cannula probe

c. Bladder thermistor

d. Oral thermometer

7-59. A perianesthesia nurse is assigned to manage the care of a patient receiving procedural sedation. The nurse refuses to participate in the procedure until:

  a. The physician has ordered the medications to be used

  b. An anesthesia provider is in the same room

  c. An anesthesia ventilator/gas machine is in the same room

  d. A second nurse is found to assist the physician

7-60. A patient has just undergone an extensive mastoidectomy with tympanoplasty. After 4.5 hours in the operating room, the patient arrives in the Phase I PACU with a temporal artery temperature reading of 39.8° C. The perianesthesia nurse can anticipate which of the following cardiac manifestations of hyperthermia?

  a. Tachycardia

  b. Hypertension

  c. Atrial flutter

  d. Bradycardia

7-61. A 32-year-old patient is admitted to the Phase I PACU after general anesthesia for an emergency hysterectomy after a vaginal delivery. Total blood loss (EBL) after delivery and during surgery was 2500 mL, BP was 90/40, HR was 100, RR was 20, and SpO_2 was 100%. The nurse questions the accuracy of the SpO_2 because of the:

  a. Duration of the procedure

  b. Relatively stable BP

  c. Oxyhemoglobin curve shift

  d. Potentially low hemoglobin

7-62. Which of the following conditions can potentiate a nondepolarizing neuromuscular blocking agent?

  a. Hyperthermia

  b. Hypothermia

  c. Overhydration

  d. Sepsis

Thirty minutes after arriving in the Phase I PACU after a cystoscopy, a 79-year-old patient becomes confused and has abnormal speech. The nurse immediately notifies the physician.

7-63. Considering this patient has received an anesthetic, is older, and may be a potential stroke victim, what is the perianesthesia nurse concerned about?

  a. Upper airway obstruction and hypoventilation

  b. Upper airway obstruction and bronchospasm

  c. Lower airway obstruction and laryngospasm

  d. Lower airway obstruction, bronchospasm

Consider this scenario for questions 7-64 and 7-65.

A 34-year-old patient has been admitted to the Phase I PACU after a 4-hour lumbar laminectomy.

7-64. Understanding the potential risks for this patient, what piece of information is the nurse most interested in hearing about during the report?

  a. Preoperative state of anxiety

  b. Number of screws inserted

  c. Surgical position of patient

  d. Type of bone graft inserted

7-65. Considering the evidence, what is the nurse certain to include in the documentation of the admission assessment for this patient?

  a. Pupil checks

  b. Swallow test

  c. Blood glucose

  d. Skin assessment

Answers and Rationales for Chapter 7, Maintenance of Normothermia, Physiologic Comfort, and the Therapeutic Environment

7-1. *Correct answer:* **b**

Heat loss by conduction involves the transfer of heat energy through direct contact between objects (e.g., cold operating room tables, chilled skin preparation products). Ways to prevent heat loss by conduction include warming objects that will be in touch with the body and warming intravenous fluids. (Odom-Forren J. *Drain's Perianesthesia Nursing: A Critical Care Approach.* 6th ed. St. Louis, MO: Saunders; 2013:741.)

7-2. *Correct answer:* **c**

Examples of active warming measures include the application of a forced-air convection warming system, as well as circulating-water mattresses, resistive heating blankets, radiant warmers, negative-pressure warming systems, and warmed humidified inspired oxygen. Passive warming measures include the application of warmed blankets, reflective blankets, socks, and head coverings. (Schick L, Windle PE. *PeriAnesthesia Nursing Core Curriculum: Preprocedure, Phase I and Phase II PACU Nursing.* 3rd ed. St. Louis, MO: Saunders; 2016:404.)

7-3. *Correct answer:* **a**

The postanesthesia plan of care for patients having pituitary procedures must include interventions to monitor and manage thermoregulation. This includes monitoring for hyperthermia, a result of hypothalamic influences, and for hypothermia due to decreased thyroid-stimulating hormone levels. (Schick L, Windle PE. *PeriAnesthesia Nursing Core Curriculum: Preprocedure, Phase I and Phase II PACU Nursing.* 3rd ed. St. Louis, MO: Saunders; 2016:729.)

7-4. *Correct answer:* **a**

According to the guideline for the promotion of perioperative normothermia, temperature measurement recommendations that are supported by strong evidence include the following statements: near-core measures of oral temperature best approximates core, the same route of temperature measurement should be used throughout the perianesthesia period for comparison purposes, and caution should be taken in interpreting extreme values from any site with near-core instruments. (Schick L, Windle PE. *PeriAnesthesia Nursing Core Curriculum: Preprocedure, Phase I and Phase II PACU Nursing.* 3rd ed. St. Louis, MO: Saunders; 2016:402-403.)

7-5. *Correct answer:* **d**

Horizontal violence, also known as lateral violence or bullying, is defined as hostile and aggressive behaviors by an individual or a group of individuals toward another member or group of members in the workplace. These behaviors can be verbal or nonverbal and are intended to be offensive and intimidating and cause the receiving individual to experience stress. (American Society of PeriAnesthesia Nurses. Position Statement 9. A position statement on workplace violence, horizontal hostility and workplace incivility in the perianesthesia settings. (*2015-2017 Perianesthesia Nursing Standards, Practice Recommendations and Interpretive Statements.* Cherry Hill, NJ: ASPAN; 2014:117-121.)

7-6. *Correct answer:* **b**

This type of behavior is a concern because "these actions disrupt relationships and create barriers to communication needed to effectively care for patients." (American Society of PeriAnesthesia Nurses. Position Statement 9. A position statement on workplace violence, horizontal hostility and workplace incivility in the perianesthesia settings. *2015-2017 Perianesthesia Nursing Standards, Practice Recommendations and Interpretive Statements.* Cherry Hill, NJ: ASPAN; 2014:117-121.)

7-7. *Correct answer:* **b**

Postoperative urinary retention is relatively common following urinary or gynecological procedures, hernia repairs and the use of regional and spinal anesthesia. Symptoms include restlessness, pelvic pain, hypertension, increased HR and RR, anxiety, and diaphoresis. (Odom-Forren J. *Drain's Perianesthesia Nursing: A Critical Care Approach.* 6th ed. St. Louis, MO: Saunders; 2013:598; Schick L, Windle PE. *PeriAnesthesia Nursing Core Curriculum : Preprocedure, Phase I and Phase II, PACU Nursing.* 3rd ed. St. Louis, MO: Saunders; 2016:1241-1242.)

7-8. *Correct answer:* **c**

Postoperative urinary retention (POUR) is defined as greater than 500 mL of bladder volume. Scanning the bladder enables the nurse to assess the patient for postoperative urinary retention. (Odom-Forren J. *Drain's Perianesthesia Nursing: A Critical Care Approach.* 6th ed. St. Louis, MO: Saunders; 2013:598.)

7-9. *Correct answer:* **c**

Convection involves the loss of body heat due to air or water moving by the skin and carrying away body heat. (Odom-Forren J. *Drain's Perianesthesia Nursing: A Critical Care Approach.* 6th ed. St. Louis, MO: Saunders; 2013:741; Schick L, Windle PE. *PeriAnesthesia Nursing Core Curriculum:*

Preprocedure, Phase I and Phase II PACU Nursing. 3rd ed. St. Louis, MO: Saunders; 2016:407.)

7-10. *Correct answer:* **b**

Patients over the age of 60 and with a prior history of renal impairment are at an increased risk of developing acute renal failure in the presence of nonsteroidal anti-inflammatory drugs (NSAIDs). This risk is increased in patients with volume depletion; therefore, it is important that the patient's volume not be restricted. (Odom-Forren J. *Drain's Perianesthesia Nursing: A Critical Care Approach.* 6th ed. St. Louis, MO: Saunders; 2013:438.)

7-11. *Correct answer:* **d**

An HR of 220 bpm or higher is characteristic of supraventricular tachycardia (SVT). The presence of a pulse directs the caregivers to follow the interventions identified by pediatric advanced life support (PALS) for the management of tachyarrhythmias. The first intervention identified for the management of stable SVT is vagal maneuvers. Due to the age of the child, ice to the face is the most appropriate vagal maneuver to use. (Chameides C, Samson R, Schexnayder S, Hazinski M. *Recognition and management of tachycardia.* In: *Pediatric Advanced Life Support Provider Manual.* Dallas, TX: American Heart Association; 2011:121-140.)

7-12. *Correct answer:* **b**

In addition to environmental sources of hypothermia (e.g., operating room temperature, patient transport between levels of care), other potential causes of hypothermia include vasodilating anesthetic agents (e.g., isoflurane, desflurane), neuromuscular blocking agents, and administration of cool IV fluids. (Schick L, Windle PE. *PeriAnesthesia Nursing Core Curriculum: Preprocedure, Phase I and Phase II PACU Nursing.* 3rd ed. St. Louis, MO: Saunders; 2016:232.)

7-13. *Correct answer:* **a**

All of these are risk factors that should be taken into consideration when assessing a patient for potential development of postoperative nausea and vomiting (PONV); however, nausea accompanied by vertigo and nystagmus often accompanies ear surgery. These patients should be instructed to avoid any quick movements. (Odom-Forren J. *Drain's Perianesthesia Nursing: A Critical Care Approach.* 6th ed. St. Louis, MO: Saunders; 2013:452.)

7-14. *Correct answer:* **d**

Scopolamine prevents the transmission of signals between the vestibule in the inner ear and the vomiting center of the brain, which occurs especially in those susceptible to motion sickness. (Odom-Forren J. *Drain's Perianesthesia Nursing: A Critical Care Approach.* 6th ed. St. Louis, MO: Saunders; 2013:408t.)

7-15. *Correct answer:* **a**

According to studies related to nursing and fatigue, medical error rates can triple after workers perform 12.5 hours of sustained activity. Inadequate sleep and the ensuing fatigue have implications on health, safety, and the economics of the workplace. (American Society of PeriAnesthesia Nurses. Position Statement 3. A position statement on "On call/Work Schedule." (*2015-2017 Perianesthesia Nursing Standards, Practice Recommendations and Interpretive Statements.* Cherry Hill, NJ: ASPAN; 2014:97-99.)

7-16. *Correct answer:* **c**

Granisetron is a serotonin 5-HT3 receptor antagonist used to prevent nausea and vomiting, as is dolasetron. Haloperidol is an antidopaminergic used as an antiemetic, whereas lorazepam is a benzodiazepine used primarily to relieve anxiety. Lorazepam has been effective in the treatment of nausea related to chemotherapy and/or radiation. (Odom-Forren J. *Drain's Perianesthesia Nursing: A Critical Care Approach.* 6th ed. St. Louis, MO: Saunders; 2013:405; Kizior RJ, Hodgson BB. *Saunders Nursing Drug Handbook 2015.* St. Louis, MO: Saunders; 2016: 384-386, 559-561, 566-568, 720-722.)

7-17. *Correct answer:* **b**

The pneumoperitoneum resulting from the insufflation of the abdomen by CO_2 can create increased intraabdominal pressures. These pressures can lead to increased airway pressures and decreased lung volumes. The reduction of lung volumes can affect oxygenation. (Odom-Forren J. *Drain's Perianesthesia Nursing: A Critical Care Approach.* 6th ed. St. Louis, MO: Saunders; 2013:669.)

7-18. *Correct answer:* **c**

The body maintains its core temperature at a narrow range between 36° C and 38° C. This is the definition of normothermia. (Odom-Forren J. *Drain's Perianesthesia Nursing: A Critical Care Approach.* 6th ed. St. Louis, MO: Saunders; 2013:740.)

7-19. *Correct answer:* **a**

Side effects of scopolamine include confusion, disorientation, hallucination, and dysphoria, as well as sedation, dry mouth, and visual disturbances. (Odom-Forren J. *Drain's Perianesthesia Nursing: A Critical Care Approach.* 6th ed. St. Louis, MO: Saunders; 2013:407t-408t.)

7-20. *Correct answer:* **d**

A sudden decrease in end-tidal CO_2 (ETCO$_2$) indicates that CO_2 in inhaled gases is no longer being detected. Possible causes include a completely blocked endotracheal tube, esophageal intubation, a disconnection in the breathing circuit, and inadvertent extubation. The prudent perianesthesia nurse will auscultate the lungs to confirm adequate ventilations. (Odom-Forren J. *Drain's Perianesthesia Nursing: A Critical Care Approach.* 6th ed. St. Louis, MO: Saunders; 2013:482.)

7-21. *Correct answer:* **b**

Although a gradual increase in $ETCO_2$ level may be an indication of a small ventilator leak or partial airway obstruction that impacts minute ventilation, a large increase in $ETCO_2$ can be an early sign of malignant hyperthermia. (Odom-Forren J. *Drain's Perianesthesia Nursing: A Critical Care Approach.* 6th ed. St. Louis, MO: Saunders; 2013:359-360.)

7-22. *Correct answer:* **b**

There is increasing evidence that indicates family-centered care is beneficial to all. Allowing a family presence creates a diversion for the patient that decreases anxiety and dissatisfaction for both the patient and the family. Visitation should be centered on the needs of the patient while taking into consideration activities occurring in the unit. (Odom-Forren J. *Drain's Perianesthesia Nursing: A Critical Care Approach.* 6th ed. St. Louis, MO: Saunders; 2013:772-773.)

7-23. *Correct answer:* **d**

Behavioral signs such as fidgeting and guarding and facial expressions such as grimacing are much better indicators of pain in patients with intellectual disabilities. The Chronic Pain Scale for Nonverbal Adults with Intellectual Disabilities (CPS-NAID) is a good example of an alternative numerical rating scale appropriate for special populations. (Pasero C, McCaffery M. *Pain Assessment and Pharmacologic Management.* St. Louis, MO: Mosby; 2011:152-153.)

7-24. *Correct answer:* **c**

When providing postoperative discharge instructions, the patient and family should be taught about surgical complications and when to call the surgeon for questions. These include pain not relieved by prescribed pain medication, bleeding, fever with temperature above $38.3°$ C ($101°$ F), urinary retention, uncontrolled nausea and vomiting, extreme swelling or redness around the surgical wound or drainage that has changed to yellow or green, and if the intravenous catheter site shows signs of redness or drainage. (Schick L, Windle PE. *PeriAnesthesia Nursing Core Curriculum: Preprocedure, Phase I and Phase II PACU Nursing.* 3rd ed. St. Louis, MO: Saunders; 2016:1282.)

7-25. *Correct answer:* **a**

When providing for a safe and therapeutic environment, preanesthesia patients should be separated from patients undergoing procedures and/or recovering from anesthesia or sedation. (American Society of PeriAnesthesia Nurses. Standard II environment of care. In: *2015-2017 Perianesthesia Nursing Standards, Practice Recommendations and Interpretive Statements.* Cherry Hill, NJ: ASPAN; 2014:21.)

7-26. *Correct answer:* **d**

Metoclopramide is a good choice for patients when gastric stasis is the cause of nausea and vomiting. Granisetron is more effective in the treatment of vomiting, and diphenhydramine is a good choice for patients with a history of motion sickness. (Odom-Forren J. *Drain's Perianesthesia Nursing: A Critical Care Approach.* 6th ed. St. Louis, MO: Saunders; 2013:407t.)

7-27. *Correct answer:* **c**

Hyperalgesia, an increased sensation of pain in response to a normally painful stimulus, can be caused by damage to nociceptors, damage to peripheral nerves, inflammation, or long-term opioid use. (Schick L, Windle PE. *PeriAnesthesia Nursing Core Curriculum: Preprocedure, Phase I and Phase II PACU Nursing.* St. Louis, MO: Saunders; 2016:437t; Pasero C, McCaffery M. *Pain Assessment and Pharmacologic Management.* St. Louis, MO: Mosby; 2011: 177, 715.)

7-28. *Correct answer:* **c**

Pain tolerance, the intensity of pain that a person is willing to endure, varies from person to person and even within the same person depending on coping skills, past experiences with pain, energy level, and motivation to endure pain. Identifying the patient's pain tolerance is critical to providing pain relief. (Schick L, Windle PE. *PeriAnesthesia Nursing Core Curriculum: Preprocedure, Phase I and Phase II PACU Nursing.* 3rd ed. St. Louis, MO: Saunders; 2016:437t; Pasero C, McCaffery M. *Pain assessment and pharmacologic management.* St. Louis, Mo.: Elsevier/Mosby; 2011: 291-293.)

7-29. *Correct answer:* **d**

Dantrolene pretreatment is no longer recommended as a standard of care. The best course of action would be to avoid all triggering agents. (Odom-Forren J. *Drain's Perianesthesia Nursing: A Critical Care Approach.* 6th ed. St. Louis, MO: Saunders; 2013:401.)

7-30. *Correct answer:* **b**

Most people who take their pain medicine as directed by their doctor do not become addicted, even if they take the medicine for a long time. However, some people may be at a higher risk of becoming addicted than others. People who have been addicted to substances in the past or those with a family member who is or has been addicted to drugs or alcohol may be at increased risk of becoming addicted to opioids; however, fear of addiction is not a reason to avoid opioids to effectively relieve pain, and drugs other than opioids can be used to manage pain. (Odom-Forren J. *Drain's Perianesthesia Nursing: A Critical Care Approach.* 6th ed. St. Louis, MO: Saunders; 2013:444.)

7-31. *Correct answer:* **d**

According to ASPAN Practice Recommendation 1, safe staffing should reflect patient acuity. Because the second patient in this question is an ASA IV and has an extensive cardiac history, the nurse should be concerned about the hemodynamic instability. The needs of the second patient may prevent the nurse from providing proper care and monitoring for the first patient. (American Society of PeriAnesthesia Nurses. Practice Recommendation 1. Patient classification/staffing recommendations. In: *2015-2017 Perianesthesia Nursing Standards, Practice Recommendations and Interpretive Statements.* Cherry Hill, NJ: ASPAN; 2014:34-38.)

7-32. *Correct answer:* **d**

Clinical practice guidelines are systematically developed statements or guides designed to provide a key link between evidence-based knowledge and health care practice. (Odom-Forren J. *Drain's Perianesthesia Nursing: A Critical Care Approach.* 6th ed. St. Louis, MO: Saunders; 2012:78.)

7-33. *Correct answer:* **c**

Hypercarbia is the most commonly presenting symptom associated with malignant hyperthermia. (Odom-Forren J. *Drain's Perianesthesia Nursing: A Critical Care Approach.* 6th ed. St. Louis, MO: Saunders; 2013:401.)

7-34. *Correct answer:* **c**

The National Patient Safety goal for 2017 published by The Joint Commission (NPSG.06.01.01) directs nurses and hospitals to "make improvements to ensure that alarms on medical equipment are heard and responded to on time." (The Joint Commission. 2017 National Patient Safety Goals. Retrieved December 5, 2016, from https://www.jointcommission.org/assets/1/6/2017_NPSG_HAP_ER.pdf; Schick L, Windle PE. *PeriAnesthesia Nursing Core Curriculum: Preprocedure, Phase I and Phase II PACU Nursing.* 3rd ed. St. Louis, MO: Saunders; 2016:34.)

7-35. *Correct answer:* **c**

Children 3 years of age and older are able to utilize the Wong-Baker Faces Scale, which consists of six cartoon faces showing increasing degrees of distress. Face 0 signifies "no hurt" and face 5 the "worst hurt you can imagine." The child chooses the face that best describes pain at the time of assessment. (Odom-Forren J. *Drain's Perianesthesia Nursing: A Critical Care Approach.* 6th ed. St. Louis, MO: Saunders; 2013:433.)

7-36. *Correct answer:* **c**

The first action that should be taken in the presentation of malignant hyperthermia is the discontinuation of all triggering agents. The patient should then be hyperventilated with 100% oxygen and the procedure should be terminated as soon as possible. (Odom-Forren J. *Drain's Perianesthesia Nursing: A Critical Care Approach.* 6th ed. St. Louis, MO: Saunders; 2013:401.)

7-37. *Correct answer:* **d**

When taking an opiate for an extended period, the patient may become less sensitive to it, which in turn necessitates an increase in dosage to obtain the same effect. Patients experiencing physical dependence can experience withdrawal syndrome caused by abrupt cessation, rapid dose reduction, decreasing blood level of the drug, and/or administration of an antagonist. It is possible to be physically dependent without being addicted. This patient should be monitored for symptoms of withdrawal such as chills, abdominal cramping, and joint pain. (Schick L, Windle PE. *PeriAnesthesia Nursing Core Curriculum: Preprocedure, Phase I and Phase II PACU Nursing.* 3rd ed. St. Louis, MO: Saunders; 2016:437; Pasero C, McCaffery M. *Pain assessment and pharmacologic management.* St. Louis, Mo.: Elsevier/Mosby; 2011: 297-298.)

7-38. *Correct answer:* **d**

There are several reasons that infants are at risk for hypothermia. These include the fact that their head and body surface area are proportionately larger, they have less subcutaneous fat, and there is a decreased ability to produce heat. An infant can lose up to 75% of body heat through exposure of head to room air. Also, there is no shiver response in infants younger than 3 months of age. (Schick L, Windle PE. *PeriAnesthesia Nursing Core Curriculum: Preprocedure, Phase I and Phase II PACU Nursing.* 3rd ed. St. Louis, MO: Saunders; 2016:201.)

7-39. *Correct answer:* **d**

Preoperative active warming has been shown to reduce the incidence of unplanned perioperative hypothermia. (Schick L, Windle PE. *Perianesthesia Nursing Core Curriculum: Preprocedure, Phase I and Phase II PACU Nursing.* 3rd ed. St. Louis, MO: Saunders; 2016:411.)

7-40. *Correct answer:* **c**

There are no objective measures of pain, which makes the assessment of the sensation completely subjective. "Pain is whatever the experiencing person says it is, existing whenever he says it does." (Schick L, Windle PE. *PeriAnesthesia Nursing Core Curriculum:*

Preprocedure, Phase I and Phase II PACU Nursing. 3rd ed. St. Louis, MO: Saunders; 2016:436.)

7-41. *Correct answer:* **a**

Tolerance is most commonly seen when a decrease in the duration of analgesia for a given opioid dose occurs. Physical dependence can happen with the chronic use of many drugs, including but not limited to opioids, and refers to a state resulting from chronic use of a drug that may produce tolerance and where negative physical symptoms of withdrawal result from abrupt discontinuation or dosage reduction. Addiction, on the other hand, is the compulsive use of a drug despite harmful consequences. It is characterized by an inability to stop using a drug and the failure to meet work, social, or family obligations. (Schick L, Windle PE. *PeriAnesthesia Nursing Core Curriculum: Preprocedure, Phase I and Phase II PACU Nursing.* 3rd ed. St. Louis, MO: Saunders; 2016:437t; Odom-Forren J. *Drain's Perianesthesia Nursing : A Critical Care Approach.* 6th ed. St Louis, Missouri: Elsevier; 2013: 444-445.)

7-42. *Correct answer:* **a**

Intravenous insulin and glucose are a standard treatment for the management of hyperkalemia in a malignant hyperthermia episode. The insulin helps to shift the potassium back into the intracellular space, lowering the overall serum concentration of potassium. (Schick L, Windle PE. *PeriAnesthesia Nursing Core Curriculum: Preprocedure, Phase I and Phase II PACU Nursing.* 3rd ed. St. Louis, MO: Saunders; 2016: 418-419.)

7-43. *Correct answer:* **b**

Around-the-clock (ATC) dosing should be considered when pain is anticipated to be continuous. Administering the pain medication around the clock prevents undertreatment of pain, which would be highly likely in a patient who is unable to communicate. Insertion of a gastrostomy tube may be painful, making it highly likely that she will experience pain for at least the next 48 hours. (Odom-Forren J. *Drain's Perianesthesia Nursing: A Critical Care Approach.* 6th ed. St. Louis, MO: Saunders; 2012:552.)

7-44. *Correct answer:* **c**

Preemptive analgesia is defined as the implementation of interventions prior to the onset of a noxious stimulus or injury in order to reduce the centrally mediated response to the stimulus. (Schick L, Windle PE. *PeriAnesthesia Nursing Core Curricu Preprocedure, Phase I and Phase II PACU Nursing.* 3rd ed. St. Louis, MO: Saunders; 2016:444-445.)

7-45. *Correct answer:* **c**

Chickenpox is an example of a disease that is transmitted by airborne droplets. (Odom-Forren J. *Drain's Perianesthesia Nursing: A Critical Care Approach.* 6th ed. St. Louis, MO: Saunders; 2013:803.)

7-46. *Correct answer:* **d**

During transport, the patient should be masked to protect persons along the route of tranport. Personnel who transport the patient need not be masked. (Odom-Forren J. *Drain's Perianesthesia Nursing: A Critical Care Approach.* 6th ed. St. Louis, MO: Saunders; 2013:48.)

7-47. *Correct answer:* **a**

According to the American Pain Society, the lowest effective dose for the shortest time needed is a key principle when developing the plan. (Odom-Forren J. *Drain's Perianesthesia Nursing: A Critical Care Approach.* 6th ed. St. Louis, MO: Saunders; 2013:427-449.)

7-48. *Correct answer:* **c**

Patients should be monitored for malignant hyperthermia recurrence for 24 to 48 hours. (Odom-Forren J. *Drain's Perianesthesia Nursing: A Critical Care Approach.* 6th ed. St. Louis, MO: Saunders; 2013:747; American Society of PeriAnesthesia Nurses., Schick L, Windle PE. *PeriAnesthesia Nursing Core Curriculum : Preprocedure, Phase I and Phase II, PACU nursing.* 3rd ed. St. Louis, MO: Saunders; 2016: 418.)

7-49. *Correct answer:* **b**

Gas flow valves on the bag should be open to allow oxygen to flow through the bag. (Chameides C, Samson R, Schexnayder S, Hazinski M. Resources for management of respiratory emergencies. In: *Pediatric Advanced Life Support Provider Manual.* Dallas, TX: American Heart Association; 2011:61-67.)

7-50. *Correct answer:* **b**

According to the American Society of PeriAnesthesia Nurses (ASPAN), the perianesthesia registered nurse uses clinical judgment and critical thinking to determine nurse-to-patient ratios, patient mix, and staffing mix that accommodate patient complexity and nursing care requirements. (American Society of PeriAnesthesia Nurses. Practice Recommendation 1. Patient classification/staffing recommendations. In: *2015-2017 Perianesthesia Nursing Standards, Practice Recommendations and Interpretive Statements.* Cherry Hill, NJ: ASPAN; 2014:34-40.)

7-51. *Correct answer:* **b**

Documented risk factors for postoperative nausea and vomiting (PONV) include female gender, nonsmoking status, postoperative opioid use, and a personal and family history of motion sickness or PONV. Other risk factors include type of surgery or procedure, type and dose of anesthetic agents used, and length of surgery or procedure. (Schick L, Windle PE. *PeriAnesthesia Nursing Core Curriculum: Preprocedure, Phase I and Phase II PACU Nursing.* 3rd ed. St. Louis, MO: Saunders; 2016:424-426.)

7-52. *Correct answer:* **b**

Extremes of ages, female gender, normal or below-normal body mass index (BMI), length and type of surgical procedure, and body surface area/wound area uncovered are all risk factors for the development of unplanned perioperative hypothermia. (Odom-Forren J. *Drain's Perianesthesia Nursing: A Critical Care Approach.* 6th ed. St. Louis, MO: Saunders; 2013:742.)

7-53. *Correct answer:* **b**

After pharmacologic interventions, physiologic comfort measures such as repositioning the patient or using heat or cold therapies are identified. The next most successful intervention to relieve or decrease pain is family visitation. The other three interventions listed in this question are not indicated as useful in the clinical practice guideline. (Odom-Forren J. *Drain's Perianesthesia Nursing: A Critical Care Approach.* 6th ed. St. Louis, MO: Saunders; 2013:773.)

7-54. *Correct answer:* **c**

Nurses working in the perianesthesia environment should be aware that some drugs are associated with the development of drug-induced parkinsonism, akathisia, acute dystonic reactions, and tardive dyskinesia. Medications that are associated with these extrapyramidal effects include chlorpromazine, haloperidol, and metoclopramide. (Odom-Forren J. *Drain's Perianesthesia Nursing: A Critical Care Approach.* 6th ed. St. Louis, MO: Saunders; 2013:108.)

7-55. *Correct answer:* **d**

Malignant hyperthermia is triggered by certain general inhalation agents, depolarizing neuromuscular blocking agents, and stress. (Odom-Forren J. *Drain's Perianesthesia Nursing: A Critical Care Approach.* 6th ed. St. Louis, MO: Saunders; 2013:744.)

7-56. *Correct answer:* **b**

Guidelines recommend that temperature be assessed every 15 minutes in the hypothermic patient. (Schick L, Windle PE. *PeriAnesthesia Nursing Core Curriculum: Preprocedure, Phase I and Phase II PACU Nursing.* 3rd ed. St. Louis, MO: Saunders; 2016:414.)

7-57. *Correct answer:* **d**

The creation of the CO_2 pneumoperitoneum has several adverse effects on the cardiovascular and respiratory systems. All these adverse effects are exacerbated by the commonly used Trendelenburg position. (Odom-Forren J. *Drain's Perianesthesia Nursing: A Critical Care Approach.* 6th ed. St. Louis, MO: Saunders; 2013:668-670.)

7-58. *Correct answer:* **a**

The most accurate core temperature measurement is obtained via a pulmonary artery catheter because the artery bathes the catheter with blood from the core compartment and its surroundings. (Schick L, Windle PE. *PeriAnesthesia Nursing Core Curriculum: Preprocedure, Phase I and Phase II PACU Nursing.* St. Louis, MO: Saunders; 2016:402.)

7-59. *Correct answer:* **d**

According to the American Society of PeriAnesthesia Nurses' Practice Recommendation 7, the nurse who is managing the care of the patient receiving sedation shall have no other responsibilities that would leave the patient unattended or compromise continuous monitoring. The second nurse is needed to assist the physician, leaving the first nurse to monitor the patient throughout the procedure. (American Society of PeriAnesthesia Nurses. Practice Recommendation 7. The role of the registered nurse in the management of patients undergoing sedation for short-term therapeutic, diagnostic or surgical procedures. In: *2015-2017 Perianesthesia Nursing Standards, Practice Recommendations and Interpretive Statements.* Cherry Hill, NJ: ASPAN; 2014:62-65.)

7-60. *Correct answer:* **a**

Tachycardia can be an indication of hemorrhage, pain, fever, and dehydration. Patients with severe hyperthermia can also present with hypotension and cardiac failure. (Schick L, Windle PE. *PeriAnesthesia Nursing Core Curriculum: Preprocedure, Phase I and Phase II PACU Nursing.* 3rd ed. St. Louis, MO: Saunders; 2016:606; Odom-Forren J. *Drain's Perianesthesia Nursing: A Critical Care Approach.* 6th ed. St Louis, MO: Saunders; 2013: 398-401.)

7-61. *Correct answer:* **d**

When a patient presents with low hemoglobin, a high SpO_2 value might not reflect adequate oxygenation. Even if well-saturated with hemoglobin, fewer hemoglobin carriers are available to transport oxygen and may be inadequate to meet tissue needs. (Odom-Forren J. *Drain's Perianesthesia Nursing: A Critical Care Approach.* 6th ed. St. Louis, MO: Saunders; 2013:356-357.)

7-62. *Correct answer:* **b**

In addition to certain medications such as antimicrobials and steroids, nondepolarizing neuromuscular blocking agent–induced paralysis can be enhanced by physiologic imbalances such as respiratory acidosis, dehydration, hypercapnia, hypokalemia, hyponatremia, hypermagnesemia, and hypothermia. (Schick L, Windle PE. *PeriAnesthesia Nursing Core Curriculum: Preprocedure, Phase I and Phase II PACU Nursing.* 3rd ed. St. Louis, MO: Saunders; 2016:386.)

7-63. *Correct answer:* **a**

Anesthesia places the patient at risk for hypoventilation. Older patients metabolize drugs at a slower rate and therefore are at increased risk for hypoventilation during the postanesthesia period. The patient with acute stroke is at risk for respiratory compromise from aspiration, upper airway obstruction, hypoventilation and (rarely) neurogenic pulmonary edema. (Sinz E, Navarro E. *Advanced Cardiovascular Life Support Provider Manual.* Dallas, TX: American Heart Association; 2011:139.)

7-64. *Correct answer:* **c**

Prudent perianesthesia nurses are aware of the potential complications related to prolonged or improper positioning during the surgical procedure. Also, during a lumbar laminectomy the surgeon does not routinely insert plates, screws, or bone grafts. (Odom-Forren J. *Drain's Perianesthesia Nursing: A Critical Care Approach.* 6th ed. St. Louis, MO: Saunders; 2013:348.)

7-65. *Correct answer:* **d**

Evidence has shown that prolonged surgery, greater than 3 hours, can precipitate the development of pressure ulcers within 4 days of surgery. This patient was lying in the same position for 4 hours without moving and was unable to sense pressure on a location of the body or change position. (Odom-Forren J. *Drain's Perianesthesia Nursing: A Critical Care Approach.* 6th ed. St. Louis, MO: Saunders; 2013: 348-351.)

8

Anesthesia and Malignant Hyperthermia

Theresa Clifford, Nancy Strzyzewski, and Vallire D. Hooper

8-1. During the anesthesia stage of delirium, the patient is at risk for:

a. Vomiting, bronchospasm, and cardiac arrest

b. Vomiting, laryngospasm, and cardiac arrest

c. Nausea, hypoxia, and cardiac dysrhythmia

d. Nausea, agitation, and cardiac dysrhythmia

8-2. While completing a Phase I PACU admission assessment, the nurse notes that the patient's respirations are irregular, RR 8, and difficult to count because they are shallow; the pupils are dilated and are not moving; the patient does not respond to verbal command; and the patient's general muscle tone appears to be slack. The nurse is concerned because it appears the patient is in which stage of anesthesia?

a. Analgesia

b. Delirium

c. Anesthesia

d. Overdose

8-3. During the preanesthesia nursing assessment, the nurse knows that malignant hyperthermia (MH) is an inherited disorder that affects:

a. The baroreceptors of the heart

b. Muscle metabolism

c. Cardiopulmonary gas exchange

d. Homeostatic thermoregulation

8-4. As the perianesthesia nurse is performing an admission assessment on a patient after general anesthesia, the patient states, "I am having trouble breathing." The BP is 180/70, RR 8, and the SpO$_2$ is 100%. During respiration, the chest wall and abdominal muscles are not working together in a coordinated effort. Considering this assessment, the nurse recognizes that the first drug the patient may need is a/an:

a. Vasoactive agent

b. Antiemetic

c. Reversal agent

d. Pain management agent

8-5. In the absence of a peripheral nerve stimulator, the best indication of a patient's readiness for extubation in the Phase I PACU is the ability to:

a. Follow verbal commands

b. Wiggle their fingers

c. Open their eyes

d. Lift the head for 5 seconds

8-6. The injection of a local anesthetic in the immediate vicinity of a major nerve plexus is termed a:

a. Conduction block

b. Infiltration anesthesia

c. Neuroaxial block

d. Peripheral nerve block

8-7. The primary role of the perianesthesia nurse when assisting the anesthesia provider during the placement of a regional anesthetic is to:

a. Assure appropriate patient position

b. Obtain adequate supplies

c. Monitor for patient response/complications

d. Administer sedation

8-8. It is important to instruct a patient in the use of slings or braces after partial motor blockade in order to:

a. Keep the surgical site protected
b. Prevent swelling in the affected extremity
c. Keep the affected extremity elevated
d. Prevent patient injury related to the insensate limb

8-9. In the same-day surgery unit, a patient expresses anxiety about the choice of anesthetics for a total knee replacement. The anesthesia provider has recommended a spinal block with sedation. The patient is concerned about being awake during the operation. The preadmission nurse offers reassurance and explains that there are medications commonly used for sedation. Drugs commonly used include all of the following EXCEPT:

a. Dexmedetomidine
b. Lorazepam
c. Flumazenil
d. Haloperidol

8-10. The Malignant Hyperthermia Association of the United States (MHAUS) recommends core temperature monitoring for all patients undergoing general anesthesia lasting more than _____ minutes.

a. 30
b. 60
c. 90
d. 120

8-11. A patient is resting with the eyes closed but responds easily to verbal commands. You would give the patient a Ramsay score of:

a. 1
b. 3
c. 5
d. 6

8-12. A 45-year-old male patient arrives in the Phase I PACU with weak peripheral reflexes and decreased ventilatory effort. The perianesthesia nurse notes that the RR is 8 and breath sounds are distant. What medications are most likely indicated for this patient?

a. Oxygen and naloxone
b. Naloxone and flumazenil
c. Glycopyrrolate and atropine
d. Neostigmine and glycopyrrolate

Consider this scenario for questions 8-13 and 8-14.

An 18-year-old patient with a history of advanced Duchenne muscular dystrophy arrived into the Phase I PACU after a brief anesthetic for a right myringotomy and tube. He has severe lower extremity contractures and has an indwelling suprapubic catheter. Anesthesia reports that the procedure was well tolerated after inhalation anesthesia using only sevoflurane.

8-13. The perianesthesia nurse completes an initial assessment noting that the patient's urine is the color of a cola beverage. This is a potential sign of:

a. Urine myoglobins
b. Ketoacidosis
c. Acute bladder injury
d. Polycystic kidneys

8-14. While calling for immediate anesthesia support to reassess the patient, the perianesthesia nurse begins to consider applying a urimeter to the suprapubic tube for more accurate urine output assessment. The renal goals for treating a patient with a malignant hyperthermia (MH) event include ensuring a urinary output of:

a. 1 mL/kg/h
b. 2 mL/kg/h
c. 3 mL/kg/h
d. 4 mL/kg/h

8-15. Assessment of temperature is essential in the patient recovering from inhalation anesthesia because inhalation agents:

a. Stimulate the pituitary
b. Depress the pituitary
c. Stimulate the hypothalamus
d. Depress the hypothalamus

8-16. A patient with known susceptibility to malignant hyperthermia (MH) has just undergone a surgical procedure using "safe" anesthetics. The patient should be monitored in the Phase II PACU for at least:

a. 1–1.5 hours
b. 2–2.5 hours
c. 3–3.5 hours
d. 4–4.5 hours

8-17. Rhabdomyolysis is an indication of:

a. Hyperthermia
b. Hypokalemia
c. Carbon dioxide retention
d. Release of dead muscle fibers into the bloodstream

8-18. Although a malignant hyperthermia (MH) event can be triggered at the first exposure of a patient to anesthesia, the average patient will demonstrate the first signs of MH after _____ anesthetics.

a. Two
b. Three
c. Four
d. Five

8-19. The three states with a high incidence of malignant hyperthermia (MH) are:

a. Alaska, Hawaii, and Oregon
b. Wisconsin, Michigan, and West Virginia
c. Maine, Massachusetts, and Rhode Island
d. Florida, Mississippi, and Louisiana

8-20. An _____ attaches to a specific receptor to block the neurotransmitter from stimulating the receptor.

a. Agonist
b. Activator
c. Antagonist
d. Actualizer

8-21. Signs that a malignant hyperthermia (MH) crisis is resolving include declining end-tidal carbon dioxide ($ETCO_2$), declining temperature, and:

a. Increasing heart rate
b. Spontaneous return of circulation
c. Spontaneous return of ventilation
d. Decreasing heart rate

8-22. The goals of therapy for a patient experiencing malignant hyperthermia (MH) include prompt administration of dantrolene, treatment of hyperkalemia, rapid cooling, and:

a. Initiation of cardiopulmonary bypass
b. Hyperventilation
c. Rapid extubation
d. Treatment of hyperglycemia

8-23. A malignant hyperthermia cart must be available wherever anesthesia is administered. Kits stored in the cart include all of the following EXCEPT:

a. Lumbar puncture kit
b. Central venous pressure sets
c. Pulmonary artery catheter kits
d. Transducer kits for arterial cannulation

8-24. A patient with a history of myasthenia gravis presents in the Phase I PACU after administration of a general anesthetic with a muscle relaxant. The primary symptom that the nurse will be monitoring for is:

a. Postoperative delirium
b. Postoperative nausea and vomiting
c. Excessive sedation
d. Prolonged muscle weakness

8-25. Given that malignant hyperthermia (MH) is a high-risk, low-frequency event, perianesthesia nurses should take advantage of several methods available for ongoing competency training. The Malignant Hyperthermia Association of the United States (MHAUS) recommends:

a. Completing a monthly MH quiz
b. Contacting MH hotline consultants for training support
c. Conducting mock MH drills
d. Reviewing case scenarios

8-26. Agents known to be safely administered to patients with malignant hyperthermia susceptibility (MHS) include:

a. Propofol
b. Desflurane
c. Sevoflurane
d. Isoflurane

8-27. Sevoflurane is known to cause:

a. Myocardial and respiratory depression
b. Myocardial and respiratory stimulation
c. Respiratory depression and rapid emergence
d. Respiratory stimulation and rapid emergence

8-28. A 45-year-old male patient is transferred from the operating room to the Phase I PACU after open rotator cuff repair. During the preanesthesia assessment, the patient reported a history of emergence delirium related to posttraumatic stress disorder. The anesthesia provider has initiated a dexmedetomidine infusion to provide sedation to allow a slower, calmer emergence. The MOST concerning side effect that the perianesthesia nurse must monitor the patient for is:

a. Respiratory depression
b. Hypothermia
c. Malignant hyperthermia
d. Bradycardia

8-29. A 16-year-old field hockey player is recovering from an open reduction of a fractured ankle. Ten minutes earlier she was given a popliteal nerve block to support a multimodal approach to pain management. The

young patient begins to complain of tinnitus and dizziness. The perianesthesia nurse anticipates the following recommended treatment for this patient:

a. Diphenhydramine 25 mg
b. Diphenhydramine 50 mg
c. Lipid emulsion 10%
d. Lipid emulsion 20%

8-30. Dantrolene belongs to the drug class:

a. Nucleoside reverse transcriptase inhibitor
b. Skeletal muscle relaxant
c. Antipyretic
d. Antihypercapnia agent

8-31. An example of a long-acting nondepolarizing neuromuscular blocking agent (NMBA) is:

a. Pancuronium bromide
b. Vecuronium bromide
c. Atracurium besylate
d. Rocuronium bromide

8-32. After flat foot reconstruction surgery on a 42-year-old middle-school teacher, the anesthesia provider orders a continuous infusion of ropivacaine via popliteal nerve block and catheter. The perianesthesia nurse understands that ropivacaine:

a. Has a duration of 6 to 8 hours
b. Produces high cardiotoxicity
c. Is classified as a low-potency amino amide
d. May have slightly less effect on motor nerves

8-33. A 24-year-old adopted male patient engaged to be married in the fall has been told that he is at risk for malignant hyperthermia (MH). He is understandably anxious about the possibility of passing on this susceptibility to any offspring. The nurse interviewing this patient knows that the most definitive test for MH is:

a. Serial serum lab studies
b. Allergy testing
c. Caffeine-halothane contracture test
d. Thermoregulation challenge test

8-34. Inhalation agents disrupt the regulation of body temperature by depressing the effect of the:

a. Brainstem
b. Cerebral cortex
c. Frontal lobe
d. Hypothalamus

8-35. A 35-year-old patient has been in the Phase I PACU for 90 minutes after general anesthesia. Although the plan was to extubate her immediately after surgery, she remains intubated and on a ventilator. Respiratory parameters are measured; her tidal volume is 100 mL and inspiratory force is negative 20 cm H_2O. Reversal agents were given twice. Which genetic disorder is the patient suspected to have?

a. Malignant serotonin syndrome
b. Malignant hyperthermia
c. Neuroleptic malignant syndrome
d. Atypical pseudocholinesterase

8-36. An 82-year-old patient is reintubated in the Phase I PACU. A propofol infusion is initiated. Understanding the pharmacology of propofol, the nurse closely monitors the patient for a:

a. Profound decrease in blood pressure
b. Profound increase in blood pressure
c. Increase in cardiac output
d. Sharp decrease in pulse

8-37. Upon arrival to the Phase I PACU after a total hip replacement with spinal anesthesia, the patient tells the nurse, "I don't feel well. I feel like I am going to vomit. My arms feel funny and I can't feel myself breathe." The nurse suspects:

a. Acute stroke
b. Rapid transport
c. Fluid deficit
d. High spinal block

8-38. Midazolam should be administered with caution in patients with myocardial ischemia because midazolam produces:

a. Decrease in BP, increase in HR, and reduction in SVR
b. Increase in BP, increase in HR, and no change in SVR

c. Decrease in BP, decrease in HR, and reduction in SVR
d. Increase in BP, increase in HR, and increase in SVR

8-39. A patient experiences chest wall rigidity during the administration of moderate sedation. The agent most likely associated with this incident is:

a. Fentanyl
b. Midazolam
c. Morphine
d. Propofol

8-40. Dantrolene sodium requires dilution. The most appropriate diluent is:

a. Sterile saline with a bacteriostatic agent
b. Sterile saline without a bacteriostatic agent
c. Sterile water with a bacteriostatic agent
d. Sterile water without a bacteriostatic agent

8-41. Immediate nursing interventions for a patient experiencing a high spinal block may include:

a. Oxygen and assistance with a bag valve mask
b. Oxygen and treatment for postoperative nausea
c. Oxygen, computed tomography (CT) scan, and thrombolytic therapy
d. Oxygen and fluid bolus followed by vasopressors

8-42. What is the peak action of hydromorphone?

a. 1 to 5 minutes
b. 5 to 20 minutes
c. 10 to 20 minutes
d. 15 to 20 minutes

8-43. Common signs of malignant hyperthermia that follow an increase in end-tidal carbon dioxide ($ETCO_2$) include tachycardia, tachypnea, and:

a. Masseter spasm
b. Sudden drop in $ETCO_2$
c. Piloerection
d. Complete pharyngeal relaxation

8-44. A patient becomes obtunded with RR of 6 after intravenous administration of 50 mcg of fentanyl. The most appropriate reversal agent for this patient would be:

a. Atropine
b. Flumazenil
c. Naloxone
d. Neostigmine

8-45. Complications after an acute malignant hyperthermia (MH) crisis include:

a. Acute renal failure
b. Cardiomyopathy
c. Permanent muscle contractures
d. Acute hepatic failure

8-46. A patient experiences fixed chest syndrome after the administration of fentanyl. The FIRST thing that the nurse should do is:

a. Elevate the head of the bed
b. Encourage the patient to cough
c. Obtain an order for naloxone
d. Anticipate the need for succinylcholine

8-47. Temperature elevation associated with malignant hyperthermia (MH):

a. Often occurs immediately
b. Occurs after the patient is brought to the Phase I PACU
c. Occurs as a late sign of an MH event
d. Occurs before a rise in end-tidal carbon dioxide ($ETCO_2$) but after masseter spasms

8-48. Ketamine is contraindicated in patients who are at risk for:

a. Cardiovascular shock
b. Increased intracranial pressure
c. Reactive airway disease
d. Decreased intracranial pressure

8-49. During the preoperative assessment, the patient tells the nurse, "I don't react well to anesthesia. The last time I had surgery, I had horrible muscle pain in my neck and back the next day. It even hurt to blink my eyes and smile." The nurse suspects this discomfort was due to:

a. Surgical positioning
b. Ketamine
c. Succinylcholine
d. Rocuronium

8-50. The nurse is preparing to review discharge instructions with a patient after general anesthesia during which ketamine was given. Understanding the pharmacodynamics of ketamine, what action does the nurse take before beginning the discussion?

a. Medicate the patient for pain
b. Discontinue the peripheral line
c. Ambulate the patient to the bathroom
d. Bring the family to the bedside

8-51. In an effort to reduce the severity of vivid dreaming, confusion, and hallucinations associated with intraoperative ketamine administration, the perianesthesia nurse should:

a. Avoid verbal and tactile stimulation
b. Encourage the family to awaken the patient
c. Have the patient deep-breathe and cough
d. Avoid the administration of any additional pain management agents

8-52. Adverse effects of dantrolene include transient muscle weakness, gastrointestinal upset, ventilatory compromise, and:

a. Phlebitis
b. Hyperactivity
c. Oliguria
d. Polycythemia

8-53. The nurse administers two opioid doses to a patient just arriving in the Phase I PACU before realizing that the patient received naloxone at the end of the case in the operating room. The nurse's primary focus should be to monitor the patient for:

a. Excessive pain
b. Respiratory depression
c. Hallucinations
d. Chest wall rigidity

8-54. Ketamine is a valuable anesthetic agent because:

a. Pharyngeal and laryngeal reflexes remain intact
b. Potential for postoperative nausea is increased
c. Systolic blood pressure is only slightly decreased
d. Diastolic blood pressure is only slightly decreased

8-55. A patient is suspected of having a malignant hyperthermia (MH) event. Laboratory work is drawn. Creatine kinase (CK) results are back. Elevated CK indicates:

a. Rising calcium levels
b. Falling calcium levels
c. Muscle breakdown
d. Decompensated acidosis

8-56. Laboratory tests during the acute phase of malignant hyperthermia (MH) are required. These include:

a. Creatine kinase, myoglobins, and comprehensive metabolic panel (CMP)
b. Partial thromboplastin time, glucose, and blood cultures
c. Acetylcholinesterase, C-reactive protein, and complete blood count
d. Prothrombin time, fibrinogen, and immunoglobulins

8-57. A 34-year-old patient becomes restless and agitated in the postanesthesia care unit. Midazolam 0.2 mg/kg is administered as per physician order. Understanding the pharmacology of this drug, the perianesthesia nurse ensures:

a. Postoperative nausea and vomiting (PONV) is assessed
b. Restraints are readily available
c. Family is at the bedside
d. Oxygen is available

Consider this scenario for questions 8-58 to 8-62.

A 57-year-old, 70-kg male patient presents to the ambulatory surgery unit for an elective open acromioplasty. His medical history includes type 2 diabetes, arthritis, hypertension, and hypercholesterolemia. Current medications include atorvastatin calcium, lisinopril, hydroxychloroquine, methotrexate, folic acid, and tramadol. The patient has had prior uneventful general anesthetics. Anesthesia patient classification is an American Society of Anesthesiologists (ASA) physical status II.

8-58. Within 25 minutes of premedication with midazolam 2 mg, fentanyl 100 mg, and cefazolin 1 gm, as well as anesthesia induction using succinylcholine 100 mg IV, the end-tidal carbon dioxide ($ETCO_2$) rose from 41 to 114. The most probable cause of a rapid rise in $ETCO_2$ is:

a. Obstruction of oxygen flow via airway adjuncts
b. Worsening of chronic bronchitis during intubation
c. Uncontrolled hypermetabolism
d. Cardiovascular collapse

8-59. While the perioperative circulating nurse calls the Malignant Hyperthermia Association of the United States (MHAUS), the anesthesia provider orders an initial bolus of dantrolene. Based on the stated weight of 70 kg, the first dose for this patient should be:

a. 25 mg
b. 125 mg
c. 150 mg
d. 175 mg

8-60. After a total of 45 minutes from the onset of symptoms, the cardiac monitor begins to display ventricular arrhythmias. The perianesthesia nurse anticipates preparing for the administration of:

a. Amiodarone
b. Diltiazem
c. Furosemide
d. Propranolol

8-61. After stabilization, the patient is monitored in a critical care unit for development of complications. Dantrolene will be administered to treat any recurrence of the symptoms of malignant hyperthermia (MH) for a period of:

a. 12 to 24 hours
b. 24 to 36 hours
c. 36 to 48 hours
d. 48 to 72 hours

8-62. When a malignant hyperthermia (MH) crisis is identified, it is important to suspend aggressive cooling measures to avoid hypothermia when the core temperature of the patient reaches:

a. 36° C
b. 36.5° C
c. 37° C
d. 38° C

8-63. During the report from the anesthesia provider, the postanesthesia nurse is told a remifentanil infusion was used throughout the case. What questions should the nurse ask?

a. When was the drug initiated, and how did the blood pressure respond?
b. When was the drug initiated, and how many milligrams were given?

c. When was the drug discontinued, and was any vasopressor used?
d. When was the drug discontinued, and was any other opioid given?

8-64. Following report that the patient received a neuromuscular blockade in the operating room, what assessment should the nurse perform on this patient?

a. Head lift and hand grip
b. Leg lift and hand grip
c. Facial symmetry and leg lift
d. Visual fields and leg lift

8-65. The hyperkalemia associated with a malignant hyperthermia (MH) crisis is treated with a combination of glucose and:

a. Rapid-acting insulin
b. Short-acting insulin
c. Intermediate-acting insulin
d. Long-acting insulin

Answers and Rationales for Chapter 8, Anesthesia and Malignant Hyperthermia

8-1. *Correct answer:* **b**
This stage of anesthesia begins as the patient is losing consciousness and ends with the loss of protective reflexes. These reflexes include the laryngeal and pharyngeal reflexes (gag and swallow), which protect the lungs from aspiration of gastric contents. This stage is characterized by "excitement." Several untoward responses such as vomiting, laryngospasm, and even cardiac arrest can take place during this stage. (Odom-Forren J. *Drain's Perianesthesia Nursing: A Critical Care Approach.* 6th ed. St. Louis, MO: Saunders; 2013:255.)

8-2. *Correct answer:* **c**
During the stage of analgesia, the patient is able to open the eyes on command and breathe normally. During the stages of anesthesia and overdose, respirations are erratic or absent. The stage of delirium is marked by dilated, nonmoving pupils and a regular pattern of breathing. The patient has lost consciousness as physiologically the patient is either moving toward the stage of anesthesia or emerging from anesthesia. Understanding the stages of anesthesia is essential to the perianesthesia nurse because the patient must pass through the stage of delirium during recovery from anesthesia and may be admitted to postanesthesia care while in the stage of delirium. While in the stage of delirium, the patient is at risk for vomiting, aspiration, and cardiac arrest. Therefore, the nurse must provide vigilant assessment and monitoring during this stage of anesthesia. (Odom-Forren J. *Drain's Perianesthesia Nursing: A Critical Care Approach.* 6th ed. St. Louis, MO: Saunders; 2013:254-255.)

8-3. *Correct answer:* **b**
Malignant hyperthermia (MH) is a genetic abnormality of muscle metabolism initiated by certain triggering agents and resulting in a hypermetabolic state. (Odom-Forren J. *Drain's Perianesthesia Nursing: A Critical Care Approach.* 6th ed. St. Louis, MO: Saunders; 2013:401.)

8-4. *Correct answer:* **c**
During normal respiration in the adult patient, the chest and abdomen rise and fall in one coordinated motion. This lack of coordinated muscle movement during respiration is known as *paradoxical motion* and indicates a lack of muscle strength. Hypertension and the patient's subjective complaint of difficulty breathing also indicate inadequate return of muscle strength. This patient is experiencing residual neuromuscular blockade or inadequate reversal. The priority medication for this patient is a reversal agent. (Schick L, Windle PE. *PeriAnesthesia Nursing Core Curriculum: Preprocedure, Phase I and Phase II Nursing.* 3rd ed. St. Louis, MO: Saunders; 2016:551-552.)

8-5. *Correct answer:* **d**
The ability to lift and hold one's head off a pillow for less than or equal to 5 seconds indicates adequate muscle function to independently maintain an airway. (Odom-Forren J. *Drain's Perianesthesia Nursing: A Critical Care Approach.* 6th ed. St. Louis, MO: Saunders; 2013:303.)

8-6. *Correct answer:* **a**
Per definition, a local anesthetic injected in the immediate vicinity of a major nerve plexus is a conduction block. These blocks are generally given in the brachial or lumbar plexus or as a neuraxial anesthetic. (Odom-Forren J. *Drain's Perianesthesia Nursing: A Critical Care Approach.* 6th ed. St. Louis, MO: Saunders; 2013:311.)

8-7. *Correct answer:* **c**
The primary role of the perianesthesia nurse when assisting with a regional block placement is to monitor the patient for adverse reactions. (Odom-Forren J. *Drain's Perianesthesia Nursing: A Critical Care Approach.* 6th ed. St. Louis, MO: Saunders; 2013:322.)

8-8. *Correct answer:* **d**
Patients should use slings or braces to prevent injury related to partial motor blockade and related lack of sensation and control. Patients should be advised to avoid movements that might cause injury due to the motor and sensory blockade. (Odom-Forren J. *Drain's Perianesthesia Nursing: A Critical Care Approach.* 6th ed. St. Louis, MO: Saunders; 2013:331, 335.)

8-9. *Correct answer:* **c**
Flumazenil is actually a benzodiazepine antagonist used to reverse the sedative effects of benzodiazepines such as diazepam and midazolam. (Odom-Forren J. *Drain's Perianesthesia Nursing: A Critical Care Approach.* 6th ed. St. Louis, MO: Saunders; 2013:696.)

8-10. *Correct answer:* **a**
Temperature elevation is a sign of an impending malignant hyperthermia (MH) crisis. The Malignant Hyperthermia Association of the United States (MHAUS) recommends core temperature monitoring for all patients undergoing general anesthesia lasting more than 30 minutes. Appropriate sites for continuous electronic core temperature monitoring include the esophagus, nasopharynx, bladder, and pulmonary artery. (Rosenberg H, Pollock N, Schiemann A, et al. *Malignant hyperthermia: a review.* Orphanet J Rare Dis. 2015;10(93):1-19.)

8-11. *Correct answer:* **b**
A Ramsay score of 3 indicates that the patient responds to commands. (Schick L, Windle PE. *PeriAnesthesia Nursing Core Curriculum: Preprocedure, Phase I and Phase II Nursing.* 3rd ed. St. Louis, MO: Saunders; 2016:338t.)

8-12. *Correct answer:* **d**
To restore neuromuscular transmission back to normal, an antiacetylcholinesterase is needed to block acetylcholinesterase from metabolizing acetylcholine at the neuromuscular junction. Acetylcholine displaces the competitive neuromuscular blocking agent from the muscle cell so the cell can depolarize and muscle movement can occur. Neostigmine is the anticholinesterase drug of choice. Anticholinesterase agents cause muscarinic effects such as bradycardia, salivation, miosis, and hyperperistalsis. To prevent these symptoms from occurring, an antimuscarinic drug must also be given with or immediately after an anticholinesterase drug is administered. Neostigmine is given to interfere with the breakdown of acetylcholine, and atropine or glycopyrrolate is given to treat the side effects from neostigmine. (Odom-Forren J. *Drain's Perianesthesia Nursing: A Critical Care Approach.* 6th ed. St. Louis, MO: Saunders; 2013:292-295.)

8-13. *Correct answer:* **a**
Patients with central core disease and other muscle diseases are at added risk for developing malignant hyperthermia (MH). During an evolving MH event, the urine may become dark and cola colored from the breakdown of myoglobin. Early recognition of MH is essential. (Odom-Forren J. *Drain's Perianesthesia Nursing: A Critical Care Approach.* 6th ed. St. Louis, MO: Saunders; 2013:401.)

8-14. *Correct answer:* **b**
Hydration and diuretics ensure urine output of at least 2 mL/kg/h. Urine output must be carefully monitored. (Odom-Forren J. *Drain's Perianesthesia Nursing: A Critical Care Approach.* 6th ed. St. Louis, MO: Saunders; 2013:401.)

8-15. *Correct answer:* **d**
Inhalation agents wield a depressant effect on the hypothalamus. This effect disrupts the regulation of body temperature that may lead to either hyperthermia or inadvertent hypothermia. (Odom-Forren J. *Drain's Perianesthesia Nursing: A Critical Care Approach.* 6th ed. St. Louis, MO: Saunders; 2013:262.)

8-16. *Correct answer:* **a**

In a malignant hyperthermia (MH)-susceptible patient, if no signs of MH are noted one hour postoperatively following an MH-safe anesthetic technique, it is unlikely that MH will occur. The patient should be monitored in a Phase II/step-down PACU for at least another hour to an hour and a half after the first hour in the Phase I PACU. MH-susceptible patients require close vital sign and temperature monitoring while in the PACU. (Odom-Forren J. *Drain's Perianesthesia Nursing: A Critical Care Approach.* 6th ed. St. Louis, MO: Saunders; 2013:401.)

8-17. *Correct answer:* **d**

Rhabdomyolysis refers to the breakdown of skeletal muscle, which is associated with excretion of myoglobin in the urine. Classically, malignant hyperthermia (MH) presents with hypercarbia, tachycardia, cardiac arrhythmias, pyrexia, rigidity, and metabolic acidosis, and rhabdomyolysis as a late sign. (Urden LD, Stacy KM, Lough ME. *Critical Care Nursing : Diagnosis and Management.* 7th ed. St. Louis, MO: Elsevier; 2014:704; Rosenberg H, Pollock N, Schiemann A, et al. *Malignant hyperthermia: a review.* Orphanet J Rare Dis. 2015;10(93):1-19.)

8-18. *Correct answer:* **b**

The incidence of malignant hyperthermia (MH) episodes during anesthesia is between 1:5,000 and 1:100,000 anesthetics. Even though an MH crisis may develop at first exposure to anesthesia with those agents known to trigger an MH episode, on average, patients require three anesthetics before triggering. Reactions develop more frequently in males than females (2:1). (Odom-Forren J. *Drain's Perianesthesia Nursing: A Critical Care Approach.* 6th ed. St. Louis, MO: Saunders; 2013:744-745; Rosenberg H, Pollock N, Schiemann A, et al. Malignant hyperthermia: a review. *Orphanet J Rare Dis.* 2015;10(93):1-19.)

8-19. *Correct answer:* **b**

Malignant hyperthermia (MH) averages approximately 600 cases per year in the United States. Current states with higher incidence of MH events include Wisconsin, Michigan, and West Virginia. (Odom-Forren J. *Drain's Perianesthesia Nursing: A Critical Care Approach.* 6th ed. St. Louis, MO: Saunders; 2013:744.)

8-20. *Correct answer:* **c**

An antagonist is a chemical agent that attaches to a specific receptor site for the purposes of blocking the stimulation and action of that site as opposed to activating the receptor. (Odom-Forren J. *Drain's Perianesthesia Nursing: A Critical Care Approach.* 6th ed. St. Louis, MO: Saunders; 2013:236.)

8-21. *Correct answer:* **d**

Ambulatory surgery facilities and hospitals should have a procedure and policy to transfer a stabilized malignant hyperthermia (MH) patient to an intensive or critical care unit (ICU). Signs of stability may include $ETCO_2$ declining or normal, heart rate stable or decreasing without dysrhythmias, initiation of dantrolene, declining temperature, and, if present, resolving generalized muscular rigidity. (Odom-Forren J. *Drain's Perianesthesia Nursing: A Critical Care Approach.* 6th ed. St. Louis, MO: Saunders; 2013:401.)

8-22. *Correct answer:* **b**

Immediate treatment of acute malignant hyperthermia (MH) includes discontinuation of any trigger agent, calling for help, and rapidly ventilating the patient's lungs with large tidal volumes with a bag–mask system and oxygen (total oxygen flow should exceed 15 L/min). (Odom-Forren J. *Drain's Perianesthesia Nursing: A Critical Care Approach.* 6th ed. St. Louis, MO: Saunders; 2013:401.)

8-23. *Correct answer:* **a**

Suggested supplies for a malignant hyperthermia cart include intravenous lines with assorted cannula gauges, central venous pressure sets, transducer kits for arterial and central venous cannulation, esophageal or other core temperature probes, pulmonary artery catheter, and laboratory test tubes for blood chemistry analysis. (Odom-Forren J. *Drain's Perianesthesia Nursing: A Critical Care Approach.* 6th ed. St. Louis, MO: Saunders; 2013:6,749.)

8-24. *Correct answer:* **d**

Myasthenia gravis is associated with prolonged neuromuscular blockade. (Odom-Forren J. *Drain's Perianesthesia Nursing: A Critical Care Approach.* 6th ed. St. Louis, MO: Saunders; 2013:678-679; Schick L, Windle PE. *PeriAnesthesia Nursing Core Curriculum: Preprocedure, Phase I and Phase II Nursing.* 3rd ed. St. Louis, MO: Saunders; 2016:185-188.)

8-25. *Correct answer:* **c**

Health care providers should maintain familiarity with current Malignant Hyperthermia Association of the United States (MHAUS) recommendations and guidelines. Conducting malignant hyperthermia (MH) crisis team training that includes the operating room, Phase I and Phase II PACU, and intensive or critical care teams as a part of ongoing and annual competency education will prepare the clinical team to recognize, respond to, and treat an MH crisis. Ongoing training may also include pharmacy, laboratory, and emergency medical services personnel to highlight their roles in MH preparedness, promote continued awareness, and safeguard patient safety. (American Association of Nurse Anesthetists. *Malignant Hyperthermia Crisis Preparedness and Treatment. Position Statement.* Park Ridge, IL: AANA; 2015:1-11.)

8-26. *Correct answer:* **a**

In general, ALL volatile inhalation agents, including desflurane, sevoflurane and isoflurane, are considered unsafe agents for patients with susceptibility to or known malignant hyperthermia. Agents that are considered safe for anesthesia in these patients include barbiturates and intravenous agents (e.g., propofol, ketamine, midazolam) as well as the gaseous inhalation agent nitrous oxide, opioids and anxiolytic drugs (e.g., diazepam, lorazepam, clonazepam).(Odom-Forren J. *Drain's Perianesthesia Nursing: A Critical Care Approach.* 6th ed. St. Louis, MO: Saunders; 2013:747-748.)

8-27. *Correct answer:* **c**

Although all inhalation agents, including sevoflurane, are known to cause respiratory depression, rapid emergence is the hallmark characteristic of this rapidly acting agent. (Schick L, Windle PE. *PeriAnesthesia Nursing Core Curriculum: Preprocedure, Phase I and Phase II Nursing.* 3rd ed. St. Louis, MO: Saunders; 2016:381-382.)

8-28. *Correct answer:* **d**

Intervention is necessary, including decreasing or stopping the dexmedetomidine infusion, and increasing the rate of intravenous fluid administration along with elevation of the lower extremities may be all that is needed. Other side effects may include nausea, hypotension, and dry mouth. (Odom-Forren J. *Drain's Perianesthesia Nursing: A Critical Care Approach.* 6th ed. St. Louis, MO: Saunders; 2013:145-147.)

8-29. *Correct answer:* **d**

Lipid emulsion therapy is thought to bind to local anesthetic molecules, which allows for a reduction in the amount of circulating molecules that can bind within the cardiovascular system. The current recommended preparation of lipids is a 20% emulsion. (Odom-Forren J. *Drain's Perianesthesia Nursing: A Critical Care Approach.* 6th ed. St. Louis, MO: Saunders; 2013:321-322.)

8-30. *Correct answer:* **b**

The drug dantrolene sodium effectively treats malignant hyperthermia (MH) with inhibition of further release of calcium in the skeletal muscle. It is classified as a muscle relaxant. (Odom-Forren J. *Drain's Perianesthesia Nursing: A Critical Care Approach.* 6th ed. St. Louis, MO: Saunders; 2013:747.)

8-31. *Correct answer:* **a**

Rocuronium bromide is classified as a short-acting nondepolarizing neuromuscular blocking agent (NMBA), whereas vecuronium bromide and atracurium besylate are intermediate acting. Of the drugs listed, pancuronium bromide is the only long-acting nondepolarizing NMBA. (Odom-Forren J. *Drain's Perianesthesia Nursing: A Critical Care Approach.* St. Louis, MO: Saunders; 2013:294.)

8-32. *Correct answer:* **d**

Ropivacaine is chemically similar to bupivacaine. It is a high-potency amino amide. Ropivacaine seems to be less cardiotoxic than bupivacaine; however, cardiotoxicity may still be of concern with slightly larger doses. Bupivacaine and ropivacaine both have more of an effect on sensory nerves than on motor nerves, although ropivacaine may have slightly less effect on motor nerves. (Schick L, Windle PE. *PeriAnesthesia Nursing Core Curriculum: Preprocedure, Phase I and Phase II PACU Nursing.* 3rd ed. St. Louis, MO: Saunders; 2016:352-353.)

8-33. *Correct answer:* **c**

The most definitive test for detection of malignant hyperthermia susceptibility (MHS) is the biopsy of skeletal muscle. Samples are obtained from the quadriceps muscle and are subjected to isometric contracture testing using a submersion of caffeine-halothane. (Schick L, Windle PE. *PeriAnesthesia Nursing Core Curriculum: Preprocedure, Phase I and Phase II PACU Nursing.* 3rd ed. St. Louis, MO: Saunders; 2016:417.)

8-34. *Correct answer:* **d**

Inhalation agents disrupt the regulation of body temperature through their action on the hypothalamus. (Odom-Forren J. *Drain's Perianesthesia Nursing: A Critical Care Approach.* 6th ed. St. Louis, MO: Saunders; 2013:262.)

8-35. *Correct answer:* **d**

Plasma cholinesterase is responsible for the metabolism of succinylcholine. Patients who have atypical pseudocholinesterase have a genetic variant that will either mildly or severely affect the rate at which succinylcholine is metabolized. This delay in metabolization will cause prolonged effect of the drug and may require the use of a ventilator. (Odom-Forren J. *Drain's Perianesthesia Nursing: A Critical Care Approach.* 6th ed. St. Louis, MO: Saunders; 2013:299.)

8-36. *Correct answer:* **a**

Propofol decreases blood pressure accompanied by a reduction in cardiac output or systemic vascular resistance. Because the drug has a sympatholytic or vagotonic effect, the pulse remains unchanged. The reduction in blood pressure is more pronounced in elderly patients. (Odom-Forren J. *Drain's Perianesthesia Nursing: A Critical Care Approach.* 6th ed. St. Louis, MO: Saunders; 2013:267.)

8-37. *Correct answer:* **d**

Excessive spread of local anesthesia that occurs with spinal anesthesia is a high spinal block. The symptoms the patient is experiencing are consistent with a high spinal block: upper extremity sensory and motor changes, respiratory distress, and apnea. (Odom-Forren J. *Drain's Perianesthesia Nursing: A Critical Care Approach.* 6th ed. St. Louis, MO: Saunders; 2013:330.)

8-38. *Correct answer:* **a**

Because midazolam produces a decrease in BP, an increase in HR, and a reduction in SVR, it should be used with caution in patients with myocardial ischemia because it increases the workload of the heart. (Odom-Forren J. *Drain's Perianesthesia Nursing: A Critical Care Approach.* 6th ed. St. Louis, MO: Saunders; 2013:269.)

8-39. *Correct answer:* **a**

Rapid intravenous injection of fentanyl may trigger bronchial constriction and chest wall rigidity, commonly called *fixed chest syndrome*. (Odom-Forren J. *Drain's Perianesthesia Nursing: A Critical Care Approach*. 6th ed. St. Louis, MO: Saunders; 2013:282.)

8-40. *Correct answer:* **d**

When the appropriate personnel arrive, more than one person should mix the dantrolene sodium (20 mg per 60 mL of sterile water). A note of warning is needed to ensure that the sterile water does not contain preservatives and that the entire 60 mL of sterile water will be used. (Odom-Forren J. *Drain's Perianesthesia Nursing: A Critical Care Approach*. 6th ed. St. Louis, MO: Saunders; 2013:708.)

8-41. *Correct answer:* **a**

High spinal blocks pose a threat to the patient's airway. Although the patient may also have hypotension with a high spinal block, the immediate concern is the patient's airway and inability to move the chest wall during inhalation and exhalation. The stem of this question does not mention anything about hypotension, but there is information the patient may be having respiratory issues. The best answer to this question is the one that offers airway management. (Odom-Forren J. *Drain's Perianesthesia Nursing: A Critical Care Approach*. 6th ed. St. Louis, MO: Saunders; 2013:330.)

8-42. *Correct answer:* **b**

The onset of action of hydromorphone is less than 60 seconds, and peak action is attained at 5 to 20 minutes (with an average of 30 minutes). (Odom-Forren J. *Drain's Perianesthesia Nursing: A Critical Care Approach*. 6th ed. St. Louis, MO: Saunders; 2013:242t.)

8-43. *Correct answer:* **a**

Unexpected tachycardia, tachypnea, and jaw muscle rigidity (masseter spasm) are often common signs of malignant hyperthermia (MH) that follow the significant CO_2 increase. (Odom-Forren J. *Drain's Perianesthesia Nursing: A Critical Care Approach*. 6th ed. St. Louis, MO: Saunders; 2013:745-746.)

8-44. *Correct answer:* **c**

Naloxone is the appropriate reversal agent for opioids. (Odom-Forren J. *Drain's Perianesthesia Nursing: A Critical Care Approach*. 6th ed. St. Louis, MO: Saunders; 2013:285.)

8-45. *Correct answer:* **a**

Renal failure can occur because of myoglobinuria or hypotension. Consumption coagulopathies, such as disseminated intravascular coagulation, have been reported along with acute heart failure and pulmonary edema. Because the brain is the organ most sensitive to hyperthermia (permanent brain damage can occur with temperatures greater than or equal to 41° C), brain deterioration can occur in patients who are not promptly treated. (Odom-Forren J. *Drain's Perianesthesia Nursing: A Critical Care Approach*. 6th ed. St. Louis, MO: Saunders; 2013:750.)

8-46. *Correct answer:* **d**

Symptoms of fixed chest syndrome are generally the result of the rapid injection of opioids. This leads to bronchial constriction resulting from ventilatory muscle rigidity and subsequent airway resistance. The intravenous administration of a subclinical dose of succinylcholine relieves the chest wall rigidity and allows for ventilation. (Odom-Forren J. *Drain's Perianesthesia Nursing: A Critical Care Approach*. 6th ed. St. Louis, MO: Saunders; 2013:282.)

8-47. *Correct answer:* **c**

Temperature elevation is often a late sign of malignant hyperthermia (MH). Temperature variations during MH are best detected with core temperature measurement (nasopharyngeal or oropharyngeal, esophageal, or pulmonary artery). (Odom-Forren J. *Drain's Perianesthesia Nursing: A Critical Care Approach*. 6th ed. St. Louis, MO: Saunders; 2013:746.)

8-48. *Correct answer:* **b**

As a dissociative agent, ketamine can produce a state of profound analgesia combined with a state of unconsciousness. Respiratory function is usually unimpaired, except after rapid intravenous injection, when it may become depressed for a short time. Ketamine is sympathomimetic in action and is beneficial to patients with asthma because of its bronchodilating effect. When patients receive ketamine, the pharyngeal and laryngeal reflexes remain intact. Ketamine accelerates the heart rate moderately and increases both the systolic and the diastolic pressure for several minutes, after which the pulse and blood pressure return to preinjection levels. Ketamine does increase cerebral blood flow and intracranial pressure and is therefore contraindicated in patients who are at risk for increased intracranial pressure. (Odom-Forren J. *Drain's Perianesthesia Nursing: A Critical Care Approach.* 6th ed. St. Louis, MO: Saunders; 2013:274-276.)

8-49. *Correct answer:* **c**

Typically, if succinylcholine is used during induction to prepare the patient for intubation, a single dose is given. A single dose of this drug is known to cause fasciculations or mini contractions as the muscle cell depolarizes after the drug has been given. These mini contractions or fasciculations frequently lead to muscle pain. (Odom-Forren J. *Drain's Perianesthesia Nursing: A Critical Care Approach.* 6th ed. St. Louis, MO: Saunders; 2013:300.)

8-50. *Correct answer:* **d**

Ketamine is classified as a dissociative agent. It produces dissociation of the thalamoneocortical and limbic systems. This mechanism of action interferes with the way the brain assigns meaning to everyday stimuli. Although the patient appears to be awake, the patient has no recall of surgery. This drug may be used at the beginning of anesthesia during induction or throughout the case for pain management. Use of this drug to manage pain allows the anesthesia provider to decrease the amount of opioids needed for pain management. If ketamine was administered during anesthesia, the patient may appear to understand discharge instructions, but due to the mechanism of action of this drug, the patient may not be able to understand or remember discharge instructions. Having a family member at the bedside during review of the discharge instructions will assist the nurse to provide a safe discharge for the patient. (Schick L, Windle PE. *PeriAnesthesia Nursing Core Curriculum: Preprocedure, Phase I and Phase II Nursing.* 3rd ed. St. Louis, MO: Saunders; 2016:364-366.)

8-51. *Correct answer:* **a**

The irrational behavior, hallucinations, and confusion generally associated with emergence from ketamine can be mediated by avoiding verbal and tactile stimulation of the patient. (Schick L, Windle PE. *PeriAnesthesia Nursing Core Curriculum: Preprocedure, Phase I and Phase II Nursing.* 3rd ed. St. Louis, MO: Saunders; 2016:364-366.)

8-52. *Correct answer:* **a**

Adverse effects of dantrolene in short-term administration are minor and may include phlebitis in 9% of cases, transient muscle weakness in 21%, gastrointestinal upset in 4%, and respiratory compromise in patients with preexisting muscle disorders. (Schick L, Windle PE. *PeriAnesthesia Nursing Core Curriculum: Preprocedure, Phase I and Phase II Nursing.* 3rd ed. St. Louis, MO: Saunders; 2016:417-418; Rosenberg H, Pollock N, Schiemann A, et al. *Malignant hyperthermia: a review.* Orphanet J Rare Dis. 2015;10(93):1-19.)

8-53. *Correct answer:* **b**

Because naloxone is an opioid antagonist, it blocks the action of opioids until it releases from the receptor. Once released, the patient may experience resedation and respiratory depression if there is opioid still available in the system. (Odom-Forren J. *Drain's Perianesthesia Nursing: A Critical Care Approach.* 6th ed. St. Louis, MO: Saunders; 2013: 285-286.)

8-54. *Correct answer:* **a**

Ketamine does not have an effect of the pharyngeal and laryngeal reflexes. Ketamine does accelerate the heart rate and increase both systolic and diastolic blood pressure for several minutes. (Odom-Forren J. *Drain's Perianesthesia Nursing: A Critical Care Approach.* 6th ed. St. Louis, MO: Saunders; 2013:274-276.)

8-55. *Correct answer:* **c**

Creatine kinase (CK) is an enzyme chiefly found in the brain, skeletal muscles, and the heart. Elevated CK levels indicate damage to the muscles. After the masseter muscle rigidity (MMR) often seen in malignant hyperthermia (MH), rhabdomyolysis occurs in virtually all patients, and the CK values indicate muscle breakdown. (Odom-Forren J. *Drain's Perianesthesia Nursing: A Critical Care Approach.* 6th ed. St. Louis, MO: Saunders; 2013:708; Fleisher LA, Roizen MF. Essence of anesthesia practice. 3rd ed. Philadelphia: Elsevier/Saunders; 2011: 232-233.)

8-56. *Correct answer:* **a**

During a suspected malignant hyperthermia (MH) crisis, blood samples should be drawn for immediate results on electrolyte and arterial blood gas analysis. Also obtained are samples for creatine kinase (CK), myoglobin, comprehensive metabolic panel, prothrombin time/partial thromboplastin time (PT/PTT), fibrinogen, fibrin split products, complete blood count (CBC), and platelets. (Odom-Forren J. *Drain's Perianesthesia Nursing: A Critical Care Approach.* 6th ed. St. Louis, MO: Saunders; 2013:749.)

8-57. *Correct answer:* **d**

Midazolam causes depression of the central nervous system (CNS), which results in sedation and drowsiness. This drug causes respiratory depression and therefore can potentiate other drugs the patient may have received during the course of anesthesia. (Odom-Forren J. *Drain's Perianesthesia Nursing: A Critical Care Approach.* 6th ed. St. Louis, MO: Saunders; 2013:268-269.)

8-58. *Correct answer:* **c**

The most consistent indicator of potential malignant hyperthermia (MH) in the operating room is an unanticipated increase (e.g., doubling or tripling) of end-tidal CO_2 (ETCO$_2$) when minute ventilation is kept constant. MH usually demonstrates symptoms in less than 30 minutes from the start of anesthesia in the majority of cases. (Odom-Forren J. *Drain's Perianesthesia Nursing: A Critical Care Approach.* 6th ed. St. Louis, MO: Saunders; 2013:401.)

8-59. *Correct answer:* **d**

During the acute malignant hyperthermia (MH) crisis, the initial dose of dantrolene is 2.5 mg/kg repeated pro re nata (prn) to limit MH. Equally important is the cessation of any triggering agents and active physiologic cooling by all routes available. (Odom-Forren J. *Drain's Perianesthesia Nursing: A Critical Care Approach.* 6th ed. St. Louis, MO: Saunders; 2013:401.)

8-60. *Correct answer:* **a**

Either lidocaine or amiodarone is supported by the advanced cardiac life support (ACLS) protocols for the treatment of dysrhythmias. In the case of malignant hyperthermia, calcium channel blockers like diltiazem are avoided. Calcium channel blockers may increase hyperkalemia and lead to death. (Odom-Forren J. *Drain's Perianesthesia Nursing: A Critical Care Approach.* 6th ed. St. Louis, MO: Saunders; 2013:749.)

8-61. *Correct answer:* **d**

After a malignant hyperthermia (MH) crisis, the patient may need to be treated with dantrolene for at least 48 to 72 hours. Patients should be monitored in the intensive or critical care unit (ICU) for MH complications, including a recurrence of the symptoms despite treatment with dantrolene. Twenty-five percent of MH events relapse. (Odom-Forren J. *Drain's Perianesthesia Nursing: A Critical Care Approach.* 6th ed. St. Louis, MO: Saunders; 2013:401.)

8-62. *Correct answer:* **d**

To avoid hypothermia, discontinue all the cooling interventions when the body temperature decreases to 38° C. (Odom-Forren J. *Drain's Perianesthesia Nursing: A Critical Care Approach.* 6th ed. St. Louis, MO: Saunders; 2013:749.)

8-63. *Correct answer:* **d**

Remifentanil is a highly potent synthetic narcotic with an extremely short half-life. Due to the short half-life of this drug, it is administered by IV infusion. A "sudden discontinuation of infusions of this drug after surgery may bring on sudden onset of intense pain." Understanding the properties of this drug, the nurse should ask when the infusion was stopped and what other medications were given to manage pain so as to be prepared to treat the patient's immediate pain needs. (Schick L, Windle PE. *PeriAnesthesia Nursing Core Curriculum: Preprocedure, Phase I and Phase II Nursing.* 3rd ed. St. Louis, MO: Saunders; 2016:370.)

8-64. *Correct answer:* **a**

Head lift and hand grip are standard tests of return of muscle function after neuromuscular blockade. If the patient is able to sustain a head lift unaided while supine and sustain strong hand grips, approximately 50% of the neuromuscular receptors have returned to normal. An inability to perform either head lift or strong bilateral hand grip is an indication of residual neuromuscular blockade. (Odom-Forren J. *Drain's Perianesthesia Nursing: A Critical Care Approach.* 6th ed. St. Louis, MO: Saunders; 2013:306.)

8-65. *Correct answer:* **b**

The Malignant Hyperthermia Association of the United States (MHAUS) recommends keeping regular insulin (100 units/mL) available at all times. (Odom-Forren J. *Drain's Perianesthesia Nursing: A Critical Care Approach.* 6th ed. St. Louis, MO: Saunders; 2013:749.)

9

Diversity and Psychosocial Assistance

Diane Swintek, Nancy Strzyzewski, and Theresa Clifford

9-1. Cultural competency is essential because it promotes:

a. Meaningful plans of care

b. Expedient assessments

c. Standardized care

d. Traditional practices

9-2. The perianesthesia nurse is caring for a toddler after dental surgery for multiple dental caries. The nurse knows pain behavior may be demonstrated as grimacing and:

a. Agitation

b. Passiveness

c. Contentedness

d. Whimpering

9-3. Entering a preoperative room, the nurse notes the patient and her family belong to an ethnic group the nurse has no knowledge of or experience with. Attempting to provide culturally sensitive care, the nurse:

a. Makes sincere eye contact

b. Shakes everyone's hand

c. Speaks slowly and loudly

d. Shows respect to the males

9-4. When interviewing a 17-year-old during a preoperative assessment, a successful communication strategy is to:

a. Ask sensitive questions first

b. Interview with parents present

c. Use brief yes or no questions

d. Ensure patient confidentiality

During a preoperative assessment of an 82-year-old patient, the nurse is concerned to discover the patient drinks two to three cups of chamomile tea daily. The last time the patient drank this tea was last night.

9-5. The nurse recognizes the herb may cause:

a. Anticoagulation

b. Hypotension

c. Bradycardia

d. Hypoglycemia

9-6. The preadmission nurse has just completed an assessment on a patient who reports a history of lupus erythematosus. The nurse remembers that lupus is an autoimmune disorder of connective tissues that is characterized by joint pain and swelling. Although the etiology is unknown, lupus is more common in all of the following EXCEPT:

a. Females

b. Asians

c. Caucasians

d. African Americans

9-7. A 64-year old female patient arrives for a left breast lumpectomy. She learned from the internet that vitamin E can be used to support a healthy immune system and has been taking supplements twice a day in preparation for her surgery. Her last dose of vitamin E was the day before her surgery at bedtime. What action should the nurse take?

a. Consult with the anesthesia provider

b. Notify the surgeon immediately

c. Prepare to administer platelets preoperatively

d. Nothing; vitamin E supplements are harmless

Consider this scenario for questions 9-8 to 9-12.

The ambulatory nurse is completing the preoperative admission for a 60-year-old male patient with early-onset Alzheimer's disease. After verifying with the patient and family that they followed all the preoperative instructions, the nurse verifies that the consents were signed at the surgeon's office.

9-8. To decrease anxiety for this patient, the preop nurse will:

   a. Place him in a waiting room with family

   b. Maintain a calm, unhurried, and accepting manner

   c. Distract him when placing the intravenous

   d. Have all the providers together for the admission interview

9-9. The patient's wife reports that he had to resign from his job as a service repair technician in the last 6 months because he was unable to complete his jobs. Some behavioral characteristics you would expect are impaired reading ability and:

   a. Paranoia

   b. Gentleness

   c. Depression

   d. Repetitive movements

9-10. In the Phase I PACU, to minimize the risk of aspiration, the head of the bed is raised. Other important measures to assist this Alzheimer's patient to have an uncomplicated recovery are to:

   a. Restrain him for safety until fully awake

   b. Suction frequently to remove secretions

   c. Prepare administration of antipsychotics

   d. Have a family member with him

9-11. The patient is able to transfer to the Phase II PACU in preparation for discharge. Together the Phase I PACU nurse and Phase II PACU nurse reorient the patient to surroundings, verify safe transportation, and:

   a. Let him watch TV as a distraction

   b. Verify there is a competent adult at home

   c. Give only written discharge instructions

   d. Use a numeric pain scale for consistency

9-12. When caring for a patient of advanced years, keep in mind that he or she may be experiencing sensory loss, such as presbyopia or presbycusis. In communicating with this patient the nurse must:

   a. Face the patient when speaking

   b. Speak softly to reduce overstimulation

   c. Document concurrently in the electronic health record (EHR)

   d. Have the patient remove his or her glasses

9-13. For what age range is the Face, Legs, Activity, Cry, Consolability (FLACC) scale useful to measure pain and distress in children?

   a. Infant to 5 years

   b. Infant to 7 years

   c. 2 to 7 years old

   d. 5 to 7 years old

9-14. Pediatric patients who present with disorders on the autism spectrum require watchful monitoring to keep them safe in the perianesthesia environment. In the Phase I PACU the patient may manifest:

   a. Seizure activity

   b. Garbled speech

   c. Hand flapping

   d. Dulled reflexes

9-15. A frustrated surgeon insists the Phase I PACU nurse transfuse blood into a patient who is a Jehovah's Witness. Aware of patients' rights, the nurse refuses knowing that the patient's right to refuse blood products is supported by:

   a. The Joint Commission Annual Safety Goals

   b. Patient Self-Determination Act

   c. Centers for Medicare and Medicaid Services Guidelines for Safety

   d. National Standards on Cultural Care

9-16. A 2-year-old child wakes up restless in the Phase I PACU. After assessing the child and determining he is physiologically stable, the nurse:

a. Provides explanations for experiences

b. Covers the child completely for privacy

c. Sets clear limits and boundaries

d. Reunites the child with the caregiver quickly

9-17. While considering discharge teaching for an 82-year-old Native American patient, the nurse takes into consideration that traditionally Native Americans do not:

a. Take prescription medications

b. Believe in Western medicine

c. Listen to Women

d. Believe in infection

9-18. While conducting a preoperative assessment for an older adult patient, the prudent nurse includes risk factors for:

a. Migraine

b. Hardiness

c. Anorexia

d. Delirium

9-19. While in the Phase I PACU, a 16-year-old female patient has been medicated for pain. Although her pain score has decreased from 7 to 5, she remains restless. An effective strategy to use with her is:

a. Deep breathing

b. Essential oils

c. Acupressure

d. Parental separation

9-20. During the preoperative assessment, Mr. Y answers "yes" to every question. The nurse questions the accuracy of the assessment because the patient:

a. Disrespects Western medicine

b. Is being secretive

c. Is not really listening

d. Wishes to prevent disharmony

9-21. A 32-year-old Asian female patient is ready for the operating room. She has asked her anesthesia provider permission to take a piece of jade with her to have it nearby during her surgery. The provider is aware that the reason for this request is that the Chinese Americans believe jade prevents:

a. Nausea

b. Pain

c. Harm

d. Fear

9-22. Which of the following statements concerning a Jehovah's Witness is true?

a. A Jehovah's Witness will agree to a transfusion only if life saving

b. A Jehovah's Witness may refuse surgery on Christmas

c. A Jehovah's Witness will agree to plasma and platelets

d. A Jehovah's Witness may not agree to autologous blood transfusions

9-23. While caring for a 5-year-old patient in the Phase II PACU, what approach or techniques will the nurse incorporate to enhance discharge teaching?

a. Speaking clearly to the parents

b. Hands-on experience for the child

c. Plan teaching to last 5 to 10 minutes

d. Parallel play to clarify the topic

9-24. In the African American culture, perceptions of health derive from religious and holistic beliefs and practices. Good health is defined as:

a. Reward for body and mind

b. Love and service to God

c. Harmony with nature

d. Control of evil influences

9-25. During the hour a 13-year-old female patient has been in the Phase I PACU, her pain score has decreased after pain medication administration. She has been responding politely and appropriately to the nurse. When her parents arrive at her bedside, the patient begins to sob and cries out, "This pain is killing me!" Understanding adolescent behavior, the nurse recognizes that:

a. Adolescents often lie

b. Adolescents are secretive

c. Regression is common

d. Girls are dramatic

Consider this scenario for questions 9-26, 9-27, and 9-28.

The perianesthesia nurse is assigned to admit a 19-year-old female patient coming to the same-day surgery center for a large loop excision of transformation zone (LLETZ) procedure of the cervix after an abnormal Pap smear. During the admission assessment she is busy texting with friends.

9-26. The nurse asks that she put her phone down so that the admission can be completed. Her behavior demonstrates:

a. Projecting an aura of calm and cool

b. Rejection of hospital rules

c. Indifference to the needs of others

d. Staying in control of self

9-27. In late adolescence there is more commitment to intimate relationships. Another common characteristic of late adolescence is:

a. Mature communication with parents

b. Unrealistic expectations of partners

c. Establishing own value system

d. Conforming to societal norms

9-28. In the Phase I PACU the patient does not want the nurse to check her sanitary pad. The PACU nurse knows this is related to:

a. Wanting to appear in control

b. Concern about body image

c. Intensity of pain

d. Anxiety about bleeding

9-29. A patient presents for parathyroidectomy in the preoperative area. The perianesthesia nurse knows that a preoperative calcium level is important information in providing safe postoperative care. Another important preoperative assessment is:

a. Patient teaching about position

b. Patient voice quality

c. History of palpitation

d. History of asthma

9-30. The perianesthesia nurse is taking care of a male patient, age 9, with a known moderate developmental delay. It is expected that his behavior would:

a. Be appropriate for his age

b. Demonstrate a flat affect after anesthesia

c. Be appropriate for a 2- to 6-year-old

d. Include making a lot of noise or talking

9-31. While on call, the perianesthesia nurse is assigned to a patient she finds ethically difficult to provide care for. What is the nurse's responsibility to the patient?

a. Provide care until another nurse can provide relief

b. Explain her ethical concerns to the patient

c. Limit communication with the patient/family

d. Continue to care for the patient until discharge

9-32. To improve communication with a developmentally delayed patient, remain calm, relaxed, and:

a. Mimic their words

b. Speak slower and louder

c. Talk to the parent or caregiver

d. Repeat the information

9-33. In the preoperative unit, a non–English-speaking mother of a 5-year-old patient becomes upset when the nurse attempts to remove a bracelet from the child. What intervention could the nurse investigate?

a. Remind the interpreter compliance is necessary

b. Notify the surgeon of the need to cancel the case

c. Call security to restrain and remove the mother

d. Secure the item elsewhere on the child's body

9-34. Taking the time to know an older patient's personal preferences will assist in prioritizing his or her care. Chronological age, however, is just one consideration. In order of importance, the perianesthesia nurse must first consider:

a. Level of understanding of instructions

b. Access to health care

c. Presence of comorbidities

d. Living situation

9-35. The substance abuse patient presents a significant challenge for the perianesthesia nurse when it comes to pain control interventions. Nonmedical use of a drug will lead to:

a. Tremulousness

b. Central nervous system (CNS) depression

c. Impaired judgment

d. Drug tolerance

9-36. The toddler's predominant age-related fear is:

a. Permanent separation

b. Dismemberment

c. Loss of privacy

d. Mutilation

9-37. While caring for patients from another culture, the culturally sensitive perianesthesia nurse would:

a. Observe family for cues regarding eye contact

b. Speak to the male family members only

c. Speak loudly to be better understood

d. Shake hands firmly to indicate acceptance

9-38. The patient with a history of multiple sclerosis presents with unpredictable sensory and motor symptoms. The perianesthesia nurse needs to be alert to the presence of motor symptoms such as paresis, bladder dysfunction, and:

a. Dysesthesia

b. Dysphagia

c. Nystagmus

d. Decreased energy

9-39. The National Standards on Culturally and Linguistically Appropriate Services mandates requirements for all organizations receiving federal funding. These requirements include:

a. Easily understood patient materials

b. Private rooms for cultural rituals

c. Native-speaking care providers

d. Traditionally prepared foods

9-40. In the Chinese culture it is thought that disease is caused by:

a. Imbalance of the organs

b. Way of life

c. Negative energy

d. Excess of emotion

9-41. The perianesthesia nurse has started an infusion of cefazolin for a 17-year-old male patient scheduled to have an anterior cruciate ligament (ACL) repair. This adolescent complains of faintness, lightheadedness, and ocular pruritus. The nurse knows the first intervention is:

a. Epinephrine

b. Fluid bolus

c. Stop the infusion

d. High-flow oxygen

9-42. Medication reconciliation is an important measure to keep patients safe after a surgical procedure. The Joint Commission has established a national patient safety goal regarding medication reconciliation to:

a. Organize the route of administration

b. Provide only those medicines routinely needed

c. Identify and resolve discrepancies

d. Obtain information on current regimens

Consider this scenario for questions 9-43 and 9-44.
The nurse caring for a 9-month-old infant in the Phase I PACU identifies the child has a quivering chin, restless legs, and a rigid body posture. The child is crying steadily and is difficult to console.

9-43. What is the child's Face, Legs, Activity, Cry, Consolability (FLACC) score?

a. 6

b. 7

c. 8

d. 9

9-44. What medication should be administered to this 9-month-old patient?

a. Morphine 0.05 to 0.1 mg/kg

b. Morphine 1 to 2 mg/kg

c. Meperidine 0.25 to 0.50 mg/kg

d. Acetaminophen 15 mg/kg

9-45. Effective pain assessment of the adolescent patient includes:

a. Watching for behavioral cues

b. Frequently questioning the patient

c. Expecting the patient to self-report

d. Using the Face, Legs, Activity, Cry, Consolability (FLACC) scale to assess

9-46. A patient afflicted with macular degeneration is being prepared for surgery by the perianesthesia nurse. What must the nurse know about macular degeneration to keep this patient safe during this admission?

a. This causes complete blindness

b. Patients can see out of one eye

c. This is loss of the center vision field

d. Patients can see only 20 feet

9-47. It is important to understand the core values of patients. The older patient has respect for authority, believes in hard work, and:

a. Wants things done his or her way

b. Lives in the moment

c. Believes in duty before reward

d. Is impatient with delay

9-48. Myasthenia gravis is a chronic, progressive autoimmune disease that causes worsening voluntary muscle weakness. The stress of surgery may cause an exacerbation of symptoms exhibited as:

a. Respiratory difficulty

b. Hypothermia

c. Urinary retention

d. Systemic inflammation

9-49. A 46-year-old male patient has arrived in the preop holding unit pending surgery for an inflamed gallbladder. The patient is a recent immigrant from Sudan, and the nurse recognizes quickly that English is not the patient's first language. Language barriers, aside from impairing good communication between providers and patients, can also lower patient satisfaction, compromise patient safety, and:

a. Lower provider satisfaction

b. Motivate patients to learn English

c. Incentivize providers to learn a second language

d. Lead to enhanced access to supportive services

9-50. An older couple comes to the ambulatory surgery center for the husband, age 76, to have a transurethral prostate biopsy to further evaluate an elevated prostate-specific antigen (PSA) (greater than 8). Their daughter has driven them to the center. The daughter chastises her father for urinary incontinence in the preoperative area while waiting for the perianesthesia nurse to perform the admission. The perianesthesia nurse is aware that elder abuse is growing in incidence. Types of elder abuse include financial, physical, and:

a. Chemical restraint

b. Social exploitation

c. Religious beliefs

d. Humiliation

Answers and Rationales for Chapter 9, Diversity and Psychosocial Assistance

9-1. *Correct answer:* **a**

Cultural competence defines the behaviors, perspectives, and policies that allow healthcare workers to provide services that are effective in all cultural situations. Knowledge of various race, ethnic, gender or sexual, cultural, or religious differences enables the perianesthesia nurse to provide meaningful interventions during the course of perianesthesia care. (Schick L, Windle PE. *PeriAnesthesia Nursing Core Curriculum: Preprocedure, Phase I and Phase II Nursing.* 3rd ed. St. Louis, MO: Saunders; 2016:120.)

9-2. *Correct answer:* **a**

Toddlers react intensely to actual or perceived painful stimuli. Some other pain behaviors of note are opening the eyes wide, rocking, rubbing, clenching teeth or lips, or trying to run away. Prepare the toddler hours or minutes before a procedure, as preparing too far in advance produces even more anxiety. (Schick L, Windle PE. *PeriAnesthesia Nursing Core Curriculum: Preprocedure, Phase I and Phase II PACU Nursing.* 3rd ed. St. Louis, MO: Saunders; 2016: 238-239.)

9-3. *Correct answer:* **d**

Show respect to the male members of the family, as they are often the decision makers in many cultures. Eye contact, shaking hands, and speaking loudly to non-English patients may be seen as disrespectful. (Schick L, Windle PE. *PeriAnesthesia Nursing Core Curriculum: Preprocedure, Phase I and Phase II Nursing.* 3rd ed. St. Louis, MO: Saunders; 2016:136.)

9-4. *Correct answer:* **d**

When interviewing adolescents, it is important to remember that privacy is of utmost importance to these patients. Successful preoperative strategies include beginning with less sensitive questions first and then proceeding to more direct or open-ended questions, interviewing the adolescent without parents present when possible, and ensuring confidentiality and privacy. (Odom-Forren J. *Drain's Perianesthesia Nursing: A Critical Care Approach.* 6th ed. St. Louis, MO: Saunders; 2013: 699; Schick L, Windle PE. *PeriAnesthesia Nursing Core Curriculum: Preprocedure, Phase I and Phase II Nursing.* 3rd ed. St. Louis, MO: Saunders; 2016:259.)

9-5. *Correct answer:* **a**

Chamomile may impair anticoagulation due to platelet inhibition. The American Society of Anesthesiologists (ASA) recommends that patients are instructed to stop ingesting chamomile (and all herbal supplments) at least 2 weeks before surgery. (Schick L, Windle PE. *PeriAnesthesia Nursing Core Curriculum: Preprocedure, Phase I and Phase II Nursing.* 3rd ed. St. Louis, MO: Saunders; 2016:145t.)

9-6. *Correct answer:* **c**

Lupus is more common in females than males and in African Americans and Asians than people of other races. People with lupus are generally aged 10 to 50. (Schick L, Windle PE. *PeriAnesthesia Nursing Core Curriculum: Preprocedure, Phase I and Phase II PACU Nursing.* 3rd ed. St. Louis, MO: Saunders; 2016:112.)

9-7. *Correct answer:* **b**
Most herbal remedies, including vitamin E, may increase bleeding. The impaired coagulation may affect the surgical procedure. (Schick L, Windle PE. *PeriAnesthesia Nursing Core Curriculum: Preprocedure, Phase I and Phase II Nursing.* 3rd ed. St. Louis, MO: Saunders; 2016:153t.)

9-8. *Correct answer:* **b**
During the admission assessment it is important that the nurse maintain a calm, unhurried, and supportive manner to put this patient and family at ease. The stimulation of the preoperative unit increases anxiety for this patient. Minimize the number of personnel who interact with the patient at one time, and consider using a topical anesthetic when inserting the intravenous. (Schick L, Windle PE. *PeriAnesthesia Nursing Core Curriculum: Preprocedure, Phase I and Phase II PACU Nursing.* 3rd ed. St. Louis, MO: Saunders; 2016:159.)

9-9. *Correct answer:* **a**
From your interactions with the patient's wife, you understand that your patient is in the confusion stage of the disease process. It is common in this stage for the patient to feel paranoia and have difficulty reading. Other idiosyncrasies of this stage of Alzheimer's disease are confusion, aggression, delusions, wandering, and difficulty managing daily activities. (Schick L, Windle PE. *PeriAnesthesia Nursing Core Curriculum: Preprocedure, Phase I and Phase II PACU Nursing.* 3rd ed. St. Louis, MO: Saunders; 2016:165.)

9-10. *Correct answer:* **d**
If possible, it is best practice to have a family member be with the patient in the Phase I PACU. This will assist you in your communications with the patient. Family can help you reorient the patient to the environment. (Schick L, Windle PE. *PeriAnesthesia Nursing Core Curriculum: Preprocedure, Phase I and Phase II PACU Nursing.* 3rd ed. St. Louis, MO: Saunders; 2016:164, Box 8-3.)

9-11. *Correct answer:* **b**
Verify that there is safe transportation to the home and a competent adult to stay with the patient in the home. Use a pain intensity scale that is appropriate for your patient, as the numeric pain scale—the scale used most often—may be difficult for the patient to understand. Show respect for your patient by reviewing the discharge instructions with him and his family member. (Schick L, Windle PE. *PeriAnesthesia Nursing Core Curriculum: Preprocedure, Phase I and Phase II PACU Nursing.* 3rd ed. St. Louis, MO: Saunders; 2016:164, Box 8-4.)

9-12. *Correct answer:* **a**
Face the patient when speaking so he or she can hear you clearly and see your mouth move. This patient may be reading lips to disguise his or her hearing loss. The decrease in acoustic acuity makes it difficult for this patient population to discern different tones. Men in particular lose the ability to hear the higher register voice. (Schick L, Windle PE. *PeriAnesthesia Nursing Core Curriculum: Preprocedure, Phase I and Phase II PACU Nursing.* 3rd ed. St. Louis, MO: Saunders; 2016:286, 294-295; Odom-Forren, J. *Drain's PeriAnesthesia Nursing: A Critical Care Approach.* 6th ed. St. Louis, MO: Saunders; 2013:716.)

9-13. *Correct answer:* **b**
The Face, Legs, Activity, Cry, Consolability (FLACC) scale is useful in assessing pain or distress in infants and children up to 7 years. (Schick L, Windle PE. *PeriAnesthesia Nursing Core Curriculum Preprocedure, Phase I and Phase II Nursing.* 3rd ed. St. Louis, MO: Saunders; 2016:239.)

9-14. *Correct answer:* **c**

Symptoms that the patient diagnosed with autism may demonstrate in the perianesthesia environment are hand flapping and body rocking. These children need the nurse to speak slowly and clearly. Do not insist on eye contact, as some children find this distressing. Provide language tools for the child to communicate, such as a communication board, sign language, or a parent/caregiver the child trusts. (Schick L, Windle PE. *PeriAnesthesia Nursing Core Curriculum: Preprocedure, Phase I and Phase II PACU Nursing.* 3rd ed. St. Louis, MO: Saunders; 2016:188-190.)

9-15. *Correct answer:* **b**

The Patient Self-Determination Act states patients have the right under state law to agree to or refuse medical or surgical treatment. (Schick L, Windle PE. *PeriAnesthesia Nursing Core Curriculum: Preprocedure, Phase I and Phase II PACU Nursing.* 3rd ed. St. Louis, MO: Saunders; 2016:28; Odom-Forren, J. *Drain's Perianesthesia Nursing: A Critical Care Approach.* 6th ed. St. Louis, MO: Saunders; 2013:90.)

9-16. *Correct answer:* **d**

Major stressors for preschoolers include separation; separation/stranger anxiety is heightened at this age. A successful nonpharmacologic strategy for pain management for the pediatric patient is to allow the parent to stay with the child and encourage the parent to talk softly to the child. (Schick L, Windle PE. *PeriAnesthesia Nursing Core Curriculum: Preprocedure, Phase I and Phase II Nursing.* 3rd ed. St. Louis, MO: Saunders; 2016:234.)

9-17. *Correct answer:* **d**

Native Americans consider the germ theory a function of modern medicine and generally do not believe in infection, communicable agents, or physiologic processes. The Native American believes illness is a result of disharmony with self and the spirit world. (Schick L, Windle PE. *PeriAnesthesia Nursing Core Curriculum: Preprocedure, Phase I and Phase II Nursing.* 3rd ed. St. Louis, MO: Saunders; 2016:133.)

9-18. *Correct answer:* **d**

The older adult should be assessed preoperatively for all the elements identified in Practice Recommendation 2, including risk factors for developing postoperative delirium. (American Society of PeriAnesthesia Nurses. Practice Recommendation 2: components of assessment and management for the perianesthesia patient. In *2015-2017 PeriAnesthesia Nursing Standards, Practice Recommendations and Interpretive Statements.* Cherry Hill, NJ: ASPAN; 2014:41-46.)

9-19. *Correct answer:* **a**

Adolescents can be taught to use nonpharmacologic coping techniques to help manage pain and promote comfort such as relaxation, deep breathing, self-comforting talk, and/or the use of imagery. (Schick L, Windle PE. *PeriAnesthesia Nursing Core Curriculum: Preprocedure, Phase I and Phase II Nursing.* 3rd ed. St. Louis, MO: Saunders; 2016:261.)

9-20. *Correct answer:* **d**

Since harmony and peacefulness are core tenets of Chinese culture, many patients will say "yes" in spite of a lack of understanding in order to maintain harmony. Thus, the nurse must question the accuracy of the assessment based on the patient's reluctance to express any misunderstanding regarding the questions asked. (Schick L, Windle PE. *PeriAnesthesia Nursing Core Curriculum: Preprocedure, Phase I and Phase II Nursing.* 3rd ed. St. Louis, MO: Saunders; 2016:130-131.)

9-21. *Correct answer:* **c**

People of Chinese American descent believe that wearing jade, whether a charm or a piece of jewelry, helps to prevent harm. (Schick L, Windle PE. *PeriAnesthesia Nursing Core Curriculum: Preprocedure, Phase I and Phase II PACU Nursing.* 3rd ed. St. Louis, MO: Saunders; 2016:131.)

9-22. *Correct answer:* **d**

Jehovah's Witnesses of deep faith are generally opposed to homologous blood transfusions; some may submit to autologous blood transfusions or may refuse surgery if a blood transfusion is required, and they do not partake in national holidays, including Christmas. Each person of the Jehovah's Witness faith must decide individually if any natural or manufactured components of blood can be used. (Schick L, Windle PE. *PeriAnesthesia Nursing Core Curriculum: Preprocedure, Phase I and Phase II PACU Nursing*. 3rd ed. St. Louis, MO: Saunders; 2016:138.)

9-23. *Correct answer:* **b**

Children between the ages of 4 and 7 have demonstrated that hands-on experiences work well. The information provided should be short and concise, and the amount of time spent on the topic should be limited to less than 5 minutes. (Schick L, Windle PE. *PeriAnesthesia Nursing Core Curriculum: Preprocedure, Phase I and Phase II Nursing*. 3rd ed. St. Louis, MO: Saunders; 2016:208.)

9-24. *Correct answer:* **c**

The basis of health culture beliefs stems from a magico-religious and holistic foundation. Good health is synonymous with harmony, with nature, and with personal good luck. The perceptions about health come from ethnomedical, biomedical, and popular beliefs. (Schick L, Windle PE. *PeriAnesthesia Nursing Core Curriculum: Preprocedure, Phase I and Phase II PACU Nursing*. 3rd ed. St. Louis, MO: Saunders; 2016:134.)

9-25. *Correct answer:* **c**

It is not unusual for adolescents to deal with pain through regressive behavior. (Schick L, Windle PE. *PeriAnesthesia Nursing Core Curriculum: Preprocedure, Phase I and Phase II Nursing*. 3rd ed. St. Louis, MO: Saunders; 2016:265.)

9-26. *Correct answer:* **a**

The late adolescent is at the crossroads of childhood and adulthood. Projecting an aura of being calm and cool is a response to the anxiety and fear they have about the scheduled surgery. Loss of control, separation anxiety, and emotional/behavioral regression also affect behavior. A scheduled versus an emergent surgical procedure allows for greater sense of control for the adolescent. (Schick L, Windle PE. *PeriAnesthesia Nursing Core Curriculum: Preprocedure, Phase I and Phase II PACU Nursing*. 3rd ed. St. Louis, MO: Saunders; 2016:256-257.)

9-27. *Correct answer:* **c**

Now is when the adolescent is separating from parents and establishing his or her own value systems. The late adolescent is less self-centered, social relationships are more mature, and his or her able to express thoughts and feelings about different aspects of life. (Schick L, Windle PE. *PeriAnesthesia Nursing Core Curriculum: Preprocedure, Phase I and Phase II PACU Nursing*. 3rd ed. St. Louis, MO: Saunders; 2016:256.)

9-28. *Correct answer:* **b**

Concern about body image causes fear and anxiety for adolescents. In the unfamiliar environment their self-concept is shaken and may cause them to regress in their behavior. (Schick L, Windle PE. *PeriAnesthesia Nursing Core Curriculum: Preprocedure, Phase I and Phase II PACU Nursing*. 3rd ed. St. Louis, MO: Saunders; 2016:256-257.)

9-29. *Correct answer:* **b**

It is safest for the patient to be in a euthyroid state before any thyroid surgery. Evaluation of the patient's voice quality provides a baseline for the postoperative nurse to be alert for laryngeal nerve damage. The laryngeal nerve may be injured during the surgery from clamping, compression, stretching, or even severing. (Odom-Forren J. *Drain's Perianesthesia Nursing: A Critical Care Approach*. 6th ed. St. Louis, MO: Saunders; 2013:577, 579.)

9-30. *Correct answer:* **c**

Although the chronologic age is 9, the moderate developmental delay alerts the nurse that this child would act more like a child of 2 to 6 years of age. Patients with this level of impairment are less verbal. (Schick L, Windle PE. *PeriAnesthesia Nursing Core Curriculum: Preprocedure, Phase I and Phase II PACU Nursing.* 3rd ed. St. Louis, MO: Saunders; 2016:158.)

9-31. *Correct answer:* **a**

According to the Perianesthesia Standards for Ethical Practice, "where the perianesthesia registered nurse's personal convictions prohibit participation, that nurse may remove himself or herself from a patient care situation, as long as such removal does not harm the patient or constitute a breach of duty. However, if an unplanned situation arises in which no other registered nurse is available to care for the patient, then the objecting nurse must ensure that the care needs of the patient are met." (American Society of PeriAnesthesia Nurses. Perianesthesia standards for ethical practice. In: *2015-2017 PeriAnesthesia Nursing Standards, Practice Recommendations and Interpretive Statements.* Cherry Hill, NJ: ASPAN; 2014:10-13.)

9-32. *Correct answer:* **d**

To improve your communication with this patient population, take the time to speak slowly and clearly, and repeat the information as many times as needed. It is important to show your respect by communicating directly with the patient and allowing him or her time to formulate and ask a question. (Schick L, Windle PE. *PeriAnesthesia Nursing Core Curriculum: Preprocedure, Phase I and Phase II PACU Nursing.* 3rd ed. St. Louis, MO: Saunders; 2016:159.)

9-33. *Correct answer:* **d**

Some cultures view jewelry as religious articles and may not be permitted to remove them from the body. If the site interferes with surgery, the mother may consent to placement of the article on another part of the body. (Schick L, Windle PE. *PeriAnesthesia Nursing Core Curriculum: Preprocedure, Phase I and Phase II Nursing.* 3rd ed. St. Louis, MO: Saunders; 2016:154.)

9-34. *Correct answer:* **c**

In treating the whole patient in a person-centered care model, the nurse must learn the physiologic functioning, presence of comorbidities, present medication regimen, and psychologic outlook of the person. All of these will have an impact on his or her response to health care interventions. (Odom-Forren J. *Drain's Perianesthesia Nursing: A Critical Care Approach.* 6th ed. St. Louis, MO: Saunders; 2013:711.)

9-35. *Correct answer:* **d**

In drug tolerance the patient requires increasingly larger doses to obtain the same effect as that of a lesser dose. One in 10 patients has a drug use disorder. The most commonly abused medication class is opioids. This leads to physical dependence, psychologic dependence, and drug tolerance. (Odom-Forren J. *Drain's Perianesthesia Nursing: A Critical Care Approach.* 6th ed. St. Louis, MO: Saunders; 2013:730.)

9-36. *Correct answer:* **a**

Major stressors for preschoolers include separation; separation/stranger anxiety is heightened at this age. (Schick L, Windle PE. *PeriAnesthesia Nursing Core Curriculum: Preprocedure, Phase I and Phase II Nursing.* 3rd ed. St. Louis, MO: Saunders; 2016:202, Box 9-6.)

9-37. *Correct answer:* **a**

Observe the patient and family for cues regarding culturally appropriate eye contact. (Schick L, Windle PE. *PeriAnesthesia Nursing Core Curriculum: Preprocedure, Phase I and Phase II Nursing.* 3rd ed. St. Louis, MO: Saunders; 2016:126.)

9-38. *Correct answer:* **b**

Loss of motor function for patients diagnosed with multiple sclerosis includes bladder dysfunction, bowel dysfunction, dysphagia, spasticity, or diplopia. Sensory function lost due to this disease can include numbness, paresthesia, pain, dysesthesia, and decreased proprioception. (Schick L, Windle PE. *PeriAnesthesia Nursing Core Curriculum: Preprocedure, Phase I and Phase II PACU Nursing.* 3rd ed. St. Louis, MO: Saunders; 2016:183.)

9-39. *Correct answer:* **a**

The National Standards on Culturally and Linguistically Appropriate Services publish provisions providing culturally competent care. According to these Standards, Standard 7 in particular, health care organizations must make available easily understood patient-related materials. (Schick L, Windle PE. *PeriAnesthesia Nursing Core Curriculum: Preprocedure, Phase I and Phase II Nursing.* 3rd ed. St. Louis, MO: Saunders; 2016:95.)

9-40. *Correct answer:* **d**

The Chinese culture believes that disease is caused by the excess or lack of emotion; anxiety; or irregularity in food or drink or cold or heat. There are three prime components of Chinese health. Tao is the way of life, virtue, heaven, and death. The chi is the vitality, the universal energy, and the fundamental concept of traditional Chinese medicine. Yin and yang represent the duality and unity of the universe and tao. (Schick L, Windle PE. *PeriAnesthesia Nursing Core Curriculum: Preprocedure, Phase I and Phase II PACU Nursing.* 3rd ed. St. Louis, MO: Saunders; 2016:130-131.)

9-41. *Correct answer:* **c**

The nurse needs to respond immediately when an allergic reaction is suspected. The first intervention is to stop the infusion of the drug thought to cause this reaction followed by the administration of 100% oxygen. (Odom-Forren J. *Drain's Perianesthesia Nursing: A Critical Care Approach.* 6th ed. St. Louis, MO: Saunders; 2013:321.)

9-42. *Correct answer:* **c**

The Joint Commission established a hospital national patient safety goal regarding medication reconciliation to compare the list of medications that the patient brought to the hospital with the medications ordered while in the hospital. It is essential that a competent individual in the hospital identify and resolve discrepancies to ensure patient safety. Important information is collected to reconcile current and newly ordered medications and to provide safe prescribing of medications. (Odom-Forren J. *Drain's Perianesthesia Nursing: A Critical Care Approach.* 6th ed. St. Louis, MO: Saunders; 2013:657-658.)

9-43. *Correct answer:* **d**

According to the FLACC score the patient receives 2 points for a quivering chin, 1 point for restless legs, 2 points for a rigid body, 2 points for a steady cry, and 2 points for difficulty to console, for a total of 9 points. (Schick L, Windle PE. *PeriAnesthesia Nursing Core Curriculum: Preprocedure, Phase I and Phase II PACU Nursing.* 3rd ed. St. Louis, MO: Saunders; 2016:239t.)

9-44. *Correct answer:* **a**

The correct dose is morphine 0.05 to 0.1 mg/kg. Meperidine is indicated for shivering, not pain. Acetaminophen is recommended at 15 mg/kg for children age two and older or 12.5 mg/kg every four hours. (Schick L, Windle PE. *PeriAnesthesia Nursing Core Curriculum: Preprocedure, Phase I and Phase II PACU Nursing.* 3rd ed. St. Louis, MO: Saunders; 2016:244t.)

9-45. *Correct answer:* **a**

Adolescents expect the nurse to know they are in pain and believe they should not have to ask for pain medication. They are able to reliably report pain using self-reporting tools. It is important to observe for behavioral signs of pain including increased muscle tension, grimacing, muscle rigidity, and reluctance to move. (Schick L, Windle PE. *PeriAnesthesia Nursing Core Curriculum: Preprocedure, Phase I and Phase II Nursing.* 3rd ed. St. Louis, MO: Saunders; 2016:265.)

9-46. *Correct answer:* **c**

Macular degeneration is a specific vision impairment that causes loss of sight in the center vision field. This disease accounts for 54% of all blindness. (Schick L, Windle PE. *PeriAnesthesia Nursing Core Curriculum: Preprocedure, Phase I and Phase II PACU Nursing.* 3rd ed. St. Louis, MO: Saunders; 2016:171.)

9-47. *Correct answer:* **c**

The older patient, aged 75 to 84 years, is also known as the silent generation. Duty before reward, respect for authority, hard work, and dedication and sacrifice are some of the core values of this population. Likewise, some personality traits associated with this patient population are discipline, conformity, logic, and consistency. (Schick L, Windle PE. *PeriAnesthesia Nursing Core Curriculum: Preprocedure, Phase I and Phase II PACU Nursing.* 3rd ed. St. Louis, MO: Saunders; 2016:284.)

9-48. *Correct answer:* **a**

Acute respiratory difficulty is a serious symptom of a myasthenia crisis. Additionally the patient may have oropharyngeal muscle weakness that is exhibited as difficulty chewing, swallowing, and talking. The severity of the progressive muscle weakness is greatest after prolonged use of affected muscles. Symptoms improve with rest and medication. (Schick L, Windle PE. *PeriAnesthesia Nursing Core Curriculum: Preprocedure, Phase I and Phase II PACU Nursing.* 3rd ed. St. Louis, MO: Saunders; 2016:185-188.)

9-49. *Correct answer:* **a**

Communication between patients with limited English abilities and their providers is affected by language barriers. These issues may result in patient and provider dissatisfaction, compromised patient safety, potential suboptimal quality of care, and health disparities for this population. (Odom-Forren J. *Drain's Perianesthesia Nursing: A Critical Care Approach.* 6th ed. St. Louis, MO: Saunders; 2013:67.)

9-50. *Correct answer:* **d**

Verbal abuse is psychologically damaging, and in elder abuse may take the form of humiliation, intimidation, or the threat of physical abuse. Physical abuse may be sexual, beating, slapping, kicking, or neglect. Withholding food, care, and company are equally abusive to the elderly. (Schick L, Windle PE. *PeriAnesthesia Nursing Core Curriculum: Preprocedure, Phase I and Phase II PACU Nursing.* 3rd ed. St. Louis, MO: Saunders; 2016:296-297.)

10

Patient and Family Education

Susan Norris and Theresa Clifford

10-1. While preparing a patient who will be undergoing infiltration of local anesthesia, the nurse instructs the patient to report all of the following EXCEPT:

a. Metallic taste in the mouth
b. Tingling of the lips
c. Ringing in the ears
d. Sweet taste in the mouth

10-2. To help reduce the incidence of surgical site infections, the perianesthesia nurse can teach the preoperative patient simple principles to support lowering the risk. These include how to observe wounds, how to change dressings, how to clean wounds, and:

a. To report excessive bleeding
b. Knowledge of postoperative medications
c. The importance of hand washing
d. The need for adequate carbohydrate intake

10-3. Preoperative education for the patient contemplating bariatric surgery includes information about preparation and the surgical procedure itself. The education includes postoperative instructions related to:

a. Diet, lifestyle changes, and potential complications
b. Increasing dietary intake of carbohydrates to provide energy for healing
c. Decreasing postoperative activity to minimize the risk of thrombophlebitis
d. Prolonged fasting and bowel rest to promote wound healing

10-4. The advantages of using simulation for the clinical training of health care providers include all of the following EXCEPT:

a. Mistakes do not harm patients
b. Personnel can work with actual equipment
c. Simulation scenarios can be simplified
d. Role playing can help develop critical thinking

10-5. According to the American Society of Anesthesiologists' (ASA's) fasting guidelines, a healthy adult patient undergoing an elective procedure may be instructed to continue to consume clear liquids until:

a. 2 hours preoperatively
b. 4 hours preoperatively
c. 6 hours preoperatively
d. 8 hours preoperatively

10-6. A hospital is located in an area with a large population of immigrants. As a result of the wide diversity of patients cared for in the day surgery unit, the staff demonstrate competencies in:

a. An additional language besides English
b. Multigenerational thinking
c. Cultural sensitivity
d. Gender differences

10-7. According to the American Society of Anesthesiologists' (ASA's) fasting guidelines, a healthy 8-month-old patient undergoing an elective procedure may be instructed to continue to consume formula until:

a. 2 hours preoperatively
b. 4 hours preoperatively
c. 6 hours preoperatively
d. 8 hours preoperatively

10-8. When interviewing a patient for pre-anesthesia and nursing assessments, it is helpful to remember that generational differences affect an individual's ability to learn and participate in care. The perianesthesia nurse knows that the patient who is born between 1980 and 2000 is known as:

a. Generation W

b. Generation Y

c. Generation X

d. Generation Z

10-9. Preoperatively patients may be instructed to hold the following medications on the day of surgery as determined by the surgeon or anesthesia provider:

a. Beta blockers

b. Anticonvulsants

c. Oral hypoglycemic medications

d. Chronic pain medications

10-10. The incidence of postoperative nausea and vomiting (PONV) is higher in the ophthalmic surgical patient than in other surgical procedures. The patient has asked for complementary therapy recommendations. The perianesthesia nurse is aware that the following therapy is very popular:

a. Ginger

b. St. John's wort

c. Licorice

d. Ginseng

10-11. A family member notices a nurse's name tag and the credentials "CAPA" on the tag. The perianesthesia nurse explains to the family that certification in perianesthesia nursing:

a. Is a validation of specialty knowledge

b. Is a validation of a specialty job description

c. Is a validation of the clinical ladder

d. Is a requirement of a magnet institution

10-12. Preoperative instructions should include information regarding the need to stop herbal supplements that can increase bleeding. These include the following EXCEPT:

a. Feverfew

b. Garlic

c. Goldenseal

d. Ginseng

10-13. Patient education is more effective when the content and methods are:

a. Individualized for the patient and family

b. Generic and scripted

c. Standardized

d. Incorporating medical and technical terminology

10-14. The goals of patient education are all of the following EXCEPT:

a. Decreased anxiety

b. Increased patient's sense of self-worth

c. Reduced facility liability

d. Increased patient satisfaction scores

10-15. According to the American Society of Anesthesiologists' (ASA's), patients should be instructed to stop taking herbal medications:

a. At least 3 days preoperatively

b. Only on the day of surgery

c. At least 7 days preoperatively

d. At least 14 days preoperatively

10-16. Marvin is a 44-year-old patient who is scheduled for a surgical repair of a badly fractured patella sustained from a fall. He admits to a recent history of opioid-related drug abuse but states he has been "sober" for a few months. His urine drug screen from six days ago was negative. During the preparation for surgery he discloses his intention to "man up" and refuse any opioids for fear of relapse. The nurse in this situation tries to reassure the patient that:

a. There is no research indicating that opioids for analgesia worsen the disease of addiction

b. Opioids will be withheld to support detoxification and rehabilitation from drug abuse

c. Providing opioids during acute pain will lead to decreased cravings for drugs of abuse

d. Toleration of significant pain will strengthen a patient's conviction to refrain from opioids

10-17. When teaching a patient to deep-breathe and cough after surgery, the nurse has the patient:

a. Take a rapid deep breath and cough once as he or she lets the breath out quickly

b. Take a rapid deep breath and cough multiple times as he or she lets the breath out at decreasing lung volumes

c. Take slow deep breaths and cough once as he or she lets the breath out slowly

d. Take slow deep breaths and cough multiple times as he or she lets the breath out quickly

10-18. Parents of a 7-year-old male patient who fell off the monkey bars at the playground and broke his left arm are anxious about his postoperative care. The patient will have a temporary cast after surgery (bright green, per patient's request). When providing discharge instructions the perianesthesia nurse includes all of the following EXCEPT:

a. Elevate the limb on pillows

b. Once dry, apply dry heat to the cast to stimulate circulation

c. Once dry, apply ice to the area of the fracture

d. Avoid putting any objects between the cast and skin

10-19. A 42-year-old healthy male patient has undergone endoscopic sinus surgery, and in preparing for discharge, the nurse instructs the patient to:

a. Notify the surgeon if having to change the mustache dressing more than once per hour

b. Attempt to keep swallowing secretions

c. Blow the nose gently with extreme caution

d. Apply a heating pad to the frontal sinus area

10-20. Within 20 minutes of admission to the PACU after a uvulopalatopharyngoplasty, a previously responsive but drowsy patient is observed to have decreasing SpO_2 and shallow respiratory effort. Prompt intervention includes which of the following?

a. Draw up naloxone because the patient is overnarcotized

b. Prepare for probable intubation with a size 8 endotracheal tube

c. Stimulate the patient and prepare to apply continuous positive airway pressure

d. Wake the patient to teach use of the incentive spirometer

10-21. It is a very busy day in the Phase II PACU area of a same-day surgery center. Staffing is adequate, but due to high patient complexity, the unlicensed assistive personnel (UAP) are supporting the RN staff. The RN can delegate all of the following activities to trained UAP EXCEPT:

a. Provide a review of discharge instructions to the patient and family

b. Collect a urine sample for laboratory studies

c. Obtain and document vital signs

d. Check a postoperative finger-stick blood glucose

10-22. The primary purpose of teaching a postoperative elective outpatient to "stay on top of their pain" is to:

a. Prevent recurrence of the original source of pain

b. Enhance the ability to meet functional goals

c. Avoid having to call the surgeon for additional prescriptions

d. Enhance the ability of the body to rest and heal

10-23. A 74-year-old female patient, anxious for a vacation cruise, has scheduled an elective blepharoplasty. Postoperative instructions for the patient will include the application of intermittent ice compresses, resuming a regular diet, and minimal bending or heavy lifting. The patient should also be instructed to avoid which of the following for the first 24 hours?

a. Analgesics, as they will not be necessary

b. Applying antibiotic ointment to the incisions

c. Cold liquids with meals

d. Hot liquids with meals

10-24. The best way to evaluate patient and family understanding of instructions given is:

a. Ask if they understand the information

b. Ask them to teach the information back to you

c. Provide the patient and family with a written quiz based on the information given

d. Have them sign an attestation form

10-25. An otherwise healthy 52-year-old male patient has just had a laparoscopic-assisted removal of a cancerous bowel lesion. Discharge teaching includes timely reporting of unresolved fevers, unrelieved pain, and nausea and vomiting. The nurse is aware that this information is MOST crucial to optimize patient outcomes and early identification of problems related to:

a. Vascular injuries

b. Neurologic injuries

c. Bladder injuries

d. Bowel injuries

10-26. Patient teaching regarding the proper method of instillation of eye drops includes all of the following EXCEPT:

a. Wash hands before using the drops

b. Rub the eyes gently to disperse the medication

c. Tilt the head back with eyes open

d. Pull down the tissue below the lower lid

10-27. Discharge instructions for most surgeries should include encouragement to contact a provider or go to the nearest emergency room for any of the following EXCEPT:

a. Uncontrolled pain

b. Heavier than expected bleeding

c. Presence of a low grade fever

d. Shortness of breath

10-28. Based on theories of growth and development, school-aged children:

a. Experience separation anxiety

b. Fear body mutilation

c. Learn through play

d. Have short attention spans

10-29. A 25-year-old female patient is being admitted for ear surgery. Knowing the procedure predisposes the patient to nausea and vertigo, the nurse instructs the patient in all of the following EXCEPT:

a. Move slowly and avoid sudden, jerky movements

b. Take slow, deep breaths through the mouth

c. Sneeze with the mouth closed

d. Prevent water in the ears

10-30. The BEST time to provide discharge instructions is:

a. Just before discharge to enhance retention of information

b. Just before going to the operating room to distract from the preop anxiety

c. During the preoperative nursing assessment for early review

d. During the postoperative follow-up visit with the surgeon

10-31. Following a total knee replacement, the patient arrives in the Phase I PACU with a wound drainage device in place. When teaching the family about the wound drainage, which of the following statements is true?

a. Gravity devices are often used to prevent excess pressure to the wound

b. Wound drainage blood loss should not exceed 500 mL in 8 hours

c. Closed suction devices increase the risk of a hematoma

d. Blood loss over the first hour can be 250-300 mL

10-32. A 75-year-old female patient is brought to the surgery center by her daughter for an outpatient biopsy of the left breast. The patient is a poor historian and was diagnosed with early dementia approximately 3 years ago. She still has recognition of her daughter and can easily follow commands. Her current deficit is short-term memory. The preoperative nurse includes the daughter in any postoperative teaching. With regard to pain assessment in the cognitively impaired, all of the following tips are useful EXCEPT:

a. Attempt to obtain the patient's self-report

b. If the procedure is assumed to be painful, assume the person has pain

c. Limit the number of questions about pain to avoid suggestion

d. Look for nonverbal signs of pain like crying, restlessness, and increased agitation

10-33. The HIGHEST order of participation in perianesthesia patient teaching is a function of:

a. Ethical practice

b. Performance improvement

c. Regulatory requirements

d. Preemptive problem solving

10-34. Patients undergoing peripheral nerve blocks should be instructed on all of the following EXCEPT:

a. The expected length of the blockade

b. Support of the extremity while moving due to impaired muscle control

c. Avoidance of smoking and handling hot liquids until the block has resolved

d. Application of continuous ice to prevent thermal injury

10-35. Which of the following descriptions does NOT generally apply to the learning style of an adult?

a. Self-directed

b. Relies on experience

c. Problem centered

d. Tactile oriented

10-36. To help prevent surgical site infection, the patient should be instructed to avoid:

a. Showering or bathing with an antibacterial soap before the procedure

b. Shaving the skin near the incision area

c. Too much preoperative fluids and proteins

d. Close contact with anyone with a cold or the flu

10-37. The nurse needs to adjust information to account for barriers to learning to ensure the patient and family benefit from the education delivered. The educator should do all of the following EXCEPT:

a. Be knowledgeable about cultural diversity

b. Present information at a grade 7 level or lower

c. Provide written as well as verbal information

d. Provide for an interpreter if necessary

10-38. A young African American male patient presents for an elective tonsillectomy. He relates a history of sickle cell disease. Once determining that the patient is afebrile and hemodynamically stable, the perianesthesia nurse teaches the patient to expect that the staff will be working to prevent a sickle cell crisis by:

a. Inducing acidosis

b. Inducing mild hypoxia

c. Maintaining mild hypothermia

d. Providing intravenous hydration

10-39. To ensure safety in the surgical setting, the patient should be instructed to do all of the following EXCEPT:

a. Be sure everyone who cares for you identifies you by asking you to state your name and date of birth and checking your armband

b. Ask questions or verbalize concerns if you do not understand a test or procedure

c. Provide a list of only prescription medications when asked about medications you take

d. Ask team members who have direct contact with you if they have washed their hands

10-40. An anxious parent is concerned about the safety of her 4-year-old child being prepared for an open reduction internal fixation (ORIF) of a radial fracture on the right forearm. The perianesthesia nurse in the preoperative unit reassures the parent that the nurses in the Phase I PACU are competent to provide care to children. In addition to having basic perianesthesia education, the perianesthesia nurse caring for pediatrics has:

a. Demonstrated pediatric airway management

b. Documented courses in pediatric electrocardiogram (ECG) interpretation

c. Pediatric Advanced Life Support provider status

d. Postnatal emergency assessment and intervention

10-41. A 51-year-old female patient with diabetes is undergoing elective surgery of her right shoulder. To avoid hypoglycemia during surgery, the Phase I PACU nurse anticipates all of the following methods EXCEPT:

a. Administering dextrose 5% in Lactated Ringer's solution at 125 mL/hr

b. Administering regular insulin in 5-unit increments as needed to keep the patient's blood glucose level equal to or greater than 200 mg/dl

c. Instructing the patient to take the usual dose of long-acting or intermediate-acting insulin

d. Administering 500 to 1000 mL of 5% dextrose and water before surgery and at least 1000 mL of 5% dextrose and water during surgery

10-42. Benefits of initiating patient education before the day of surgery include decreasing all of the following EXCEPT:

a. Preoperative anxiety

b. Postoperative complications

c. Recovery time

d. Postoperative nausea

10-43. A 45-year-old athletic businessman is consenting to surgery for a herniated intervertebral lumbar disk. His injury is likely a result of aggressive physical preparation for a local marathon; however, his current symptoms prohibit him from the active lifestyle he enjoys. While preparing him for the surgical experience, the nurse describes the immediate postoperative assessments. These will include all of the following EXCEPT:

a. Bilateral pedal pulses

b. Presence of numbness in the legs

c. Limb movement and symmetry

d. Skin integrity of the lower extremities

10-44. The MOST effective method for teaching the preschooler 5-year-old what to expect when coming to the hospital for surgery is:

a. Videos

b. Puppets

c. Drawings

d. Photographs

10-45. The BEST way to encourage patient feedback is to:

a. Ask open-ended questions to validate the patient's understanding

b. Use technical terminology

c. Provide detailed information so there are no possible questions

d. Provide limited information so the patient will ask questions

10-46. Pete, age 26, is scheduled for an elective hernia repair. He is an American Society of Anesthesiologists's (ASA's) I, never having had surgery before. While considering options for supporting preoperative education, the perianesthesia nurse is aware that a person Pete's age prefers learning by:

a. Detailed explanations

b. Talking points

c. Just the facts

d. Visual stimulation

10-47. Before providing education for patients, the perianesthesia nurse completes a self-assessment reflecting strengths and weaknesses that include all of the following EXCEPT:

a. Knowledge base

b. Understanding of the information to be taught

c. Whether he or she likes or dislikes teaching

d. Language spoken

Consider this scenario for questions 10-48 and 10-49.

A 32-year-old schoolteacher is preparing for a total hip replacement due to avascular necrosis of the left femoral head after a traumatic fall from her hybrid bicycle six months earlier. Her primary care physician had recently seen her for an annual physical and had ordered a routine panel of blood tests based on the patient's family history of hypercholesterolemia and early onset of diabetes type II.

10-48. Her hemoglobin A1-C (HbA1c) is reported as 6.4%. The nurse explains to the patient that this test measures:

a. An average of the serum glucose levels over the past 30 days

b. An average of the serum glucose levels over the past 2 to 3 months

c. An average of the serum glucose levels over the past 3 to 4 months

d. An average of the serum glucose levels over the past 6 months

10-49. Although the results of her tests were explained to her by her physician, the patient asks the perianesthesia nurse to explain them in "easy" terms. The nurse teaches that a glycosylated hemoglobin (HbA1c) of 6.4% is considered:

a. Below normal

b. Normal

c. Prediabetes

d. Diabetes

10-50. Ms. H has undergone a laparoscopically assisted vaginal hysterectomy and is being discharged home from the Phase II PACU. Discharge instructions include notifying the surgeon immediately if she develops any of the following EXCEPT:

a. Shortness of breath

b. Severe abdominal pain

c. Pain in the shoulder

d. Bleeding heavier than a period

Answers and Rationales for Chapter 10, Patient and Family Education

10-1. *Correct answer:* **d**
Toxicity from local anesthetic administration includes early direct central nervous system effects, such as ringing in the ears, metallic taste, and/or circumoral tingling. (Odom-Forren J. *Drain's Perianesthesia Nursing: A Critical Care Approach.* 6th ed. St. Louis, MO: Saunders; 2013:321-322; Clark MK. Lipid emulsion as rescue for local anesthetic-related cardiotoxicity. *J Perianesth Nurs.* 2008; 23(2):111-121.)

10-2. *Correct answer:* **c**
Hand hygiene remains the most important means of preventing the spread of disease-causing germs in the perianesthesia setting. Recommendations include washing with soap and water for at least 15 to 20 seconds using liquid or foam soaps that are hospital-approved. For less visible soiling, alcohol-based hand rubs are effective in reducing the overall number of microorganisms on the skin. (Odom-Forren J. *Drain's Perianesthesia Nursing: A Critical Care Approach.* 6th ed. St. Louis, MO: Saunders; 2013:45.)

10-3. *Correct answer:* **a**
Surgical treatment for the bariatric patient requires the patient understanding the need to modify diet and lifestyle. Early ambulation and mobility are important to prevent thrombophlebitis and deep vein thromboembolism. Clear liquids are started immediately postoperatively when tolerated. (Putrycus B, Ross J. *Certification Review for Perianesthesia Nursing.* 3rd ed. St. Louis, MO: Elsevier Saunders; 2013:220, 224; Schick L, Windle PE. *PeriAnesthesia Nursing Core Curriculum: Preprocedure, Phase I and Phase II PACU Nursing.* 3rd ed. St. Louis, MO: Saunders; 2016: 1167-1169.)

10-4. *Correct answer:* **c**
Although simulation can be used to debrief real situations, a "real" situation is far more complex than an artificial scenario can capture. Simulation does provide a safe place for training health care providers in as much as the mistakes made during simulation sessions do not harm actual patients, repetition is possible, personnel can work with the actual unit equipment, and the simulator can be used to practice rarely performed procedures and learn new skills. (Odom-Forren J. *Drain's Perianesthesia Nursing: A Critical Care Approach.* 6th ed. St. Louis, MO: Saunders; 2013:40.)

10-5. *Correct answer:* **a**
Patients ingesting clear liquids 2 to 4 hours preoperatively have been shown to have smaller gastric volumes and higher gastric pH than patients fasting more than 4 hours. (Odom-Forren J. *Drain's Perianesthesia Nursing: A Critical Care Approach.* 6th ed. St. Louis, MO: Saunders; 2013:195.)

10-6. *Correct answer:* **c**
As communities become more multicultural, it is important for health care workers to become competent in cultural sensitivity. Many programs are available to in-service staff on multicultural issues that prepare the nurse to care for diverse populations. The goal is that through the provision of respectful, meaningful, and competent care to people of diverse cultures, health and well-being are achievable. Cultural caring rituals of patients are powerful forces to know, understand, assess, and use respectfully. (American Society of PeriAnesthesia Nurses. *2015-2017 PeriAnesthesia Nursing Standards, Practice Recommendations and Interpretive Statements.* Cherry Hill, NJ: ASPAN; 2014:12.)

10-7. *Correct answer:* **c**

American Society of Anesthesiologists (ASA) members and consultants agree that fasting from the intake of infant formula at least 6 hours preoperatively should be maintained. (Odom-Forren J. *Drain's Perianesthesia Nursing: A Critical Care Approach.* 6th ed. St. Louis, MO: Saunders; 2013:195.)

10-8. *Correct answer:* **b**

"Nexters," or Generation Y, describes individuals generally born between 1980 and 2000. (Schick L, Windle PE. *PeriAnesthesia Nursing Core Curriculum: Preprocedure, Phase I and Phase II PACU Nursing.* 3rd ed. St. Louis, MO: Saunders; 2016:270.)

10-9. *Correct answer:* **c**

Oral hypoglycemic medications are held on the day of surgery to avoid hypoglycemia caused by inadequate caloric intake. (Schick L, Windle PE. *PeriAnesthesia Nursing Core Curriculum: Preprocedure, Phase I and Phase II PACU Nursing.* 3rd ed. St. Louis, MO: Saunders; 2016:113-114.)

10-10. *Correct answer:* **a**

As the patient emerges from general or regional anesthesia with sedation, the incidence of postoperative nausea and vomiting (PONV) is higher in the ophthalmic surgical patient than in other surgical procedures. Ginger is a popular complementary therapy known to have a possible antiemetic effect, although the exact mechanism is unknown. (Schick L, Windle PE. *PeriAnesthesia Nursing Core Curriculum: Preprocedure, Phase I and Phase II PACU Nursing.* 3rd ed. St. Louis, MO: Saunders; 2016:433.)

10-11. *Correct answer:* **a**

The goal of advanced certification is to validate the specialty knowledge of the perianesthesia nurse. The certification verifies the perianesthesia nurse's knowledge of prerequisites, such as anatomy and physiology, medication administration and complications, anesthesia

techniques and complication management, advanced assessment skills, critical care evaluations, and the ability to adapt to changing patient conditions. (Odom-Forren J. *Drain's Perianesthesia Nursing: A Critical Care Approach.* 6th ed. St. Louis, MO: Saunders; 2013:16-17.)

10-12. *Correct answer:* **c**

Feverfew, garlic, and ginseng inhibit platelet aggregation. Garlic increases bleeding time and decreases platelet viscosity. Ginseng inhibits platelet-activating factor. (American Society of PeriAnesthesia Nurses. *A Competency-Based Orientation and Credentialing Program for the Registered Nurse in the Perianesthesia Setting.* Cherry Hill, NJ: ASPAN; 2014; Schick L, Windle PE. *PeriAnesthesia Nursing Core Curriculum: Preprocedure, Phase I and Phase II PACU Nursing.* 3rd ed. St. Louis, MO: Saunders; 2016:72.)

10-13. *Correct answer:* **a**

Individualized patient education is most effective. The content and methods should be modified for the patient and family. The nurse should determine what the patient and family want and need to know and design the teaching plan accordingly. Learner characteristics to consider include age; primary language; reading level; sensory limitations; physical condition; developmental level; mental, emotional, or educational limitations; and motivation and attitude. (Odom-Forren J. *Drain's Perianesthesia Nursing: A Critical Care Approach.* 6th ed. St. Louis, MO: Saunders; 2013:382.)

10-14. *Correct answer:* **d**

The goals of patient education are to increase the patient's sense of self-worth, decrease anxiety, and reduce facility and provider liability by ensuring that the patient and family or companion receive information in a form that they can comprehend and use to enhance the operative experience. (Odom-Forren J. *Drain's Perianesthesia Nursing: A Critical Care Approach.* 6th ed. St. Louis, MO: Saunders; 2013:381.)

10-15. *Correct answer:* **d**

The American Society of Anesthesiologists' (ASA's) advises that patients stop herbal medications at least 2 weeks before surgery. (Odom-Forren J. *Drain's Perianesthesia Nursing: A Critical Care Approach.* 6th ed. St. Louis, MO: Saunders; 2013:250.)

10-16. *Correct answer:* **a**

Opioids, when indicated, should not be withheld from patients with pain who also have addictive disease. During the experience of acute pain, any attempt to detoxify or rehabilitate an active addict should be delayed until a later time. Current research does not support the notion that administration of opioids to patients with addiction actually makes the addiction worse. By the same token, avoiding opioids will not prevent a patient from experiencing a relapse. Untreated pain may actually lead to increased cravings for drugs. (Odom-Forren J. *Drain's Perianesthesia Nursing: A Critical Care Approach.* 6th ed. St. Louis, MO: Saunders; 2013:444-445.)

10-17. *Correct answer:* **b**

Cough effectiveness depends on the inspired tidal volume and the velocity of expired airflow. The cascade cough is the most effective method. The patient should be taught to take a rapid deep inspiration to increase the volume of air in the lungs, allowing the air to pass beyond the retained secretions. On exhalation, the patient should perform multiple coughs at subsequently lower lung volumes. (Odom-Forren J. *Drain's Perianesthesia Nursing: A Critical Care Approach.* 6th ed. St. Louis, MO: Saunders; 2013:482.)

10-18. *Correct answer:* **b**

Several important points should be covered when providing instructions for cast care to prevent or identify complications early. Key are assessments for skin breakdown, neurovascular compromise, and compartment syndrome. Keeping the cast clean and dry and free of foreign objects is important. Maintaining an elevated position and applying ice when the cast is dry will help reduce neurovascular compromise and the development of compartment syndrome. (Schick L, Windle PE. *PeriAnesthesia Nursing Core Curriculum: Preprocedure, Phase I and Phase II PACU Nursing.* 3rd ed. St. Louis, MO: Saunders; 2016:1010.)

10-19. *Correct answer:* **a**

Changing the mustache dressing two to three times in 4-hour period is to be expected. Swallowing secretions can lead to nausea and vomiting. Blowing the nose can lead to increased bleeding, as can the application of heat; ice packs are preferred. (Odom-Forren J. *Drain's Perianesthesia Nursing: A Critical Care Approach.* 6th ed. St. Louis, MO: Saunders; 2013:454.)

10-20. *Correct answer:* **c**

Uvulopalatopharyngoplasty is a surgical intervention for obstructive sleep apnea and snoring. Postoperatively, patients are prone to hypoventilation and hypoxia related to operative tissue swelling and edema. Before considering reintubation, the patient should be stimulated, and continuous positive airway pressure should be applied. (Putrycus B, Ross J. *Certification Review for Perianesthesia Nursing.* 3rd ed. St. Louis, MO: Saunders; 2013:234-235, 241; Schick L, Windle PE. *PeriAnesthesia Nursing Core Curriculum: Preprocedure, Phase I and Phase II PACU Nursing.* 3rd ed. St. Louis, MO: Saunders; 2016:1066.)

10-21. *Correct answer:* **a**

There are commonly accepted rules of delegation, which mandate that the delegated activity involves the right task, circumstances, person, communication, and feedback. In addition, tasks that require nursing judgment or application of the nursing process should not be delegated to UAP. UAP may be trained to collect and report on data, such as urine samples and vital signs, but not interpret it. (American Society of PeriAnesthesia Nurses. *2015-2017 Perianesthesia Nursing Standards, Practice Recommendations and Interpretive Statements.* Cherry Hill, NJ: ASPAN; 2014:94.)

10-22. *Correct answer:* **b**

Patients should be taught to maintain adequate pain control after discharge by taking pain medications before pain is severe or out of control. The rationale is that functional goals (such as physical therapy and activities of daily living) can be best met when the patient is more comfortable. (Odom-Forren J. *Drain's Perianesthesia Nursing: A Critical Care Approach.* 3rd ed. St. Louis, MO: Saunders; 2013:441.)

10-23. *Correct answer:* **d**

Blepharoplasty is a procedure performed to correct deformities of the upper or lower eyelids. In general, this is accomplished by excising redundant skin or protruding fat. The procedure is usually performed with local anesthesia with supplemental intravenous sedation. Postoperatively, ice and cold compresses minimize swelling and bleeding and enhance comfort. Certainly activities such as bending and heavy lifting should be avoided and any acute pain should be assessed and managed with appropriate analgesics. Drugs that may lead to incisional bleeding should be avoided. Antibiotic ointment is often used for lubrication of the healing tissues. The patient may resume a regular diet after surgery; however, hot liquids are contraindicated for 24 hours to prevent vasodilation and bleeding. (Odom-Forren J. *Drain's Perianesthesia Nursing: A Critical Care Approach.* 6th ed. St. Louis, MO: Saunders; 2013:636.)

10-24. *Correct answer:* **b**

Asking the patient or caregiver to teach the instructions back to the nurse in his or her own words allows the nurse to check for understanding of the material and re-explain if necessary. (Schick L, Windle PE. *PeriAnesthesia Nursing Core Curriculum: Preprocedure, Phase I and Phase II PACU Nursing.* 3rd ed. St. Louis, MO: Saunders; 2016:1277-1279; American Society of PeriAnesthesia Nurses.

A Competency-Based Orientation and Credentialing Program for the Registered Nurse in the Perianesthesia Setting. Cherry Hill, NJ: ASPAN; 2014.)

10-25. *Correct answer:* **d**

Patients undergoing outpatient laparoscopic procedures should be taught to report early signs of bowel injuries. While relatively rare, bowel injuries are a potential complication. Typically the injury involves perforation of the small intestines which are micro in nature. These can go unrecognized while in the operating room and eventually develop into peritonitis and subsequent sepsis. Patients must be educated to report unrelieved pain, prolonged nausea and vomiting and unanticipated fevers to the surgeon. (Odom-Forren J. *Drain's Perianesthesia Nursing: A Critical Care Approach.* 6th ed. St. Louis, MO: Saunders; 2013:619.)

10-26. *Correct answer:* **b**

Eye drop instillation should be performed as follows: wash hands, tilt the head back, keep the eyes open and look upward, pull down the tissue below the lower lid, close the eyes and avoid blinking or squeezing for several minutes, and gently blot away the excess fluids from under the eye. (Schick L, Windle PE. *PeriAnesthesia Nursing Core Curriculum: Preprocedure, Phase I and Phase II PACU Nursing.* 3rd ed. St. Louis, MO: Saunders; 2016:965.)

10-27. *Correct answer:* **c**

On occasion, a patient may develop a serious postoperative complication. If patients develop shortness of breath, severe pain, or bleeding that is heavier than expected, they should be instructed to contact their physician immediately or go to the nearest emergency room. (Odom-Forren J. *Drain's Perianesthesia Nursing: A Critical Care Approach.* 6th ed. St. Louis, MO: Saunders; 2013:619.)

10-28. *Correct answer:* **b**

School-age children fear other body parts may be hurt during the operation. Offering a simple explanation of what body part will be affected and having the child indicate his or her understanding by marking the surgical site on a picture or doll allows the nurse to evaluate the child's understanding. (Schick L, Windle PE. *PeriAnesthesia Nursing Core Curriculum: Preprocedure, Phase I and Phase II PACU Nursing.* 3rd ed. St. Louis, MO: Saunders; 2016:203, Box 9-6; American Society of PeriAnesthesia Nurses. *A Competency-Based Orientation and Credentialing Program for the Registered Nurse in the Perianesthesia Setting.* Cherry Hill, NJ: ASPAN; 2014.)

10-29. *Correct answer:* **c**

Sudden turns should be avoided. Slow, deep breaths through the mouth can minimize nausea. Education should include not allowing water in the ears and opening the mouth if sneezing occurs so that the force of the sneeze has a larger exit opening. (Odom-Forren J. *Drain's Perianesthesia Nursing: A Critical Care Approach.* 6th ed. St. Louis, MO: Saunders; 2013:452.)

10-30. *Correct answer:* **c**

Ideally, discharge instructions are provided before the day of surgery to help prepare the patient and family for any home requirements, needed supplies, or alterations (e.g., removal of rugs that increase fall risk, sleeping area moved closer to the bathroom). This provides for minimization of safety concerns or enhancement of care. In addition, discharge instructions are reviewed with the patient and family or companion before the patient is discharged. (Odom-Forren J. *Drain's Perianesthesia Nursing: A Critical Care Approach.* 6th ed. St. Louis, MO: Saunders; 2013:384.)

10-31. *Correct answer:* **d**

Often with total joint replacement, it is common to have a large amount of blood loss in the immediate postoperative period—250 to 300 mL in the first hour—and as a result, careful monitoring of blood loss is required. Closed suction devices are often used and help reduce hematoma formation. Gravity devices are rarely used. (Odom-Forren J. *Drain's Perianesthesia Nursing: A Critical Care Approach.* 6th ed. St. Louis, MO: Saunders; 2013:549; Schick L, Windle PE. *PeriAnesthesia Nursing Core Curriculum: Preprocedure, Phase I and Phase II PACU Nursing.* 3rd ed. St. Louis, MO: Saunders; 2016:1034.)

10-32. *Correct answer:* **c**

In terms of assessing pain in patients with cognitive impairment, it is important to try to solicit a pain description and report from the patient. Otherwise, assume pain is present and verify with nonverbal pain behaviors such as crying, frowning, increased restlessness, and agitation. It is also important to provide instructions and questions repeatedly, allowing ample time for a response. (Odom-Forren J. *Drain's Perianesthesia Nursing: A Critical Care Approach.* 6th ed. St. Louis, MO: Saunders; 2013:434.)

10-33. *Correct answer:* **a**

The perianesthesia nurse has an ethical responsibility to patients that includes the provision of dignified, confidential, and competent care. Duties within this responsibility include advocating for safe patient care, respect for diversity, and participation in perianesthesia patient teaching. (American Society of PeriAnesthesia Nurses. *2015-2017 PeriAnesthesia Nursing Standards, Practice Recommendations and Interpretive Statements.* Cherry Hill, NJ: ASPAN; 2014:11.)

10-34. *Correct answer:* **d**

Information on the expected length of the blockade will decrease patient anxiety. Limb support while the block is resolving is critical for minimizing movement of the extremity to prevent injury. The ability to determine temperature and pressure points may be impaired. Cold therapy should be used intermittently until the block resolves. (Odom-Forren J. *Drain's Perianesthesia Nursing: A Critical Care Approach.* 6th ed. St. Louis, MO: Saunders; 2013:334-339; American Society of PeriAnesthesia Nurses. *A Competency-Based Orientation and Credentialing Program for the Registered Nurse in the Perianesthesia Setting.* Cherry Hill, NJ: ASPAN; 2014.)

10-35. *Correct answer:* **d**

In general, the adult learner is motivated internally, self-directed, and self-governed. This learner will use past experiences as a resource and may have difficulty accepting new concepts. The adult learner often has a problem-centered orientation to learning. The child learner does not assume responsibility for learning, is totally dependent on adults, relies on a transmittal method of learning (often a hands-on approach), is open to new concepts, and is subject centered. (Odom-Forren J. *Drain's Perianesthesia Nursing: A Critical Care Approach.* 6th ed. St. Louis, MO: Saunders; 2013:382.)

10-36. *Correct answer:* **b**

Patients should be instructed to avoid shaving the skin near the incision area before surgery to prevent micro-abrasions and cuts in the skin that could harbor bacteria. (Odom-Forren J. *Drain's Perianesthesia Nursing: A Critical Care Approach.* 6th ed. St. Louis, MO: Saunders; 2013:651, 654.)

10-37. *Correct answer:* **b**

Learning is influenced by personal factors such as past experiences, culture, age, ability to learn, and beliefs about health care.

Written materials should be readable at a grade 5 level or lower. (Odom-Forren J. *Drain's Perianesthesia Nursing: A Critical Care Approach.* 6th ed. St. Louis, MO: Saunders; 2013:384; Schick L, Windle PE. *PeriAnesthesia Nursing Core Curriculum: Preprocedure, Phase I and Phase II PACU Nursing.* 3rd ed. St. Louis, MO: Saunders; 2016: 89.

10-38. *Correct answer:* **d**

The goal of anesthesia for the patient with sickle cell anemia is to avoid acidosis secondary to hypoventilation. Prevention includes efforts to maintain oxygenation, prevent circulatory stasis, provide hydration, and maintain body temperature. (Schick L, Windle PE. *PeriAnesthesia Nursing Core Curriculum: Preprocedure, Phase I and Phase II PACU Nursing.* 3rd ed. St. Louis, MO: Saunders; 2016:826.)

10-39. *Correct answer:* **c**

Patients should be instructed to include EVERY medication they are taking/using, including creams, vitamins, herbs, diet supplements, all prescription and over-the-counter medications, and street drugs. Many of these substances may have serious interactions with anesthetic agents and other medications given during surgery. (Odom-Forren J. *Drain's Perianesthesia Nursing: A Critical Care Approach.* 6th ed. St. Louis, MO: Saunders; 2013:651.)

10-40. *Correct answer:* **c**

According to the American Society of PeriAnesthesia Nurses (ASPAN) Standards, the perianesthesia registered nurse providing Phase I level of care will maintain a current advanced cardiac life support (ACLS) and/or pediatric advanced life support (PALS) provider status, as appropriate to the patient population served. (American Society of PeriAnesthesia Nurses. *2015-2017 PeriAnesthesia Nursing Standards, Practice Recommendations and Interpretive Statements.* Cherry Hill, NJ: ASPAN; 2014:23.)

10-41. *Correct answer:* **c**

The goal of perioperative management for a patient with diabetes is maintenance of the serum glucose level at less than 200 mg/dL. Equally important is the prevention of hypoglycemia and severe fluid loss. (Odom-Forren J. *Drain's Perianesthesia Nursing: A Critical Care Approach.* 6th ed. St. Louis, MO: Saunders; 2013: 683-684.)

10-42. *Correct answer:* **d**

Patients benefit from learning before the surgery when they have time to review the information and ask questions. Education also increases patient compliance with instructions and improves coping mechanisms for the patient. (Odom-Forren J. *Drain's Perianesthesia Nursing: A Critical Care Approach.* 6th ed. St. Louis, MO: Saunders; 2013:648.)

10-43. *Correct answer:* **d**

The postoperative neurologic examination should include assessment of sensation in the lower extremities, as well as an assessment of the presence of tingling, numbness, or paralysis. The pedal pulses, color, temperature, and capillary refill of the lower extremities should also be assessed. (Odom-Forren J. *Drain's Perianesthesia Nursing: A Critical Care Approach.* 6th ed. St. Louis, MO: Saunders; 2013:576.)

10-44. *Correct answer:* **b**

For children, factors that affect the choice of teaching method include the child's age and developmental level, the family's available resources, and the cognitive ability of the child and parent. The preschool child (ages 3–6) responds well when there are opportunities to offer choices. Use play, picture books, storybooks, and puppets to explain procedures and activities. Speak in simple sentences and be concise. (Schick L, Windle PE. *PeriAnesthesia Nursing Core Curriculum: Preprocedure, Phase I and Phase II PACU Nursing.* 3rd ed. St. Louis, MO: Saunders; 2016:206t.)

10-45. *Correct answer:* **a**

Asking open-ended questions encourages the learner to express the content in his or her own words and allows the nurse to evaluate the patient's understanding of the information taught and correct any misunderstandings. (Schick L, Windle PE. *Perianesthesia Nursing Core Curriculum: Preprocedure, Phase I and Phase II PACU Nursing.* 3rd ed. St. Louis, MO: Saunders; 2016:89; American Society of PeriAnesthesia Nurses. *A Competency-Based Orientation and Credentialing Program for the Registered Nurse in the Perianesthesia Setting.* Cherry Hill, NJ: ASPAN; 2014.)

10-46. *Correct answer:* **d**

In terms of individuals who are the "Nexters," this group of adults is considered racially and ethnically diverse and tolerant, indulged as children by parents who spent a good deal of time with them, are blunt with opinions and expressions, carry a sense of entitlement, are tech-savvy, are good multitaskers, and are adaptable to situations and change. (Schick L, Windle PE. *PeriAnesthesia Nursing Core Curriculum: Preprocedure, Phase I and Phase II PACU Nursing.* 3rd ed. St. Louis, MO: Saunders; 2016:270.)

10-47. *Correct answer:* **d**

In order to more efficiently provide patient education, perianesthesia nurses should be self-aware of any biases they may have towards patients. Appreciation for one's own strengths and acknowledgment of opportunities for improvement are necessary for the provision of high quality and effective patient education. (Odom-Forren J. *Drain's Perianesthesia Nursing: A Critical Care Approach.* 6th ed. St. Louis, MO: Saunders; 2013:381-382.)

10-48. *Correct answer:* **b**

Serum glucose adheres to hemoglobin to make a 'glycosylated hemoglobin' molecule, called hemoglobin A1C or HbA1C. The more glucose in the blood, the more hemoglobin A1C or HbA1C will be present in the blood. The average red cell lives for 6-12 weeks before being replaced. A measurement of the HbA1c is an indicator of the average blood glucose level over the last 2 to 3 months. (Odom-Forren J. *Drain's Perianesthesia Nursing: A Critical Care Approach.* 6th ed. St. Louis, MO: Saunders; 2013:681-682.)

10-49. *Correct answer:* **c**

The criteria for diabetes, based on the glycosylated hemoglobin (HbA1c) alone, include a normal range between 4% and 5.7%, a prediabetes range between 5.8% and 6.5%, and a diabetic range greater than 6.5%. (Odom-Forren J. *Drain's Perianesthesia Nursing: A Critical Care Approach.* 6th ed. St. Louis, MO: Saunders; 2013:681-682.)

10-50. *Correct answer:* **c**

If patients have shortness of breath, severe pain, or bleeding heavier than a period, they should contact their physician immediately. Referred pain in the shoulder is a common occurrence with laparoscopic surgery. (Odom-Forren J. *Drain's Perianesthesia Nursing: A Critical Care Approach.* 6th ed. St. Louis, MO: Saunders; 2013:616-619.)

11

ASPAN Standards, Documentation, Regulatory Guidelines, and Patient Safety Needs

Sylvia Baker, Denise O'Brien, and Theresa Clifford

11-1. While caring for the Phase I PACU patient, the perianesthesia nurse ensures patient safety by providing 1:1 care until critical elements are met. Critical elements include an initial nursing assessment, ensuring that the patient has a stable airway and hemodynamic stability, the patient is free from restlessness or combative behaviors, and:

   a. The patient is able to deep-breathe and cough

   b. The patient can comply with a stir-up regimen

   c. Transfer of care has taken place

   d. Clinical monitors have been applied

11-2. In preparation for extubation, the perianesthesia nurse assesses and documents adequate muscle strength. All of these criteria are indications of adequate muscle strength EXCEPT the ability to:

   a. Lift the head from the bed for at least 5 seconds

   b. Lift the head from the bed for at least 15 seconds

   c. Open eyes widely

   d. Swallow

11-3. A right-handed, 36-year-old male patient with a history of chronic pain treated with long-acting opioids has gone to the operating room for a closed reduction of a right wrist fracture. The perianesthesia nurse considers all of the following when determining this patient's length of stay after the administration of intravenous opioid medications EXCEPT:

   a. Medication half-life

   b. Drug hypersensitivity

   c. Cumulative effects

   d. Surgical procedure

11-4. Patient and family education includes preparing the patient for surgery. To avoid postoperative infection, the patient should be taught to:

   a. Request that staff wash their hands

   b. Shave surgical site at home

   c. Avoid harsh antimicrobial soaps

   d. Prepare for a high carbohydrate diet postoperatively

11-5. Standard III of ASPAN's *2015-2017 Perianesthesia Nursing Standards,* Staffing and Personnel Management, identifies that the professional perianesthesia nurse providing Phase I level of care maintains certain competencies concerning advanced cardiac life support (ACLS) and pediatric advanced life support (PALS). This standard identifies that:

   a. An ACLS equivalency course can be provided by each facility

   b. Current ACLS or PALS provider status is maintained appropriate to patient population served

   c. PALS is only required when the pediatric population exceeds 15 cases/day

   d. Current ACLS and PALS provider status is strongly encouraged

11-6. To aid in ensuring patient safety, the Centers for Medicare & Medicaid Services (CMS) requires that a postanesthesia evaluation be completed in accordance with state law and procedures that have been approved by the medical staff and that reflect current standards of anesthesia care. This evaluation must be performed by:

a. Any advanced practitioner

b. A perianesthesia nurse

c. A practitioner who is qualified to administer anesthesia

d. An anesthesiologist on staff

11-7. As a perianesthesia nurse, the MOST important element of the American Society of Peri-Anesthesia Nurses (ASPAN) Staffing and Personnel Management Standard is:

a. The standard is endorsed by ASPAN

b. Staffing patterns reflect patient acuity, census, and workflow

c. The staffing matrix should be based on a formula incorporating adjusted patient days

d. Staffing schedules should be addressed within an organization's service standards

11-8. The perianesthesia nurse is preparing to administer packed red cells to a patient. To identify the patient, the nurse will:

a. Check the room number and procedure of the patient

b. Review the operating room number, procedure, and surgeon's name

c. Ask the patient to state his mother's name and maiden name

d. Use identifiers such as the patient's name, identification number, or birth date

11-9. When discharging a 6-month-old after a bilateral myringotomy and tube placement, the Phase II PACU nurse evaluates all of the following EXCEPT:

a. Interactions between the child and parent or significant other

b. Patient and home care provider knowledge of discharge instructions

c. Ability of home care provider to demonstrate how to measure temperature

d. Transportation plans to include a second responsible person to sit with the child

11-10. The practice of applying sequential compression devices during the perioperative phase of patient care is an example of:

a. Clinical inquiry

b. Process improvement

c. Research utilization

d. Research design

11-11. According to the Occupational Safety and Health Administration Bloodborne Pathogens (OSHA BPP) standard, institutional plans to reduce employee needlestick injuries must include input from:

a. Employees responsible for direct patient care

b. Registered clinical pharmacists and pharmacy technicians

c. Nurse managers

d. Employee health directors

11-12. When caring for a medical-surgical overflow patient in the Phase I PACU or the Phase II ambulatory surgery unit (ASU), the perianesthesia nurse:

a. Demonstrates appropriate competencies required for the patient populations

b. Groups the Phase I and medical-surgical patients in order to provide appropriate nursing ratios

c. Advocates for a modified surgical schedule to accommodate the overflow

d. Contacts the director of anesthesia services for medical management of the patient

11-13. Critical elements of the Phase I PACU admission include all of the following EXCEPT:

a. Report has been received, questions have been answered, and transfer of care has taken place

b. The patient has a stable/secure airway

c. The patient is able to answer questions

d. The patient is hemodynamically stable and free from agitation, restlessness, and combative behaviors

11-14. When participating in a study to delineate the use of a perianesthesia scoring tool, the perianesthesia nurse knows that the outcome of this study will have the most impact on the nurse's:

a. Clinical role

b. Educational role

c. Management role

d. Collaborative role

11-15. The Phase II perianesthesia nurse is caring for the following patients: one 9-year-old patient with parents at bedside, one 54-year-old patient just returning from the operating room as an initial admission, and one 45-year-old patient who is preparing for discharge (IV is discontinued and the patient is dressed in street clothes). This situation:

a. Is below the American Society of Peri-Anesthesia Nurses (ASPAN) Standard for staffing

b. Meets the ASPAN Standard for staffing

c. Exceeds the ASPAN Standard for staffing

d. Has never been tried as a staffing pattern

11-16. The perianesthesia nurse reviews The Joint Commission (TJC) National Patient Safety Goals, acknowledging that:

a. The goals are only applicable in the hospital setting

b. TJC revises the goals only when new safety issues arise

c. The goals are updated annually

d. TJC does not require adherence to the goals

11-17. Factors that influence the level of opioid-induced sedation include the dose of medication, the route of administration, the patient's opioid tolerance, current medical conditions and comorbidities, and:

a. Age 15 and younger

b. Age between 15 and 40

c. Age between 40 and 55

d. Age 55 and older

11-18. An 85-year-old male patient is being prepared for surgery to repair a fractured hip. The perianesthesia nurse assigned to care for him is aware that older patients are at an increased risk of unwanted sedation secondary to a reduction in tissue perfusion, drug metabolism, drug clearance, and:

a. Total body water

b. Bone density

c. Circulating hormones

d. Cerebral blood flow

11-19. Patient safety is primarily defined as:

a. The highest priority of perianesthesia practice

b. An updated resource for evidence-based policies and procedure

c. Having a surgical team that is collaborative

d. Sustaining no injury from a near-miss event

11-20. The most important criteria to be assessed and documented regarding the patient with a right-sided chest tube include all of the following EXCEPT:

a. Vital signs to include blood pressure, heart rate, and rhythm

b. Fluctuations in the water seal chamber

c. Frequency of Trendelenburg positioning for fluid drainage

d. Condition of dressing and surrounding tissue

11-21. The Phase II PACU nurse assesses his patient's readiness for discharge. When the patient reports that she has no transportation and no one to stay with her at home, the Phase II nurse:

a. Keeps the patient in the department an extra 4 to 6 hours

b. Notifies the surgeon/primary care provider and follows the department procedures and policies

c. Calls the patient's nearest neighbor to request assistance and to check on the patient

d. Obtains a taxi/bus voucher and accompanies the patient to the appropriate exit

11-22. The perianesthesia Phase I nurse has worked a hectic 10-hour shift, and the current schedule implies there will be at least 8 more hours of surgery and recovery time ahead. The schedule indicates this nurse will begin an "on-call" status in 2 hours. The perianesthesia nurse taking a call knows the following criteria should be met:

a. A minimum of 2 hours provided between shifts to allow for adequate nurse recuperation

b. Staff refusing to complete "on-call" requirements are subject to discipline

c. Minimum staffing ratios are rarely necessary when working "on-call"

d. Leadership should provide a plan to augment "on-call" staff based on patient census and acuity

11-23. A new orientee is reviewing guidelines for clinical documentation in the Phase I PACU. When discussing the documentation of any phone calls made to report changes in a patient's condition, a number of important elements are identified. These include the time the call was made, the person who made the call, the individual who was called, and:

a. What the person who was called was doing at the time of the call

b. What the person who made the call was doing at the time of the call

c. All information given and received during the call

d. The number of patients and staff in the unit at the time of the call

11-24. An 18-year-old female patient is scheduled for a diagnostic laparoscopy for suspected endometriosis. She is a healthy nonsmoker, with a passion for sports and athletic training. She was recently accepted into a health coach program. She reports a history of seasickness when on watercraft. Current vital signs include a BP of 92/54 and a resting HR of 56. When documenting her risks for postoperative complications, the perianesthesia nurse notes risk factors for postoperative nausea and vomiting (PONV) to include all of the following EXCEPT:

a. Female gender

b. Smoking status

c. Motion sickness

d. Cardiac output

11-25. Providing translation services for non-English–speaking patients is required under:

a. The Civil Rights Act

b. The Centers for Medicare & Medicaid Services

c. The Joint Commission Standards

d. The Health Insurance Portability and Accountability Act

11-26. The perianesthesia nurse arrives at the bedside of the patient undergoing an operative procedure. Before entering the patient's care area, the nurse will:

a. Use an alcohol-based hand sanitizer provided by her facility

b. Obtain latex-free gloves and ensure the gloves are sized correctly

c. Answer the call light of the patient in the next bay

d. Wipe off the keyboard of the bedside computer with bleach cloths

11-27. When documenting electronically, the nurse must be diligent to perform what function to protect her documentation?

 a. Use the "save" button on the keyboard

 b. Print the record for transfer of care to the next provider

 c. Sign in and out with user name and password

 d. Electronically sign name after completing documentation

11-28. The American Society of PeriAnesthesia Nurses (ASPAN) Standards state "two registered nurses, one of whom is a RN competent in Phase I Postanesthesia Nursing are in the same room/unit where the patient is receiving Phase I level of care." The PRIMARY intent is that the second nurse is:

 a. Anywhere in the hospital itself

 b. A phone call away

 c. Within the surgery department

 d. In the same room where the patient is

11-29. A patient arrives at the same-day unit before surgery complaining that the elevator doors shut too quickly, knocking the patient to the floor. After appropriate assessment, investigation of the complaint, and communication of the event to nursing leadership, the perianesthesia nurse prepares to chart the event. Documentation of the patient incident should be factual and objective but should NOT include which of the following?

 a. Patient subjective description of an event

 b. Description of any injuries sustained

 c. Outcomes of the event investigation

 d. The completed incident report

11-30. The perianesthesia nurse caring for the perinatal patient develops care plans, protocols, and clinical practices that support the unique needs of the childbearing family during surgical birth that include topics such as bringing the newborn into the Phase I PACU, providing early skin-to-skin contact with the newborn, and:

 a. Allowing for music therapy as part of the birthing plan

 b. Encouragement to breastfeed

 c. Keeping opioid therapy to a minimum

 d. Bringing the doula for active uterine management

11-31. The frequency with which the Phase II perianesthesia nurse documents on a patient is:

 a. Every 5 minutes

 b. Every 10 minutes

 c. Every 15 minutes

 d. As per institutional policy

11-32. The perianesthesia nurse understands that the sources of standards include all of the following EXCEPT:

 a. Accrediting organizations

 b. State boards of nursing

 c. Specialty nursing organizations

 d. Health care nurse executives

11-33. When caring for the patient with increased intracranial pressure, the perianesthesia nurse assesses and documents all of the important nursing interventions, including:

 a. Maintaining the head of the bed at 15 degrees

 b. Inducing hourly Valsalva maneuvers to keep pressure low

 c. Spacing all nursing care to allow frequent rest periods

 d. Obtaining adequate support to turn the patient from supine to prone every 2 hours

11-34. The perianesthesia nurse accompanies the patient being transported if the patient requires all of the following EXCEPT:

a. Evaluation during transport

b. Continuous intravenous infusions

c. A higher level of care

d. Treatment during transport

11-35. Ms. Z, 54 years old, arrives in the Phase I PACU after an inguinal hernia repair. Ms. Z's history includes obesity, diabetes mellitus, a previous cerebrovascular accident (CVA) with residual right-sided weakness, and a myocardial infarction (MI) within the past 9 months. Ms. Z arrives slightly diaphoretic, with respirations regular and facial color ruddy. Initial vital signs are BP 108/54 (preoperative BP was 147/91), HR 67, RR 16, T 96.2° F, and SpO$_2$ of 97% with O$_2$ at 5 L/nasal cannula. The inguinal dressing is clean and dry, and the abdomen is distended and firm. Your initial action for this patient is to conduct and then document:

a. Application of pulse oximetry

b. Application of cardiac monitor

c. Assessment of respiratory status

d. Assessment of neurologic status

11-36. When describing an observation regarding a patient, it is MOST important to document:

a. Immediately

b. Objectively

c. Chronologically

d. Subjectively

11-37. When caring for a patient with local anesthetic systemic toxicity (LAST), the perianesthesia nurse is prepared to document which of the following EARLY signs of cardiovascular toxicity?

a. Hypertension and atrial irritability

b. Hypotension and atrial irritability

c. Hypertension preceding hypotension

d. Atrial irritability and tachycardia

11-38. Mr. J arrived in the Phase I PACU after a renal transplant. He has a history of type 1 diabetes and end-stage renal failure, treated with hemodialysis. Laboratory tests for potassium and calcium were drawn approximately 15 minutes after his arrival. Forty-five minutes later, the laboratory technician is calling with critical results, and the clerk asks the nurse to take the phone call. The perianesthesia registered nurse expects:

a. The results are out of the normal range

b. The patient will need insulin for hyperglycemia

c. The tests need to be redrawn due to hemolysis

d. Treatment for an abnormal value will not be necessary

11-39. An 85-year-old male patient is recovering from spinal anesthesia after a repair of a fractured hip. The patient is relatively healthy for his age, having fractured his hip while climbing a ladder. The perianesthesia nurse knows that in order to document the first indication that the block is resolving, the patient will need to be assessed for:

a. Return of sensation to sharp stimulus

b. Return of temperature sensation

c. Resolution of hypotension

d. Ability to move lower extremities

11-40. The patient awakens in the operating room under the observation of the anesthesia care provider. To ensure patient safety and proceed directly to Phase II care, the perianesthesia nurse understands the MOST important element for safe fast tracking is that the patient must:

a. Meet Phase I discharge criteria in the OR

b. Be pain free at the end of surgery

c. Meet Phase I discharge criteria within minutes of arrival to Phase II

d. Be free of postoperative nausea and vomiting (PONV) at the end of surgery

11-41. The perianesthesia nurse working the early shift has left for the day. About 45 minutes after she clocked out, she calls on her cell phone to report that she forgot to chart a medication that was given to a patient who was transferred to Phase II just before she left. What should be done?

a. Take down the exact information (drug, dose, and time given) and chart it on the patient's chart

b. File an incident report and ask her to come back to work immediately and chart this information

c. Report the information to the nurse caring for the patient and save the chart for a late entry to be made

d. Refer the call to the manager and let her decide what to do

11-42. An 8-month-old patient has been brought to the same-day surgery unit for a hernia repair under general anesthesia. When collecting preanesthesia data on the pediatric patient of this age, the perianesthesia nurse considers additional components of assessment and management beyond the adult components, which include:

a. Birth history and gestational age

b. Current favorite play objects

c. Birth order of the child compared with siblings

d. Condition of the posterior fontanel

11-43. The perianesthesia nurse follows documentation guidelines that include charting accurately, comprehensively, and promptly and:

a. Providing honest critique of events

b. Offering carefully described subjective findings

c. Charting with common nursing abbreviations

d. Charting objectively to describe only what is observed

11-44. Mr. G is preparing for discharge after an uneventful laparoscopic cholecystectomy. With knowledge that right shoulder pain after laparoscopic surgery is common, the Phase II perianesthesia nurse teaches and documents patient education to include:

a. Sleeping at a 45-degree angle to eliminate the pain

b. Calling 911 if the shoulder pain is not resolved within 12 hours

c. Reassurance that the temporary pain is from surgical positioning

d. Instructions to use oral analgesics for the shoulder pain

11-45. Site marking is done when there is more than one possible location for the procedure and when performing the procedure in a different location could harm the patient. The following statements are correct regarding site marking, according to The Joint Commission, EXCEPT:

a. The mark is unambiguous and is used consistently throughout the organization

b. The mark is sufficiently permanent to be visible after skin preparation and draping

c. Alternative processes may be needed for mucosal surfaces and minimal access procedures

d. The mark is the signature of the licensed independent practitioner (LIP)

11-46. The perianesthesia nurse supervises and delegates to unlicensed assistive perianesthesia (UAP) support staff. Competencies recommended for the UAP include:

a. Unsterile dressing changes as needed

b. PEARS (pediatric emergency assessment recognition and stabilization) training

c. Basic airway support

d. Interpretation of monitor alarms

11-47. Standards of care for which perianesthesia nurses are held accountable are those standards that a reasonably prudent nurse would follow. These standards are set forth in all of the following ways EXCEPT:

a. Standards established by institutional policies and procedures

b. Standards that may vary from community to community

c. Standards established by the national nursing organizations

d. Standards that are integrated into annual performance evaluations

11-48. The competent perianesthesia nurse demonstrates teamwork, collaboration, and effective communication and will participate in:

a. Professional development

b. Multidisciplinary rounds

c. Policy implementation

d. Nursing grand rounds

11-49. To promote positive outcomes, perianesthesia nurses seek knowledge of and develop skills in the care of the pediatric patient. To provide optimal care of the pediatric patient, the perianesthesia nurse demonstrates a commitment to:

a. Nurse-managed care (NMC)

b. Value-based pediatric care (VBPC)

c. Accountable care (AC)

d. Family-centered care (FCC)

11-50. Mr. S is undergoing an open reduction and internal fixation of a tibial and fibular fracture of his left leg after a motor vehicle accident. He is awake and alert and complaining of severe leg pain. The procedure site will be marked:

a. After the patient is in the operating room and asleep

b. By the preoperative nurse using a skin marker while the patient confirms the site

c. By the licensed independent practitioner (LIP) who is performing the procedure

d. With an adhesive marker at or near the procedure site

11-51. The perianesthesia nurse understands that a policy exists to ensure safe transportation of patients. This nurse determines the:

a. Mode of transportation, number of accompanying personnel, and disposition of patient

b. Number and competency of accompanying personnel and disposition of patient

c. Mode of transportation, number, and competency of accompanying personnel

d. Mode of transportation, disposition of patient, and competency level of accompanying personnel

11-52. When caring for a Muslim perianesthesia patient, the practice of care is based on philosophical and ethical concepts that recognize and maintain privacy, dignity, and:

a. Seclusion

b. Confidentiality

c. Enmity

d. Dependence

11-53. Perianesthesia nurses implement safe medication practices by reviewing allergies and being alert to look-alike/sound-alike medications. Another example includes:

a. Proper labeling of multivial drugs

b. Using prefilled saline flushes to carefully titrate doses

c. Following institutional policy that overrides physician orders

d. Maintaining free-flow capacity of infusion devices

11-54. To ensure safe medication administration to patients, the perianesthesia nurse is responsible for all of the following EXCEPT:

  a. Proper labeling with the name of the medication, dose, and/or concentration

  b. Storage of controlled medications per institutional policy

  c. Witnessed discard of any unused opioids and/or sedatives

  d. Transfer of unused opioids to a relief nurse only if properly labeled

11-55. The perianesthesia nurse knows the best way to prevent the spread of drug-resistant organisms (DROs) is to follow standard precautions. To prevent the spread of DROs, the perianesthesia nurse does the following:

  a. Uses only industrial-strength hand soap when hand hygiene is necessary

  b. Maintains one-to-one nurse:patient ratio throughout the PACU Phase I period

  c. Accepts a second patient when there is sufficient time for donning and removing personal protective equipment (PPE)

  d. Groups two patients to allow one nurse to use the same PPE barriers between patients with similar DROs

11-56. The Phase I PACU perianesthesia nurse receives a patient from the operating room. This nurse knows that a report must be received from the anesthesia provider, vital signs must be obtained, an initial assessment must be completed, and:

  a. Electronic documentation must be initiated

  b. Clinical monitors must be connected

  c. Thorough skin and wound assessment must be conducted

  d. Transfer of care must be accepted or acknowledged

11-57. As the perianesthesia nurse accepts a patient from interventional radiology, hand-off of care includes the accurate transmittal of patient information, including treatment, current condition, and anticipated changes. According to the postprocedure plan of care, a patient having a gastrostomy tube (GT) placed should be observed for which of the following?

  a. Sepsis or peritonitis

  b. Embolization syndrome

  c. Hypotension

  d. Pseudothrombosis

11-58. The perianesthesia nurse serves as an advocate, not only for her patient, but also for peers and other members of the health care team. Characteristics of a healthy work environment when working with an impaired professional include all of the following EXCEPT:

  a. Provision of treatment options

  b. Education to promote the early identification of nurses with substance impairment

  c. Punitive reporting practices

  d. Mandatory board of nursing reporting

11-59. In the Phase I PACU, the nurse changes alarm parameters and disables alarm signals for the clinical monitoring system. The nurse makes these changes because:

  a. Loud and frequent alarm signals wake up the patient

  b. Policies address changing alarm parameters or disabling of alarm signals

  c. Nursing staff change alarm parameters and disable alarm signals without orders

  d. Nursing staff are authorized to make changes in alarm parameters or signals

11-60. A 57-year-old male patient is stabilized after emergent surgery to repair an arterial laceration of the right lower extremity sustained during an industrial accident. His preoperative and intraoperative course was complicated by an estimated blood loss of 1500 mL and wide variability in hemodynamics, including suspicious changes in his cardiac tracings. He's currently being prepared for transfer to intermediate care with the final unit of packed cells infusing. The Phase I perianesthesia nurse will accompany this patient because:

a. This patient is at risk of cardiopulmonary compromise

b. The Phase I nurse should accompany all transfers to the floor

c. The distance to intermediate care is too far for transport personnel

d. The automated external defibrillator (AED) is unavailable

11-61. Professional regulations vary by state and govern professional nursing practice and licensing. Nursing boards and state nurse practice acts provide for all of the following EXCEPT:

a. Protect the autonomy of the professional nurse

b. Protect public health

c. Require that ethical and professional conduct standards be met

d. Support reciprocity across all states

11-62. The American Society of PeriAnesthesia Nurses (ASPAN) is highly committed to a culture of safety in all perianesthesia practice settings. ASPAN's core values for a culture of safety include communication, advocacy, competency, timeliness, teamwork, and:

a. Is patient-centered

b. Assertiveness

c. Efficiency/timeliness

d. Balance

11-63. Emergency readiness requires consistent response plans for staff to follow when addressing all of the following emergencies EXCEPT:

a. Medical emergencies

b. Severe weather

c. Fire and evacuation plans

d. Equipment failure

11-64. A busy postanesthesia Phase II PACU utilizes unlicensed assistive personnel (UAP) as part of the daily staffing matrix. The perianesthesia nurse in charge for the day is familiar with the American Society of PeriAnesthesia Nurses' (ASPAN's) position on the utilization of UAP. The nurse knows that:

a. Institutional policy for scope of practice will supersede state regulations for nursing assistants

b. Delegation of tasks within the unit must be driven by the credentials of the UAP

c. The nurse in charge uses professional judgment to determine tasks to delegate

d. The UAP does not have to disclose his or her role to patients/families/significant others

11-65. For the purpose of the American Society of PeriAnesthesia Nurses' (ASPAN's) Standards of Perianesthesia Practice, the word "family" is BEST defined as:

a. The legal guardian of a 4-year-old foster child

b. A patient's oldest adult child

c. A newlywed's spouse

d. Whoever the patient says it is

11-66. A 64-year-old female patient is admitted to the Phase I PACU after general anesthesia for a fractured ankle. The repair took much longer than expected, with an overall anesthesia time of 248 minutes. During surgery she received 1400 mL crystalloid fluids intravenously, hydromorphone 1.5 mg, and ondansetron 4 mg. General anesthesia was maintained with propofol and desflurane. The FIRST priority for perianesthesia nursing assessments and documentation is:

a. Cardiovascular status, including telemetry rhythm

b. Respiratory and ventilation status

c. Surgical site assessment to include color, sensation, and circulation

d. Pain and comfort management

11-67. A 65-year-old patient has arrived in the Phase II unit after total intravenous anesthesia (TIVA) for a manipulation of a total knee replacement that was done 6 weeks previously. Although waking quickly from the TIVA, the patient is moaning and writhing in the stretcher, complaining of surgical pain 10/10 on the verbal analog scale. The Phase II perianesthesia nurse caring for this patient is aware that more vigilant monitoring for sedation and respiratory depression will be necessary after rapid administration of intravenous opioid to help minimize current pain. While providing discharge instructions, the nurse plans to teach the patient and family about other risk factors for an adverse event that can include all of the following EXCEPT:

a. When the medication peaks

b. During the hours of 11 p.m. and 7 a.m.

c. During the first 6 hours after anesthesia

d. During the first 12 hours after surgery

11-68. To prevent liability, the purposes of documentation include all of the following EXCEPT:

a. Communication of patient's condition to other health professionals

b. Use of care provider's time and time utilization of health providers' efforts

c. Assessment of improvements that might be needed by risk management and quality management

d. A legal document and use of data for quality-of-care review

11-69. Three weeks before surgery for treatment of endometriosis, an otherwise healthy 35-year-old patient reports a history of vancomycin-resistant *Enterococcus* (VRE). While documenting this history, the preoperative nurse:

a. Submits a request for increased room air exchanges

b. Notifies housekeeping that the patient care area will need terminal cleaning

c. Anticipates the need for contact precautions

d. Reserves the isolation suite for the pre- and postoperative care of the patient

11-70. Upon discharge of a patient from a Phase I PACU, the most important component of cleaning the patient care area is to:

a. Perform simple surface cleaning of all reusable and stationary items

b. Wipe down all surfaces with a hospital-approved bleach disinfectant

c. Collaborate with environmental services for routine cleaning

d. Clean all equipment according to manufacturer's instructions

11-71. A 24-year-old male patient arrives in the emergency department after a motor vehicle accident. His identity is not yet established, but his injuries are life threatening and require immediate surgical attention. In this situation, which principle of consent is considered?

a. Informed consent

b. Implied consent

c. Emergent consent

d. Assumed consent

11-72. Preprocedure verification includes:

a. Patient name and fasting status

b. Patient name, procedure site, and type of procedure

c. Procedure time, surgeon name, and anesthesia care provider name

d. Patient age, name, and procedure

11-73. A perianesthesia nurse integrates best practices to promote safe and quality patient care by advocating for:

a. Standardized electronic documentation

b. A "just" workplace culture

c. Evidence-based care

d. Patient-centered planning

11-74. After a brief operative procedure, Mr. B arrives in the Phase I PACU, and the perianesthesia nurse receives the handover report from the anesthesia care provider. Upon hearing that the patient has a history of type 1 diabetes, the nurse obtains an order to perform a bedside glucometer test. To complete the test, the nurse recognizes:

a. Any health care worker may run the bedside test

b. The required controls have been completed for the glucometer

c. Accreditation for the testing is from The Joint Commission

d. Only the anesthesia care provider is competent to run the test

11-75. The perianesthesia nurse planning for discharge of the patient with obstructive sleep apnea (OSA) from the Phase I PACU:

a. Anticipates a minimum observation period of 2 to 6 hours

b. Monitors for signs of desaturation when left undisturbed

c. Provides supplemental oxygen when administering basal opioid infusions

d. Keeps the patient stimulated and awake to maintain baseline room air saturations

11-76. When it is necessary to admit intensive care unit (ICU) overflow patients or prolong the stay of the surgical ICU patient in Phase I, the following criteria should be met:

a. The Phase I plan for overflow patients must be developed and approved by the department of anesthesia

b. All overflow patients must have nursing care provided by nurses from the ICU to ensure appropriate critical care

c. Management should provide a plan that separates the PACU and ICU patients within the unit to provide more effective acuity-related care

d. Appropriate medical management of the patient needs to be established

11-77. Advantages of ambulatory surgery that promote patient safety for the elderly patient include decreased incidence of mental confusion, decreased disruption of personal routine, and decreased:

a. Incidence of wound infections

b. Confusion with new medications

c. Risk of urinary tract infections

d. Potential for falls

11-78. The perianesthesia nurse is caring for an immediate postoperative patient in the Phase I PACU. The nurse understands that for patient safety the following staffing mix is most appropriate:

a. Two RNs, one of whom is an RN competent in Phase I perianesthesia nursing and present within the department while the patient is receiving Phase I level of care

b. Two RNS, one of whom is an RN competent in Phase I postanesthesia nursing and present in the same room/unit where the patient is receiving Phase I level of care

c. One RN is sufficient as long as emergency care can be easily summoned and rendered in the Phase I level of care area

d. One RN who is competent in Phase I perianesthesia nursing and is present in the room and constantly observing/assessing the patient while receiving Phase I level of care

11-79. Mrs. K arrives in the preoperative holding area accompanied by her husband. She presents a copy of an advance directive for her record. Advance directives are:

 a. Observed even if the patient is cognitively intact and able to answer questions

 b. Required by all patients for operative procedures

 c. Supported by the Patient Self-Determination Act

 d. Only valid when witnessed by a family member

11-80. You are the Phase I perianesthesia nurse on call with another RN who has no previous perianesthesia experience but is advanced cardiac life support (ACLS) prepared. This situation:

 a. Is below the ASPAN Standard for staffing

 b. Meets the ASPAN Standard for staffing

 c. Exceeds the ASPAN Standard for staffing

 d. Has never been tried as a staffing pattern

Answers and Rationales for Chapter 11, ASPAN Standards, Documentation, Regulatory Guidelines, and Patient Safety Needs

11-1. *Correct answer:* **c**

The critical elements are defined by ASPAN Standards as "report has been received from the anesthesia care provider, questions answered and the transfer of care has taken place; patient has a stable/secure airway; initial assessment is complete; patient is hemodynamically stable; patient is free from agitation, restlessness, combative behaviors." (American Society of PeriAnesthesia Nurses. *2015-2017 Perianesthesia Nursing Standards, Practice Recommendations and Interpretive Statements.* Cherry Hill, NJ: ASPAN; 2014:35.)

11-2. *Correct answer:* **b**

Extubation criteria for the patient in the Phase I PACU include the return of muscle strength after muscle relaxants, demonstrated by equal hand grasps and ability to head lift for 5 sustained seconds. In addition, the patient should have appropriate respiratory parameters with a rate greater than 10 bpm; adequate tidal volume and inspiratory force; and the ability to respond to commands, open eyes, cough, and swallow. (Schick L, Windle PE. *Peri-Anesthesia Nursing Core Curriculum: Preprocedure, Phase I and Phase II PACU Nursing.* 3rd ed. St. Louis, MO: Saunders; 2016:476.)

11-3. *Correct answer:* **b**

In ASPAN's position statement on safe medication administration, perianesthesia nurses are advised to be aware of the pharmacokinetics of various medications that cause respiratory depression, unwanted sedation, and alterations in hemodynamic stability. Factors to consider when determining a patient's length of stay after administration of medications include but are not limited to the amount, type, and timing of medication; the patient's response; medication half-life and peak; drug interactions; and cumulative effects. (American Society of PeriAnesthesia Nurses. *2015-2017 Perianesthesia Nursing Standards, Practice Recommendations and Interpretive Statements.* Cherry Hill, NJ: ASPAN; 2014:109.)

11-4. *Correct answer:* **a**

Educate patients, and their families as needed, who are undergoing a surgical procedure about surgical site infection prevention. This education should include instructions to shower with antimicrobial soaps, avoid shaving the area preoperatively, plan for a high protein diet, take all antibiotics as ordered. In addition, patients should expect and be able to request that their healthcare providers wash their hands prior to providing care. (Odom-Forren J. *Drain's Perianesthesia Nursing: A Critical Care Approach.* 6th ed. St. Louis, MO: Saunders; 2013:651.)

11-5. *Correct answer:* **b**

Under the Personnel Management section of the Staffing and Personnel Management Standard, it is written, "The perianesthesia registered nurse providing Phase I level of care will maintain a current advanced cardiac life support (ACLS) and/or pediatric advanced life support (PALS) provider status, as appropriate to the patient population served." (American Society of PeriAnesthesia Nurses. *2015-2017 Perianesthesia Nursing Standards, Practice Recommendations and Interpretive Statements.* Cherry Hill, NJ: ASPAN; 2014:23.)

11-6. *Correct answer:* **c**

The Centers for Medicare & Medicaid Services (CMS) requires a postanesthesia evaluation, which must be completed in accordance with state law and hospital policies and procedures. These policies and procedures must be approved by the institutional medical staff and reflect current standards of anesthesia care. According to CMS, this evaluation must be completed by a practitioner who is qualified to administer anesthesia. (American Society of PeriAnesthesia Nurses. *2015-2017 Perianesthesia Nursing Standards, Practice Recommendations and Interpretive Statements.* Cherry Hill, NJ: ASPAN; 2014:109.)

11-7. *Correct answer:* **b**

The American Society of PeriAnesthesia Nurses (ASPAN) recommends that staffing patterns be based on acuity, census, patient flow process, and physical facility. (American Society of PeriAnesthesia Nurses. *2015-2017 Perianesthesia Nursing Standards, Practice Recommendations and Interpretive Statements.* Cherry Hill, NJ: ASPAN; 2014:23.)

11-8. *Correct answer:* **d**

Wrong patient errors occur throughout the care continuum. The use of at least two patient identifiers when providing care, treatment, and services will reliably identify the person for whom the treatment is intended and match the service or treatment to that individual. (American Society of PeriAnesthesia Nurses. *2015-2017 Perianesthesia Nursing Standards, Practice Recommendations and Interpretive Statements.* Cherry Hill, NJ: ASPAN; 2014:42.)

11-9. *Correct answer:* **c**

According to Practice Recommendation 2, data collected and documented to evaluate the patient's status for discharge include, but are not limited to, usual discharge criteria (stability of vitals, pain and comfort management, etc.). In addition, discharge assessment should include assessment of child–parent/significant others interactions, home care provider knowledge of discharge instructions, and arrangements for safe transportation from the institution. The Practice Recommendation for safe transportation of the child to home includes the recommendation that if the pediatric patient requires a car seat, two adults should be in the vehicle: one to drive and the other to be seated with the child. (American Society of PeriAnesthesia Nurses. *2015-2017 Perianesthesia Nursing Standards, Practice Recommendations and Interpretive Statements.* Cherry Hill, NJ: ASPAN; 2014:47, 60.)

11-10. *Correct answer:* **c**

Although research, research design, clinical inquiry, and process improvement are important standards to apply to clinical practice, research utilization and application of best available evidence to perianesthesia knowledge and interventions are crucial for validation of perianesthesia nursing practice and the delivery of safe patient care. (American Society of PeriAnesthesia Nurses. *2015-2017 Perianesthesia Nursing Standards, Practice Recommendations and Interpretive Statements.* Cherry Hill, NJ: ASPAN; 2014:27.)

11-11. *Correct answer:* **a**

The Occupational Safety and Health Administration requires that institutions obtain input from non-managerial staff actively participating in patient care when developing plans for a safer workplace. (Odom-Forren J. *Drain's Perianesthesia Nursing: A Critical Care Approach.* 6th ed. St. Louis, MO: Saunders; 2013:51-53.)

11-12. *Correct answer:* **a**

In the position statement for medical-surgical overflow in the Phase I PACU, competencies for the care of all types of patients in the perianesthesia setting must be developed and shared, particularly in the care of the overflow patient managed in the PACU and ambulatory surgery unit (ASU). Overflow patients should be grouped in close proximity based on their level-of-care requirements, the flow of the surgical schedule should remain intact as much as possible, and the medical management of the patient needs to be established by providers primarily responsible for the patient's care. (American Society of PeriAnesthesia Nurses. *2015-2017 Perianesthesia Nursing Standards, Practice Recommendations and Interpretive Statements.* Cherry Hill, NJ: ASPAN; 2014:105.)

11-13. *Correct answer:* **c**

The critical elements are defined by the American Society of PeriAnesthesia Nurses (ASPAN) Standards as "report has been received from the anesthesia care provider, questions answered and the transfer of care has taken place; patient has a stable/secure airway; initial assessment is complete; patient is hemodynamically stable; patient is free from agitation, restlessness, and combative behaviors." (American Society of PeriAnesthesia Nurses. *2015-2017 Perianesthesia Nursing Standards, Practice Recommendations and Interpretive Statements.* Cherry Hill, NJ: ASPAN; 2014:35.)

11-14. *Correct answer:* **a**

According to the American Society of PeriAnesthesia Nurses' (ASPAN's) Standard V, Research and Clinical Inquiry, research and evidence-based findings guide decision making in the nurse's clinical, educational, and management roles. In this example, the benefit of the application of a scoring tool specific to perianesthesia practice applies to the nurse in the clinical bedside role. (American Society of PeriAnesthesia Nurses. *2015-2017 Perianesthesia Nursing Standards, Practice Recommendations and Interpretive Statements.* Cherry Hill, NJ: ASPAN; 2014:27.)

11-15. *Correct answer:* **a**

According to the practice recommendation for staffing, the nurse–patient ratio in Phase II would be 1:2 when there is an initial admission of a patient after a procedure. (American Society of PeriAnesthesia Nurses. *2015-2017 Perianesthesia Nursing Standards, Practice Recommendations and Interpretive Statements.* Cherry Hill, NJ: ASPAN; 2014:35.)

11-16. *Correct answer:* **c**

The Joint Commission's (TJC's) National Patient Safety Goals are updated annually and available specific to the facility type (hospital, ambulatory, home health, etc.). (Schick L, Windle P. *PeriAnesthesia Nursing Core Curriculum: Preprocedure, Phase I and Phase II PACU Nursing.* 3rd ed. St. Louis, MO: Saunders; 2016:33.)

11-17. *Correct answer:* **d**

According to the practice recommendation for preventing unwanted sedation, among the risk factors for the development of unwanted sedation and/or respiratory depression is being aged 55 or older. (American Society of PeriAnesthesia Nurses. *2015-2017 Perianesthesia Nursing Standards, Practice Recommendations and Interpretive Statements.* Cherry Hill, NJ: ASPAN; 2014:81.)

11-18. *Correct answer:* **a**

According to the American Society for Pain Management's guidelines on monitoring for opioid-induced sedation and respiratory depression cited in the American Society of PeriAnesthesia Nurses' (ASPAN's) Practice Recommendation for the Prevention of Unwanted Sedation, older patients are at an increased risk of unwanted sedation secondary to increased sensitivity to the effects of opioids. This is a result of a reduction in total body water and overall body mass, tissue perfusion, and drug metabolism and clearance from the body. (American Society of PeriAnesthesia Nurses. *2015-2017 Perianesthesia Nursing Standards, Practice Recommendations and Interpretive Statements.* Cherry Hill, NJ: ASPAN; 2014:80.)

11-19. *Correct answer:* **a**

Patient safety is not only the core of standard practice of perianesthesia nurses, but is also considered the highest priority. It is also defined as the freedom from accidental injury caused by medical care or medical error. In general, safety is defined as a condition of being safe from undergoing or causing hurt or loss and as protection against failure, breakage, or accident. (Schick L, Windle PE. *PeriAnesthesia Nursing Core Curriculum: Preprocedure, Phase I and Phase II PACU Nursing.* 3rd ed. St. Louis, MO: Saunders; 2016:32-33.)

11-20. *Correct answer:* **c**

Assessment and documentation of chest tubes include vital signs, presence of air leaks and fluctuations, suction level (if used), dressings and drainage, presence of crepitus, and the patient positioning. The semi-Fowler position is the preferred position to facilitate drainage of chest fluids and to support optimal chest expansion. (Schick L, Windle PE. *PeriAnesthesia Nursing Core Curriculum: Preprocedure, Phase I and Phase II PACU Nursing.* 3rd ed. St. Louis, MO: Saunders; 2016:557-558.)

11-21. *Correct answer:* **b**

In the American Society of PeriAnesthesia Nurses (ASPAN) Standard II, Environment of Care, the criteria for safe patient care includes the verification that a patient has safe transportation from an institution. The practice recommendation for handoff specifies that when patients lack appropriate transportation, care management or discharge planning services, as well as patient providers, should be involved in communications regarding this gap in care. (American Society of PeriAnesthesia Nurses. *2015-2017 Perianesthesia Nursing Standards, Practice Recommendations and Interpretive Statements.* Cherry Hill, NJ: ASPAN; 2014:47, 60.)

11-22. *Correct answer:* **d**

According to the American Society of PeriAnesthesia Nurses' (ASPAN's) position statement regarding "on-call" hours, the following criteria are recommended: the number and length of "on-call" shifts should be coordinated with the number of sustained work hours and provide for adequate recuperation periods (defined as a rest period of 5 hours of uninterrupted sleep for duty exceeding 16 hours); minimum staffing is provided in accordance with ASPAN's Standards; there is a plan in place to augment "on-call" staff based upon patient census and acuity; and there is a plan in place to relieve the "on-call" nurse in the event that the manager and/or nurse determines there is potential for compromise in the delivery of safe, competent care without fear of reprisal or disciplinary action. (American Society of PeriAnesthesia Nurses. *2015-2017 Perianesthesia Nursing Standards, Practice Recommendations and Interpretive Statements.* Cherry Hill, NJ: ASPAN; 2014:98.)

11-23. *Correct answer:* **c**

Best practice regarding the documentation of any phone calls related to patient care include the following: the specific time the call was made, the person who made the call, the person called, the person to whom information was given, and all information given and received concerning the content of the call. (Schick L, Windle P. *Perianesthesia Nursing Core Curriculum: Preprocedure, Phase I and Phase II PACU Nursing.* 3rd ed. St. Louis, MO: Saunders; 2016:26.)

11-24. *Correct answer:* **d**

Known risk factors for the development of PONV include, but are not limited to, the following: female gender, history of motion sickness, nonsmoker status, use of postoperative opioids, age, anxiety, pain, and type of surgery. (Schick L, Windle PE. *PeriAnesthesia Nursing Core Curriculum: Preprocedure, Phase I and Phase II PACU Nursing.* 3rd ed. St. Louis, MO: Saunders; 2016:424.)

11-25. *Correct answer:* **a**

Under Title VI, Prohibition Against National Origin Discrimination Affecting Limited English Proficient Persons, all recipients of assistance must take reasonable steps to provide meaningful access to limited English proficient persons. This act describes examples of language assistance measures, including translation either in person or by telephone language interpreter lines. (Schick L, Windle P. *PeriAnesthesia Nursing Core Curriculum: Preprocedure, Phase I and Phase II PACU Nursing.* 3rd ed. St. Louis, MO: Saunders; 2016:95.)

11-26. *Correct answer:* **a**

Hand hygiene, contact precautions, and cleaning and disinfecting patient care equipment and the patient's environment are essential strategies for preventing the spread of health care–associated infections (HAIs). Each year, millions of people acquire an infection while receiving care, treatment, and services in a health care organization. HAIs are a patient safety issue. Improving the hand hygiene of health care staff is one of the most important ways to address HAIs. Compliance with hand hygiene guidelines will reduce the transmission of infectious agents by staff to patients, thereby decreasing the incidence of HAIs. (The Joint Commission (2016). National Patient Safety Goals. Retrieved from https://www.jointcommission.org/assets/1/6/NPSG_Chapter_HAP_Jan2017.pdf; Schick L, Windle PE. *PeriAnesthesia Nursing Core Curriculum: Preprocedure, Phase I and Phase II PACU Nursing.* 3rd ed. St. Louis, MO: Saunders; 2016:51.)

11-27. *Correct answer:* **c**

Strategies for the protection of confidential health care information must be in place when implementing a computerized documentation and information system. Passwords need to be of sufficient complexity with regular changes to ensure confidentiality. Policies must be in place requiring signing in and out of the patient record, and sufficient penalties must be in place for breaches of the security system. (Schick L, Windle PE. *PeriAnesthesia Nursing Core Curriculum: Preprocedure, Phase I and Phase II PACU Nursing.* 3rd ed. St. Louis, MO: Saunders; 2016:25.)

11-28. *Correct answer:* **d**

According to the interpretive statement for the safe staffing recommendation, the intent of this standard is that a nurse providing care to a Phase I patient is not left alone with the patient. The second nurse should be able to directly hear a call for assistance and be immediately available to assist. (American Society of PeriAnesthesia Nurses. *2015-2017 Perianesthesia Nursing Standards, Practice Recommendations and Interpretive Statements.* Cherry Hill, NJ: ASPAN; 2014:35.)

11-29. *Correct answer:* **d**

Incident reporting is a very important aspect of patient care, but incident reports should NOT become a portion of the medical record. Documentation is to be factual and objective; the medical record should record facts about the event. (Schick L, Windle PE. *PeriAnesthesia Nursing Core Curriculum: Preprocedure, Phase I and Phase II PACU Nursing.* 3rd ed. St. Louis, MO: Saunders; 2016:26.)

11-30. *Correct answer:* **b**

Many perinatal patients arrive prepared with birthing plans that include music therapy, doulas, and other labor adjuncts to maintain focus and ease the pain associated with labor, and many have preferences for minimizing pharmacologic interventions. Certain postdelivery actions are priorities for the perinatal patient and the newborn. These include allowing the newborn in the Phase I PACU, providing early skin-to-skin contact, encouraging breastfeeding, and bringing the support person into the PACU. (American Society of PeriAnesthesia Nurses. *2015-2017 Perianesthesia Nursing Standards, Practice Recommendations and Interpretive Statements.* Cherry Hill, NJ: ASPAN; 2014:127-128.)

11-31. *Correct answer:* **d**

General guidelines for defensive charting include the following: documentation should be accurate, comprehensive, objective, and legible. Charting should be done as promptly as possible after care is given, but no current recommendations exist regarding specific time frames. The prudent perianesthesia nurse will be aware of institutional policies and procedures that define documentation requirements. (Schick L, Windle PE. *PeriAnesthesia Nursing Core Curriculum: Preprocedure, Phase I and Phase II PACU Nursing.* 3rd ed. St. Louis, MO: Saunders; 2016:25-26.)

11-32. *Correct answer:* **d**

Specialty standards have been evolving since the mid-1970s. Sources of standards include examples such as accrediting organizations, state boards of nursing, the American Nurses Association, specialty organizations like the American Society of PeriAnesthesia Nurses (ASPAN), hospital or ambulatory surgery facility rules and procedures, and common practice. (Schick L, Windle PE. *PeriAnesthesia Nursing Core Curriculum: Preprocedure, Phase I and Phase II PACU Nursing.* 3rd edSt. Louis, MO: Saunders; 2016:13.)

11-33. *Correct answer:* **c**

Patient positioning is critical to minimize intracranial pressure changes. The head of the bed should be elevated between 30 and 45 degrees and the head should be maintained in a neutral position. Positioning the patient prone should be avoided, and any Valsalva maneuvers should be prevented. (Schick L, Windle PE. *PeriAnesthesia Nursing Core Curriculum: Preprocedure, Phase I and Phase II PACU Nursing.* 3rd ed. St. Louis, MO: Saunders; 2016:687.)

11-34. *Correct answer:* **b**

The American Society of PeriAnesthesia Nurses (ASPAN) recommends that perianesthesia registered nurses accompany patients who require a higher level of care or ongoing evaluation or treatment during transport and those who are at risk of cardiopulmonary compromise during transport. (American Society of PeriAnesthesia Nurses. *2015-2017 Perianesthesia Nursing Standards, Practice Recommendations and Interpretive Statements.* Cherry Hill, NJ: ASPAN; 2014:60.)

11-35. *Correct answer:* **c**

The safest order of assessment and intervention upon arrival to the Phase I PACU begins with the simultaneous application of oxygen and the assessment of the respiratory status. This is then followed by a more complete assessment of body systems. (Schick L, Windle PE. *PeriAnesthesia Nursing Core Curriculum: Preprocedure, Phase I and Phase II PACU Nursing.* 3rd ed. St. Louis, MO: Saunders; 2016:1227.)

11-36. *Correct answer:* **b**

Comprehensive documentation provides accurate information on which care can be based, and the old adage "Not charted means not done" often rings true. Accurate and objective charting of nursing actions and interventions is necessary and opinions or perceptions of events are inappropriate. It is important to chart what is observed, what was done, and what the outcomes were. The medical record is used in litigation in which professional negligence is alleged; it must be viewed as a viable way by which to defend against allegations of professional negligence. The entry should be factual, complete, and objective, containing observations, clinical signs and symptoms, patient quotes, interventions, and patient responses. (Schick L, Windle PE. *PeriAnesthesia Nursing Core Curriculum: Preprocedure, Phase I and Phase II PACU Nursing.* 3rd ed. St. Louis, MO: Saunders; 2016:25.)

11-37. *Correct answer:* **c**

The cardiovascular cascade of symptoms related to local anesthetic toxicity begins with hypertension leading to hypotension, premature ventricular beats, prolonged PR intervals and QRS on electrocardiogram (ECG), followed by cardiovascular collapse if untreated. (Schick L, Windle P. *PeriAnesthesia Nursing Core Curriculum: Preprocedure, Phase I and Phase II PACU Nursing.* 3rd ed. St. Louis, MO: Saunders; 2016: 348-349.)

11-38. *Correct answer:* **a**

Critical results of tests and diagnostic procedures are expected to be reported to responsible licensed caregivers within an established time frame so the patient may be promptly treated. Institutional written procedures will address which results are defined as critical, to whom the results are reported, and timing of the reporting. (The Joint Commission (2016). National Patient Safety Goals. Retrieved from https://www.jointcommission.org/assets/1/6/NPSG_Chapter_HAP_Jan2017.pdf; Schick L, Windle PE. *PeriAnesthesia Nursing Core Curriculum: Preprocedure, Phase I and Phase II PACU Nursing.* 3rd ed. St. Louis, MO: Saunders; 2016:25.)

11-39. *Correct answer:* **b**

Loss of sensation precedes loss of motor function when a neuraxial block is administered. Resolution of the block is assessed in reverse order. The first indication that a sensory block is resolving is the return of temperature sensation assessed by using either an alcohol wipe or an ice pack. (Schick L, Windle PE. *PeriAnesthesia Nursing Core Curriculum: Preprocedure, Phase I and Phase II PACU Nursing.* 3rd ed. St. Louis, MO: Saunders; 2016:359.)

11-40. *Correct answer:* **a**

According to the American Society of PeriAnesthesia Nurses' (ASPAN's) Fast Tracking Practice Recommendation, appropriate patient assessment must be conducted in the operating room at the end of the procedure by the anesthesia provider. These assessments must include the same criteria which determine readiness for discharge from "Phase I level of care." Discharge criteria as created by the department of anesthesia must be clear and defined in writing. (American Society of PeriAnesthesia Nurses. *2015-2017 Perianesthesia Nursing Standards, Practice Recommendations and Interpretive Statements.* Cherry Hill, NJ: ASPAN; 2014:66.)

11-41. *Correct answer:* **c**

Two documentation issues are discussed in this question. The first issue is that something needs to be added to the patient chart that occurred at an earlier time. The second issue is that a nurse is asking another nurse to make that entry. When it is necessary to add omitted information to an already existing entry, policies and procedures should be consulted and followed. Usually, the addition of information is coded on the next available line or space as a "late entry" or "addition to nursing note _____." The date and time of the information that is being added are documented, and the additional information is placed in the record. Some facilities also call this an addendum. No nurse should document in the medical record for another person unless that practice is "standard" practice, as in an emergency code. Even so, when documenting for another in an emergency, the nurse "scribe" must accurately reflect who is providing care and who is documenting. However, under no circumstances should the nurse sign another nurse's name in any portion of the record. (Schick L, Windle PE. *PeriAnesthesia Nursing Core Curriculum: Preprocedure, Phase I and Phase II PACU Nursing.* 3rd ed. St. Louis, MO: Saunders; 2016:25-26.)

11-42. *Correct answer:* **a**

Additional preanesthesia assessment elements for the pediatric patient include, but are not limited to, birth history, gestational age, developmental milestones, level of cognitive functioning, and patient/child interactions. The posterior fontanel closes by age 4 months. (American Society of PeriAnesthesia Nurses. *2015-2017 Perianesthesia Nursing Standards, Practice Recommendations and Interpretive Statements.* Cherry Hill, NJ: ASPAN; 2014:43.)

11-43. *Correct answer:* **d**

Documentation guidelines include charting with accuracy but avoiding criticism and complaints, avoiding terms such as "seems" or "appears," using standard abbreviations defined by the institution, and charting objectively (only what is observed by the nurse). (Schick L, Windle PE. *PeriAnesthesia Nursing Core Curriculum: Preprocedure, Phase I and Phase II PACU Nursing.* 3rd ed. St. Louis, MO: Saunders; 2016:25.)

11-44. *Correct answer:* **d**

Right shoulder pain after laparoscopic procedures is due to retained gases used to provide insufflation. These gases tend to irritate the peritoneal surface and diaphragm. The pain can last several days and can be managed with analgesics, as well as by sleeping with 15 degrees of elevation of the head and shoulders. (Odom-Forren J. *Drain's Perianesthesia Nursing: A Critical Care Approach.* 6th ed. St Louis, MO: Saunders; 2013:593; Schick L, Windle PE. *PeriAnesthesia Nursing Core Curriculum: Preprocedure, Phase I and Phase II PACU Nursing.* 3rd ed. St. Louis, MO: Saunders; 2016:887.)

11-45. *Correct answer:* **d**

Whatever mark is used to identify the procedure site must be used consistently by the organization. There is no requirement by The Joint Commission that the mark must be the signature of the licensed independent practitioner (LIP). (The Joint Commission (2016). National Patient Safety Goals. Retrieved from https://www.jointcommission.org/assets/1/6/NPSG_Chapter_HAP_Jan2017.pdf; Schick L, Windle PE. *PeriAnesthesia Nursing Core Curriculum: Preprocedure, Phase I and Phase II PACU Nursing.* 3rd ed. St. Louis, MO: Saunders; 2016:33.)

11-46. *Correct answer:* **c**

Under the supervision of the perianesthesia nurse, the competent perianesthesia support staff (unlicensed assistive personnel or UAP) demonstrate knowledge, skills, and behaviors to maintain a consistent level of practice. Among the most important basic skills that the UAP should demonstrate are basic life support (BLS) and basic airway support competencies. (American Society of PeriAnesthesia Nurses. *2015-2017 Perianesthesia Nursing Standards, Practice Recommendations and Interpretive Statements.* Cherry Hill, NJ: ASPAN; 2014:57.)

11-47. *Correct answer:* **b**

According to the *2015-2017 Perianesthesia Nursing Standards, Practice Recommendations and Interpretive Statements,* the specialty of perianesthesia nursing practice is regulated in part by policies and procedures dictated by the individual hospital/institution, state and federal regulatory agencies, and national accreditation organizations. (American Society of PeriAnesthesia Nurses. *2015-2017 Perianesthesia Nursing Standards, Practice Recommendations and Interpretive Statements.* Cherry Hill, NJ: ASPAN; 2014:7.)

11-48. *Correct answer:* **a**

According to the American Society of PeriAnesthesia Nurses' (ASPAN's) Recommended Competencies for the Perianesthesia Nurse, the competent nurse in perianesthesia practice demonstrates professional development in addition to teamwork, collaboration, and effective communication. (American Society of PeriAnesthesia Nurses. *2015-2017 Perianesthesia Nursing Standards, Practice Recommendations and Interpretive Statements.* Cherry Hill, NJ: ASPAN; 2014:54.)

11-49. *Correct answer:* **d**

The American Society of PeriAnesthesia Nurses' (ASPAN's) position statement on the pediatric patient describes expected outcomes for the perianesthesia nurse caring for the pediatric patient and his or her family/caregiver. Optimal care in this environment is best demonstrated through a commitment to family-centered care (FCC). FCC is defined as care provided to include the whole family throughout the health care system. (American Society of PeriAnesthesia Nurses. *2015-2017 Perianesthesia Nursing Standards, Practice Recommendations and Interpretive Statements.* Cherry Hill, NJ; ASPAN; 2014:115.)

11-50. *Correct answer:* **c**

The purpose of the site mark is to serve as a communication tool about the patient for members of the procedural team. The Joint Commission states that the individual who knows the most about the patient should mark the site. In most cases, that will be the person performing the procedure; however, it may be delegated to advanced practice registered nurses (APRNs) or physician assistants (PAs) who have collaborative or supervisory agreements with LIPs. (The Joint Commission (2016). National Patient Safety Goals. Retrieved from https://www.jointcommission.org/assets/1/6/NPSG_Chapter_HAP_Jan2017.pdf; Schick L, Windle PE, eds. *PeriAnesthesia Nursing Core Curriculum: Preprocedure, Phase I and Phase II PACU Nursing.* 3rd ed. St. Louis, MO: Saunders; 2016:33.)

11-51. *Correct answer:* **c**

With regard to the safe transportation of patients, the current recommendation is that the perianesthesia registered nurse determine the mode, number, and competency level of accompanying personnel based on patient needs. The actual disposition of the patient will be determined by the medical providers. (American Society of PeriAnesthesia Nurses. *2015-2017 Perianesthesia Nursing Standards, Practice Recommendations and Interpretive Statements.* Cherry Hill, NJ: ASPAN; 2014:60.)

11-52. *Correct answer:* **b**

According to the American Society of PeriAnesthesia Nurses (ASPAN) Standard I, patient rights are supported and upheld by perianesthesia nurses. This results in planning for and consideration of the individual patient's autonomy, confidentiality, privacy, and worth. (American Society of PeriAnesthesia Nurses. *2015-2017 Perianesthesia Nursing Standards, Practice Recommendations and Interpretive Statements.* Cherry Hill, NJ: ASPAN; 2014:20.)

11-53. *Correct answer:* **c**

Several goals exist with regard to safe medication practices. These goals include review and verify allergies; be alert and take action on look-alike/sound-alike medications; label medications, containers, and solutions; pay attention to anticoagulant therapy, insulin, cardiac medications, etc.; verify unclear orders; and avoid distraction and interruptions during medication administration. In addition, perianesthesia nurses are accountable for knowing their scope of practice and requirements of their institution for safe medication administration. (The Joint Commission (2016). National Patient Safety Goals. Retrieved from https://www.jointcommission.org/assets/1/6/NPSG_Chapter_HAP_Jan2017.pdf; Schick L, Windle PE. *PeriAnesthesia Nursing Core Curriculum: Preprocedure, Phase I and Phase II PACU Nursing.* St. Louis, MO: Saunders; 2016:332-333; American Society of PeriAnesthesia Nurses. *Perianesthesia Nursing Standards, Practice Recommendations and Interpretive Statements 2015-2016.* Cherry Hill, NJ: ASPAN; 2014:107-110.)

11-54. *Correct answer:* **d**

Unused opioids should never be accepted by a nurse who did not retrieve, prepare, or administer partial doses of opioids. (American Society of PeriAnesthesia Nurses. *2015-2017 Perianesthesia Nursing Standards, Practice Recommendations and Interpretive Statements.* Cherry Hill, NJ: ASPAN; 2014:107-110.)

11-55. *Correct answer:* **c**

According to the staffing recommendation when caring for the patient on precautions, the American Society of PeriAnesthesia Nurses (ASPAN) supports the recommendations from the Occupational Safety and Health Administration (OSHA) as well as the Centers for Disease Control and Prevention (CDC). Nurse-to-patient ratio should be one to one upon arrival of the patient; however, ratios may advance based on ASPAN's staffing recommendations, providing that the preoperative, Phase I, and Phase II care needs of the patients allow sufficient time for donning and removing respiratory protection and other protective barriers, as well as hand washing, between patients. (American Society of PeriAnesthesia Nurses. *2015-2017 Perianesthesia Nursing Standards, Practice Recommendations and Interpretive Statements.* Cherry Hill, NJ: ASPAN; 2014:39.)

11-56. *Correct answer:* **d**

The first American Society of PeriAnesthesia Nurses (ASPAN) Practice Recommendation, Patient Classification/Staffing Recommendations, defines the critical elements of accepting a patient into Phase I to include the handoff report. This element includes the receipt of the report from the anesthesia care provider, as well as the opportunity to have any questions answered. The Safe Transfer of Care Practice Recommendation further defines that the handoff concludes when the staff receiving the report accept the information and care of the patient. (American Society of PeriAnesthesia Nurses. *2015-2017 Perianesthesia Nursing Standards, Practice Recommendations and Interpretive Statements.* Cherry Hill, NJ: ASPAN; 2014:35, 59.)

11-57. *Correct answer:* **a**

The Association for Radiologic and Imaging Nursing (ARIN) has provided the American Society of PeriAnesthesia Nurses (ASPAN) with a resource titled "Handoff Communication Concerning Patients undergoing a Radiological Procedure with General Anesthesia." The patient undergoing the placement of a GT should be monitored for 2 to 4 hours for insertion site pain as well as signs of potential peritonitis. Embolization syndrome includes fever, nausea, vomiting, and pain and can result from biologic embolization of tissues. Thrombosis is actual, not pseudo, and is often associated with arterial punctures. (American Society of PeriAnesthesia Nurses. *2015-2017 Perianesthesia Nursing Standards, Practice Recommendations and Interpretive Statements.* Cherry Hill, NJ: ASPAN; 2014:142.)

11-58. *Correct answer:* **c**

Recommendations from the position statement on substance abuse include, but are not limited to, the following: recognition and nonpunitive reporting of the problem, knowledge of mandatory reporting requirements, institutional policies for management of controlled substances, and provision of treatment options to the impaired professional. (American Society of PeriAnesthesia Nurses. *2015-2017 Perianesthesia Nursing Standards, Practice Recommendations and Interpretive Statements.* Cherry Hill, NJ: ASPAN; 2014:122-123.)

11-59. *Correct answer:* **b**

Clinical alarm systems are intended to alert caregivers of potential patient problems, but if they are not properly managed, they can compromise patient safety. A systematic, coordinated approach to clinical alarm system management contributes to safe care. Elements of performance include establishing policies and procedures for managing alarms, including clinically appropriate settings for alarm signals; when alarm signals can be disabled; when alarm parameters can be changed; who in the organization has the authority to set alarm parameters; who in the organization has the authority to change alarm parameters; who in the organization has the authority to set alarm parameters to "off"; monitoring and responding to alarm signals; and checking individual alarm signals for accurate settings, proper operation, and detectability. (American Society of PeriAnesthesia Nurses. *2015-2017 Perianesthesia Nursing Standards, Practice Recommendations and Interpretive Statements.* Cherry Hill, NJ: ASPAN; 2014:14; The Joint Commission (2016). National Patient Safety Goals. Retrieved from https://www.jointcommission.org/assets/1/6/NPSG_Chapter_HAP_Jan2017.pdf.)

11-60. *Correct answer:* **a**

The Practice Recommendation for Safe Transfer of Care addresses both the hand-off process and the actual transportation of the patient from one phase of care to another. The basis of this recommendation is that the perianesthesia registered nurse should determine the mode and method of patient transport. Based on patient acuity, the perianesthesia registered nurse should accompany patients who have a potential for bleeding, airway compromise, or vomiting or require a higher level of monitoring and care. (American Society of PeriAnesthesia Nurses. *2015-2017 Perianesthesia Nursing Standards, Practice Recommendations and Interpretive Statements.* Cherry Hill, NJ: ASPAN; 2014:59-61.)

11-61. *Correct answer:* **d**

Nursing boards and state nurse practice acts vary from state to state, allowing some reciprocity of requirements but separate licensing. Currently there is no single license that allows practice by the registered professional nurse in all states of the United States. (Schick L, Windle PE. *PeriAnesthesia Nursing Core Curriculum: Preprocedure, Phase I and Phase II PACU Nursing.* 3rd ed. St. Louis, MO: Saunders; 2016:45-46.)

11-62. *Correct answer:* **c**

A culture of safety is defined as an environment whereby the sharing and implementation of knowledge and shared beliefs promote safety in the practice setting. This is supported by an environment of caring and is guided by principles of research and evidence-based practices. All core values included in this list are characteristics of a culture of safety as stated in "Principles of Safe Perianesthesia Practice American Society of PeriAnesthesia Nurses." (American Society of PeriAnesthesia Nurses. *2015-2017 Perianesthesia Nursing Standards, Practice Recommendations and Interpretive Statements.* Cherry Hill, NJ: ASPAN; 2014:14.)

11-63. *Correct answer:* **d**

Emergency readiness includes the preparation of consistent response plans for medical emergencies, fire and evacuation plans, bomb threat, infant abduction, severe weather, and violent intruder. Staff practice via drills and review of staff actions and education/training utilized to identify behaviors/activities for improvement. Also included are the role of emergency response teams and the location of emergency equipment and supplies. (Schick L, Windle PE. *PeriAnesthesia Nursing Core Curriculum: Preprocedure, Phase I and Phase II PACU Nursing.* 3rd ed. St. Louis, MO: Saunders; 2016:36.)

11-64. *Correct answer:* **c**

It is the position of the American Society of PeriAnesthesia Nurses (ASPAN) that in addition to having responsibility and accountability for all nursing care, the perianesthesia nurse also uses professional judgment to determine appropriate delegation. (American Society of PeriAnesthesia Nurses. *2015-2017 Perianesthesia Nursing Standards, Practice Recommendations and Interpretive State* Cherry Hill, NJ: ASPAN; 2014:94-95.)

11-65. *Correct answer:* **d**

The word "family" refers to two or more persons who are related in any way: biologically, legally, or emotionally. Patients and families define their families. (American Society of PeriAnesthesia Nurses. *2015-2017 Perianesthesia Nursing Standards, Practice Recommendations and Interpretive Statements.* Cherry Hill, NJ: ASPAN; 2014:25.)

11-66. *Correct answer:* **b**

Although simultaneous evaluation and observation of the patient's condition is conducted upon arrival to Phase I, the priority for assessment and documentation begins with respiratory effort/ventilation, oxygen saturation (SpO$_2$), and condition of the airway. Cardiac rate, rhythm, and vital signs, as well as pain severity and residual effect of anesthesia, are also evaluated. (Schick L, Windle PE. *PeriAnesthesia Nursing Core Curriculum: Preprocedure, Phase I and Phase II PACU Nursing.* 3rd ed. St. Louis, MO: Saunders; 2016:1227.)

11-67. *Correct answer:* **d**

According to the American Society of PeriAnesthesia Nurses' (ASPAN's) Practice Recommendation for the Prevention of Unwanted Sedation, patients are at greatest risk for adverse events during the following times: peak of medication effect, first 24 hours after surgery, after dose of opioid is increased, within the first 6 hours after anesthesia, and during the hours of 11 p.m. and 7 a.m., to name a few. (American Society of PeriAnesthesia Nurses. *2015-2017*

Perianesthesia Nursing Standards, Practice Recommendations and Interpretive Statements. Cherry Hill, NJ: ASPAN; 2014:85.)

11-68. *Correct answer:* **b**

Documentation should not be used as a means of proving how the care provider uses his time. Clinical documentation must be objective in nature. Timing is documented for activities related to the patient, not the health provider. (Schick L, Windle PE. *PeriAnesthesia Nursing Core Curriculum: Preprocedure, Phase I and Phase II PACU Nursing.* 3rd ed. St. Louis, MO: Saunders; 2016:25.)

11-69. *Correct answer:* **c**

Examples of diseases that require contact precautions include vancomycin-resistant *Enterococcus* (VRE), methicillin-resistant *Staphylococcus aureus* (MRSA), *Clostridium difficile* (C Diff), lice, and scabies. Gowns and gloves are standard personal protective equipment when caring for patients on contact precautions. (Odom-Forren J. *Drain's Perianesthesia Nursing: A Critical Care Approach.* 6th ed. St. Louis, MO: Saunders; 2013:49.)

11-70. *Correct answer:* **d**

In order to reduce the risk of hospital acquired infections, the environment of care must be kept clean. Since the majority of equipment used within the perianesthesia unit is considered to have a low risk of infection transmission, simple surface cleaning is all that is necessary to ensure safety between uses (e.g., electrodes, stethoscopes, pulse oximeter devices, blood pressure cuffs, the outside surfaces of equipment). However, some surfaces, depending on the situation, may carry a higher risk for contamination, disinfectants with detergents that are approved by the institution may be required. All manufacturers' instructions for cleaning and disinfection should be obtained, and the appropriate personnel responsible for this task should be trained initially and regularly thereafter. (Odom-Forren J. *Drain's Perianesthesia Nursing: A Critical Care Approach.* 6th ed. St. Louis, MO: Saunders; 2013:44.)

11-71. *Correct answer:* **b**

Informed consent is a legal document representing a patient's understanding and approval for care. Implied consent is not expressly written or spoken, but implied when circumstances exist that lead a reasonable person to believe that consent had been given, such as when an individual is physically or mentally incapacitated and people assume that consent would be expressed if able. (Odom-Forren J. *Drain's Perianesthesia Nursing: A Critical Care Approach.* 6th ed. St. Louis, MO: Saunders; 2013:89-90.)

11-72. *Correct answer:* **b**

Hospitals are expected to ensure that procedures are performed for the correct person and that it is the correct procedure at the correct site. Also, relevant documentation (including history and physical examination, signed procedure consent form, nursing assessment, preanesthesia assessment); diagnostic and radiology test reports; and any equipment, blood products, implants, or devices should be available for the procedure. (Schick L, Windle PE. *PeriAnesthesia Nursing Core Curriculum: Preprocedure, Phase I and Phase II PACU Nursing.* 3rd ed. St. Louis, MO: Saunders; 2016:33.)

11-73. *Correct answer:* **c**

The American Society of PeriAnesthesia Nurses (ASPAN) is a highly committed advocate for a culture of safety in all perianesthesia practice settings. ASPAN's core values for a culture of safety include communication, advocacy, competency, efficiency, timeliness, and teamwork. A culture of safety is supported by an environment of caring and is guided by principles of research and evidence-based practices. (American Society of PeriAnesthesia Nurses. *Perianesthesia Nursing Standards, Practice Recommendations and Interpretive Statements 2015-2016.* Cherry Hill, NJ: ASPAN; 2014:14-17.)

11-74. *Correct answer:* **b**

The Clinical Laboratory Improvement Amendments Program (CLIA) of 1988 provides federal regulatory standards in the United States that apply to all clinical laboratory testing; the Centers for Medicare & Medicaid Services (CMS) regulates all laboratory testing to ensure quality. Laboratory departments must be certified to receive Medicare or Medicaid reimbursement. CLIA waivers for specific point-of-care testing apparatus include the need to meet competency requirements and to complete the required controls for test equipment. (Schick L, Windle PE. *PeriAnesthesia Nursing Core Curriculum: Preprocedure, Phase I and Phase II PACU Nursing.* 3rd ed. St. Louis, MO: Saunders; 2016:50.)

11-75. *Correct answer:* **b**

The recommendations for planning the discharge of a patient with known or suspected obstructive sleep apnea (OSA) from Phase I include observing the patient undisturbed in the Phase I PACU to determine if there are signs of desaturation. In addition, the perianesthesia nurse caring for the patient in Phase I can anticipate an extended stay. (American Society of PeriAnesthesia Nurses. *2015-2017 Perianesthesia Nursing Standards, Practice Recommendations and Interpretive Statements.* Cherry Hill, NJ: ASPAN; 2014:75.)

11-76. *Correct answer:* **d**

In terms of intensive care unit (ICU) overflow, management should develop and implement a comprehensive utilization plan with ongoing assessment that supports the staffing needs for both the PACU and ICU patients when the need for overflow admission arises. In addition, the plans for utilization of PACU as overflow should include multidisciplinary approaches to manage ICU beds, including nursing assignments, competencies, and medical management of the patient. (American Society of PeriAnesthesia Nurses. *2015-2017 Perianesthesia Nursing Standards, Practice Recommendations and Interpretive Statements.* Cherry Hill, NJ: ASPAN; 2014:102.)

11-77. *Correct answer:* **a**

There are numerous advantages to ambulatory surgery for the elderly. They include a decreased risk of nosocomial infections, including wound and respiratory; decreased incidence of mental confusion; and minimized length of stay away from the home environment, to name a few. The disadvantages, however, include inability to comply with a plan of care due to forgetfulness and difficulty adjusting to changes. There is also an increased risk for confusion with new medications, as well as for postoperative falls. (Schick L, Windle PE. *PeriAnesthesia Nursing Core Curriculum: Preprocedure, Phase I and Phase II PACU Nursing.* 3rd ed. St. Louis, MO: Saunders; 2016:298.)

11-78. *Correct answer:* **b**

According to the practice recommendation for staffing, two registered nurses, one of whom is an RN competent in Phase I postanesthesia nursing, are in the same room/unit where the patient is receiving Phase I level of care. (American Society of PeriAnesthesia Nurses. *2015-2017 Perianesthesia Nursing Standards, Practice Recommendations and Interpretive Statements.* Cherry Hill, NJ: ASPAN; 2014:35.)

11-79. *Correct answer:* **c**

The Patient Self-Determination Act of 1990 requires hospitals, nursing homes, home health agencies, hospice providers, health maintenance organizations, and other health care institutions to provide information about advance health care directives to adult patients upon their admission to the health care facility. (Schick L, Windle PE. *PeriAnesthesia Nursing Core Curriculum: Preprocedure, Phase I and Phase II PACU Nursing.* 3rd ed. St. Louis, MO: Saunders; 2016:28.)

11-80. *Correct answer:* **b**

According to the practice recommendation for staffing, two registered nurses, one of whom is an RN competent in Phase I postanesthesia nursing, are in the same room/unit where the patient is receiving Phase I level of care. (American Society of PeriAnesthesia Nurses. *2015-2017 Perianesthesia Nursing Standards, Practice Recommendations and Interpretive Statements.* Cherry Hill, NJ: ASPAN; 2014:35.)

Answer Key

CHAPTER 2: Respiratory, Cardiovascular, Peripheral Vascular, and Hematologic Systems

2-1.	d
2-2.	b
2-3.	c
2-4.	b
2-5.	d
2-6.	d
2-7.	c
2-8.	a
2-9.	b
2-10.	b
2-11.	d
2-12.	c
2-13.	c
2-14.	a
2-15.	c
2-16.	b
2-17.	c
2-18.	a
2-19.	d
2-20.	d
2-21.	b
2-22.	c
2-23.	b
2-24.	b
2-25.	d
2-26.	b
2-27.	b
2-28.	c
2-29.	c
2-30.	a
2-31.	d
2-32.	c
2-33.	c
2-34.	c
2-35.	d
2-36.	b
2-37.	d
2-38.	b
2-39.	d
2-40.	b
2-41.	c
2-42.	a
2-43.	b
2-44.	c
2-45.	d
2-46.	a
2-47.	c
2-48.	c
2-49.	b
2-50.	d
2-51.	d
2-52.	a
2-53.	a
2-54.	b
2-55.	a
2-56.	b
2-57.	c
2-58.	b
2-59.	c
2-60.	b

2-61.	a		3-15.	c
2-62.	b		3-16.	a
2-63.	c		3-17.	b
2-64.	c		3-18.	a
2-65.	a		3-19.	d
2-66.	a		3-20.	d
2-67.	b		3-21.	a
2-68.	a		3-22.	c
2-69.	a		3-23.	d
2-70.	a		3-24.	c
2-71.	c		3-25.	c
2-72.	c		3-26.	a
2-73.	b		3-27.	b
2-74.	c		3-28.	b
2-75.	c		3-29.	b
2-76.	b		3-30.	c
2-77.	d		3-31.	a
2-78.	d		3-32.	b
2-79.	d		3-33.	c
2-80.	a		3-34.	a
			3-35.	b

CHAPTER 3: Neurologic and Gastrointestinal Systems

3-1.	d		3-36.	d
3-2.	b		3-37.	b
3-3.	b		3-38.	c
3-4.	a		3-39.	b
3-5.	c		3-40.	c
3-6.	c		3-41.	a
3-7.	c		3-42.	b
3-8.	a		3-43.	c
3-9.	b		3-44.	c
3-10.	b		3-45.	a
3-11.	c		3-46.	a
3-12.	d		3-47.	c
3-13.	c		3-48.	d
3-14.	c		3-49.	b
			3-50.	b

3-51.	b		4-20.	c
3-52.	c		4-21.	a
3-53.	b		4-22.	c
3-54.	a		4-23.	a
3-55.	b		4-24.	c
3-56.	b		4-25.	c
3-57.	b		4-26.	b
3-58.	d		4-27.	d
3-59.	c		4-28.	d
3-60.	a		4-29.	d
3-61.	b		4-30.	a
3-62.	b		4-31.	c
3-63.	c		4-32.	b
3-64.	a		4-33.	d
3-65.	a		4-34.	a

CHAPTER 4: Renal and Integumentary Systems

			4-35.	a
			4-36.	b
4-1.	b		4-37.	a
4-2.	d		4-38.	d
4-3.	d		4-39.	c
4-4.	d		4-40.	d
4-5.	c		4-41.	b
4-6.	b		4-42.	b
4-7.	c		4-43.	a
4-8.	d		4-44.	b
4-9.	d		4-45.	c
4-10.	d		4-46.	b
4-11.	c		4-47.	d
4-12.	a		4-48.	a
4-13.	d		4-49.	a
4-14.	c		4-50.	d
4-15.	b		4-51.	a
4-16.	c		4-52.	c
4-17.	b		4-53.	d
4-18.	a		4-54.	c
4-19.	b		4-55.	b

4-56.	d		5-24.	d
4-57.	b		5-25.	d
4-58.	b		5-26.	c
4-59.	d		5-27.	d
4-60.	b		5-28.	d
4-61.	c		5-29.	a
4-62.	d		5-30.	b
4-63.	d		5-31.	a
4-64.	b		5-32.	b
4-65.	d		5-33.	b

CHAPTER 5: Genitourologic, Reproductive, and Musculoskeletal Systems

			5-34.	d
			5-35.	d
5-1.	a		5-36.	c
5-2.	c		5-37.	d
5-3.	a		5-38.	b
5-4.	a		5-39.	a
5-5.	b		5-40.	c
5-6.	a		5-41.	b
5-7.	b		5-42.	a
5-8.	a		5-43.	d
5-9.	a		5-44.	a
5-10.	d		5-45.	a
5-11.	b		5-46.	b
5-12.	d		5-47.	a
5-13.	b		5-48.	d
5-14.	a		5-49.	c
5-15.	b		5-50.	c
5-16.	a		5-51.	d
5-17.	c		5-52.	a
5-18.	c		5-53.	d
5-19.	b		5-54.	c
5-20.	c		5-55.	b
5-21.	d		5-56.	d
5-22.	a		5-57.	b
5-23.	c		5-58.	c

5-59.	c
5-60.	d
5-61.	c
5-62.	a
5-63.	c
5-64.	a
5-65.	b

CHAPTER 6: Endocrine System, Fluids, and Electrolytes

6-1.	c
6-2.	d
6-3.	b
6-4.	b
6-5.	b
6-6.	c
6-7.	c
6-8.	b
6-9.	d
6-10.	d
6-11.	c
6-12.	b
6-13.	c
6-14.	b
6-15.	b
6-16.	b
6-17.	d
6-18.	c
6-19.	b
6-20.	b
6-21.	a
6-22.	a
6-23.	c
6-24.	c
6-25.	d
6-26.	a

6-27.	d
6-28.	d
6-29.	b
6-30.	c
6-31.	d
6-32.	b
6-33.	a
6-34.	c
6-35.	a
6-36.	b
6-37.	c
6-38.	b
6-39.	c
6-40.	d
6-41.	c
6-42.	b
6-43.	a
6-44.	c
6-45.	d
6-46.	c
6-47.	a
6-48.	c
6-49.	a
6-50.	b
6-51.	c
6-52.	a.
6-53.	d
6-54.	b
6-55.	b
6-56.	c
6-57.	c
6-58.	d
6-59.	c
6-60.	b
6-61.	d

6-62.	c		7-29.	d
6-63.	c		7-30.	b
6-64.	a		7-31.	d
6-65.	d		7-32.	d

CHAPTER 7: Maintenance of Normothermia, Physiologic Comfort, and the Therapeutic Environment

			7-33.	c
			7-34.	c
			7-35.	c
7-1.	b		7-36.	c
7-2.	c		7-37.	d
7-3.	a		7-38.	d
7-4.	a		7-39.	d
7-5.	d		7-40.	c
7-6.	b		7-41.	a
7-7.	b		7-42.	a
7-8.	c		7-43.	b
7-9.	c		7-44.	b
7-10.	b		7-45.	c
7-11.	d		7-46.	d
7-12.	b		7-47.	a
7-13.	a		7-48.	c
7-14.	d		7-49.	b
7-15.	a		7-50.	b
7-16.	c		7-51.	b
7-17.	b		7-52.	b
7-18.	c		7-53.	b
7-19.	a		7-54.	c
7-20.	d		7-55.	d
7-21.	b		7-56.	b
7-22.	b		7-57.	d
7-23.	d		7-58.	a
7-24.	c		7-59.	d
7-25.	a		7-60.	a
7-26.	d		7-61.	d
7-27.	c		7-62.	a
7-28.	c		7-63.	c

7-64. a

7-65. c

7-66. d

CHAPTER 8: Anesthesia and Malignant Hyperthermia

8-1. b

8-2. c

8-3. b

8-4. c

8-5. d

8-6. a

8-7. c

8-8. d

8-9. c

8-10. a

8-11. b

8-12. d

8-13. a

8-14. b

8-15. d

8-16. a

8-17. d

8-18. b

8-19. b

8-20. c

8-21. d

8-22. b

8-23. a

8-24. d

8-25. c

8-26. a

8-27. c

8-28. d

8-29. d

8-30. b

8-31. a

8-32. d

8-33. c

8-34. d

8-35. d

8-36. a

8-37. d

8-38. a

8-39. a

8-40. d

8-41. a

8-42. b

8-43. a

8-44. c

8-45. a

8-46. d

8-47. c

8-48. b

8-49. c

8-50. d

8-51. a

8-52. a

8-53. b

8-54. a

8-55. c

8-56. a

8-57. d

8-58. c

8-59. d

8-60. a

8-61. d

8-62. d

8-63. d

8-64. a

8-65. b

CHAPTER 9: Diversity and Psychosocial Assistance

9-1.	a
9-2.	a
9-3.	d
9-4.	d
9-5.	a
9-6.	c
9-7.	b
9-8.	b
9-9.	a
9-10.	d
9-11.	b
9-12.	a
9-13.	b
9-14.	c
9-15.	b
9-16.	d
9-17.	d
9-18.	d
9-19.	a
9-20.	d
9-21.	c
9-22.	d
9-23.	b
9-24.	c
9-25.	c
9-26.	a
9-27.	c
9-28.	b
9-29.	b
9-30.	c
9-31.	a
9-32.	d
9-33.	d
9-34.	c

9-35.	d
9-36.	a
9-37.	a
9-38.	b
9-39.	a
9-40.	d
9-41.	c
9-42.	c
9-43.	d
9-44.	a
9-45.	a
9-46.	c
9-47.	c
9-48.	a
9-49.	a
9-50.	d

CHAPTER 10: Patient and Family Education

10-1.	d
10-2.	c
10-3.	a
10-4.	c
10-5.	a
10-6.	c
10-7.	c
10-8.	b
10-9.	c
10-10.	a
10-11.	a
10-12.	c
10-13.	a
10-14.	d
10-15.	d
10-16.	a
10-17.	b
10-18.	b
10-19.	a
10-20.	c
10-21.	a
10-22.	b

10-23.	d		11-12.	a
10-24.	b		11-13.	c
10-25.	d		11-14.	a
10-26.	b		11-15.	a
10-27.	c		11-16.	c
10-28.	b		11-17.	d
10-29.	c		11-18.	a
10-30.	c		11-19.	a
10-31.	b		11-20.	c
10-32.	c		11-21.	b
10-33.	a		11-22.	d
10-34.	d		11-23.	c
10-35.	d		11-24.	d
10-36.	b		11-25.	a
10-37.	b		11-26.	a
10-38.	d		11-27.	c
10-39.	c		11-28.	d
10-40.	c		11-29.	d
10-41.	c		11-30.	b
10-42.	d		11-31.	d
10-43.	d		11-32.	d
10-44.	b		11-33.	c
10-45.	a		11-34.	b
10-46.	d		11-35.	c
10-47.	d		11-36.	b
10-48.	b		11-37.	c
10-49.	c		11-38.	a
10-50.	c		11-39.	b
			11-40.	a

CHAPTER 11: ASPAN Standards, Documentation, Regulatory Guidelines, and Patient Safety Needs

			11-41.	c
			11-42.	a
			11-43.	d
11-1.	c		11-44.	d
11-2.	b		11-45.	d
11-3.	b		11-46.	c
11-4.	a		11-47.	b
11-5.	b		11-48.	a
11-6.	c		11-49.	d
11-7.	b		11-50.	c
11-8.	d		11-51.	c
11-9.	c		11-52.	b
11-10.	c		11-53.	c
11-11.	a		11-54.	d

11-55.	c	11-68.	b
11-56.	d	11-69.	c
11-57.	a	11-70.	d
11-58.	c	11-71.	b
11-59.	b	11-72.	b
11-60.	a	11-73.	c
11-61.	d	11-74.	b
11-62.	c	11-75.	b
11-63.	d	11-76.	d
11-64.	c	11-77.	a
11-65.	d	11-78.	b
11-66.	b	11-79.	c
11-67.	d	11-80.	b

Index

Page numbers followed by *"b"* indicate boxes.